# SELF-CARE
# ANYWHERE

**Powerful Natural Remedies for Common Health Problems**

**Gary M. Skole C.P.T.    Scott R. Greenberg M.D.    Michael Gazsi N.D.**

**New Century Publishing 2000**

Cover by Carla Mattioli
Edited by Ruth E. Skole Ed.D.,
Medical Editor Vivienne Matalon, M.D.


Copyright ©1999 by Gary M. Skole
Revised edition 2000

ISBN 0-9701110-3-7
Library of Congress Catalog Card Number 00 134103
Categories 1. Health  2. Herbs  3. Homeopathy  4. Medicine
Printed in the United States

All listed addresses, phone numbers and fees have been reviewed and updated during production. However, the data is subject to change.

New Century Publishing 2000

Canada
60 Bullock Dr. Unit 7
Markham ON LP3 3P2
(905) 471-5711

United States
P.O. Box 36
East Canaan CT  06024
(860) 824-5301

## The Telehealth Card

The Telehealth Card was designed to give readers of Self-Care Anywhere the ability to always have access to many of the remedies featured in this book. By calling the number on the card, and then dialing in your desired remedy, you can listen to a pre-recorded message of a remedy from wherever there is a telephone. To activate your card, go to the Self-Care Anywhere website at **urhealthy.com** or send a check or money order to to address below. The cost of the prepaid phone card is $7.00 United States, or $9.25 Canadian. This entitles you to 30 minutes of access.

For your temporary card, cut along the lines, fold in half and tape together at the bottom. You must first activate your card in order to use it.

To activate, visit www.urhealthy.com or send a check or money order to:
Self-Care Anywhere
1155 Rt. 73, Ste 3
Mt. Laurel, NJ 08054 USA

### Self Care Anywhere

Call 1-800-_ _ _-_ _ _ _
Access Code SC_ _ _ _ _ _ _ _ _ _
Enter your access code
Dial in the code for the remedy you want
Listen to remedy

| | |
|---|---|
| 01 Anxiety | 11 Ear Infection |
| 02 Back Pain | 12 Gas |
| 03 Bites & Stings | 13 Hayfever |
| 04 Burns | 14 Headache |
| 05 Cold & Flu | 15 Heartburn |
| 06 Cold Sore | 16 Jet Lag |
| 07 Constipation | 17 Nausea |
| 08 Coughs | 18 Poison Ivy etc. |
| 09 Cuts | 19 Sinusitis |
| 10 Diarrhea | 20 Sore Throat |

Prices subject to change without notice.

# Contents

# Acknowledgements

Putting a book like this together takes a great team effort. A tremendous amount of research and coordination was required from the staff and the doctors who unselfishly gave of their time. In addition, Carla Mattioli deserves a world of credit for her patience and creativity in developing the book cover. A special thanks is deserved by Ruth Skole, Ed.D. for the numerous hours spent in editing and to Terry, Lauren and Jarrod for the sacrifices they endured and their total support throughout this entire project.

# Preface

Revolutionary changes are occurring in our health-care system. Conventional medicine is making important scientific and technological advances to help people live longer, healthier lives. At the same time, federal and private insurance programs, seeking to reduce costs, are limiting access to conventional care and exploring less costly alternatives to standard treatment. Patients, seeking safe, natural therapies, are spending billions of out-of-pocket dollars on non-traditional health care. Physicians, caught between constraints imposed by managed care, and escalating costs of pharmaceuticals, are seeking to provide quality care by integrating medical advances with the holistic-health modalities requested by their patients. As a result of these trends, health-care consumers must take more responsibility for their own health and wellness by becoming knowledgeable about their options and informed about self-care, prevention, and current treatment modalities.

*Self-Care Anywhere* can help you negotiate this medical maze by putting the information you need at your fingertips. The integrated approach to self-care included here combines alternative and complementary therapies with conventional medicine in an easy-to-use format that includes practical recommendations for numerous medical problems.

The human body is an amazing creation that has the ability to heal itself and function in ways once thought available to only a few select people. Since we are complex yet individually unique, our healthcare should be personalized to be most effective rather than "one right way for all." By utilizing the information in this book, you too may function at a higher level of wellness. Complicated ideas have been simplified, and are written in a style that allows each person to be an educated and self-reliant healthcare consumer. Many options are provided, but only you can decide which ones are best for you.

# INTRODUCTION

As hospitals continue to downsize and medical technology improves, people today are seeking to satisfy many of their basic health needs at home. With access to a wide array of advanced medical resources that can dramatically reduce the need for many office visits, self-care and preventive care are becoming all the more important.

Home healthcare involves more than having a nurse come to the house; it means utilizing the home as the primary place to provide, receive, and administer care. There will always be a need for professional healthcare providers, hospitals, and long-term care facilities. However, our dependence upon them can be greatly reduced if we become educated health-care consumers.

Being "independently healthy" simply means that each of us is primarily responsible for our own well-being. We can be comfortable making basic health-related choices ourselves, and, if a problem arises for which professional medical care is indicated, we will be sufficiently well-informed to become active participants in the decision-making process.

*Self-Care Anywhere* is a much-needed resource for individuals committed to healthy living, and for those wishing to eliminate persistent problems. With this book, you can take full advantage of all that modern healthcare has to offer, while retaining the power to shape your health and control your lifestyle. In this way, you will truly be ***Independently Healthy.***

### Are You Medically Dependent?

When illness strikes, "medically dependent" people rely on someone or something other than themselves to make health-related decisions, and take charge of their care because they do not feel qualified to do so. Does this definition describe how you relate to your own health? The following questions may provide you with the answer:

- If you were diagnosed with bronchitis, what would you do?
- What foods can reduce cholesterol?
- What can be done to decrease your chances of getting a cold?
- If you have a cold, what can be done to shorten its duration?
- If you take vitamin C for a cold, how much should you take and how often?
- Can taking too much vitamin C be harmful?
- How should you treat a bee sting?

- How is a sprained ankle treated?
- What remedies speed the healing process of a sprain?
- How can a sinus problem be treated without prescription medicine?
- Are antibiotics always necessary for treating an ear infection?
- Is it best to suppress a fever when sick?
- What can be done to prevent or reduce asthma and its related symptoms?

If you are unable to correctly answer most of these questions and do not know how to get the information easily, you are, like most modern Americans, medically dependent.

Prior to the mid-1800s, people around the world, including Americans, were self-sufficient regarding common healthcare. Traditional medical knowledge and folk remedies were handed down from generation to generation both orally, and later, in the form of written texts and articles. Although common folk remedies were effective in a variety of situations, bacterial infections killed one out of five people.

The introduction of penicillin and other "wonder" drugs in the late 1930s and early 1940s ushered in the era of modern medicine. Antibiotics were used frequently, but could be administered only by physicians. As people became accustomed to seeking medical help, they began to call on physicians for colds, earaches, upset stomachs, and a variety of other conditions that had previously required only self-care. Folk remedies were quickly forgotten, as society became more and more dependent on professional medical treatment for most ailments.

Most Americans assumed that this modern system was working well. However, a World Health Organization (WHO) study published in June, 2000 revealed that despite spending more money per person on healthcare than any other country ($3,700), the United States ranked only eighteenth in the world in terms of overall healthcare. Healthcare costs are staggering, and millions of people cannot afford standard care. In an effort to reduce costs and to make healthcare more accessible, managed care was introduced. However, this new healthcare delivery system has created more problems.

With the managed-care referral system, people can no longer see a medical specialist at will. Primary-care physicians are expected to provide more services in a shorter period of time, preventing them from taking time to explain basic self-care. Hospital stays are shorter, referrals are reduced, and people are being forced to take more responsibility for their own care, often at home and often without being adequately prepared. This medical bind in which most Americans find themselves has caused many people to seek alternative forms of healthcare. As a last resort, frustrated consumers are trying to relearn traditional methods of self-care practiced effectively by their ancestors.

## The Cost of Medical Dependency

In 1960, according to the National Center for Health Statistics, 67% of Americans visited a doctor's office at least once a year. In 1994, that figure jumped to nearly 80%. Despite evidence that we are receiving *more* health care, we are not necessarily receiving better health care. In fact, we are losing the battle against chronic and degenerative illnesses.

The authors of this book support the guidelines issued by health organizations for routine preventive physical examinations and screenings. Health problems that are detected at an early stage are easier and less expensive to treat successfully. It is also our position that individuals should be encouraged to practice more preventive healthcare and self-care for common problems.

According to a 1996 study by the Centers for Disease Control, Americans made 734,493,000 office visits to a physician for an average of 3.4 visits per person. If the average number of office visits could be reduced by just a small amount, billions of dollars per year in medical costs could be saved.

Prescription medication is another area in which medical dependency is costing Americans billions of dollars. In 1997, the nation's overall prescription-drug bill rose 13%, followed in 1998 by a 16% increase. That represents a total increase of 29%, while the cost of living increased by only 5%. In response to these escalating prices, managed-care companies have stopped paying for many name- brand drugs. There is now a good possibility that when we go to the drug store to pick up our prescriptions, we may be given something other than what the doctor ordered, creating a potentially dangerous situation.

Unfortunately, most patients and many of their physicians do not realize that there are alternatives. The most important one is to practice preventive medicine, since it is easier to prevent illness than to treat it after it occurs. The second is to develop basic knowledge and skill in the use of natural-healing methods.

For example, hypertension, or high blood pressure, is a growing problem in the United States. It is routinely treated with prescription medications that are expensive, can be addicting, and have numerous side effects. There are, however, natural alternatives that not only cost less but also have fewer, if any, side effects and may actually be beneficial to your health. These include stress management and relaxation techniques, changes in diet, and taking vitamins, minerals and herbs such as calcium, magnesium and garlic.

Most physicians were not taught about natural alternatives during their training, and many remain unaware of their beneficial properties. In response to growing interest by the general public, the medical community is beginning to investigate and publish information about herbal and other alternative therapies. At the present time, however, it is the responsibility of the informed consumer to find and implement viable options to standard medical treatment.


## Is This Program For You?

*Self-Care Anywhere* was designed with you, the healthcare consumer in mind. Using the brief questionnaire below, take a moment to assess your present health status.

- Do you feel that you have a high level of stress in your life?
- Are you carrying 10 or more pounds of excess body fat?
- Are you subject to frequent colds, flu, or other infections (more than two per year)?
- Do you suffer from aching joints?
- Do you feel sleepy after eating?
- Do you often feel sluggish or fatigued?
- Do you suffer from bloating, gas, indigestion, heartburn, constipation, or diarrhea?
- Do you suffer from migraines or other chronic headaches?
- Do you have trouble sleeping?
- Do you suffer from skin problems?
- Is your blood pressure or cholesterol high?
- Do you have frequent yeast infections?
- Do you have food allergies, asthma, or hayfever?
- Do you have a blood- sugar disorder, such as hypoglycemia or diabetes?
- Do you often use painkillers?
- Do you use antacids frequently?
- Do you suffer from premenstrual syndrome (PMS)?

Above are just a few of the common problems from which people regularly suffer. In fact, many believe that these symptoms are a normal part of life, simply ignoring them until they demand attention. Unfortunately, health problems are then more difficult to treat.

If we settle for living with marginal health today, we have already lost half the battle for a long and healthy life. When we ignore physical symptoms, we are actually ignoring the body's warning of a possible problem. Would you ignore your car if the "check engine light" came on? Let this questionnaire be *your* "check engine light."

## You and Your Car: An analogy

While the automobile is a piece of machinery and the human body a living, complex organism, there are some similarities in the way we age. Comparing a car's mileage and human chronology can vividly illustrate our aging process.

## Life Cycle of an Automobile

The first few thousand miles a new car is driven are considered to be its break-in period. Minor problems are corrected, and adjustments made so that the car runs properly and is prepared for its future "life".

For the next 20,000 to 30,000 miles, the car is in the prime of its life; it is expected to run well and have very few problems. This is the time to develop the habit of preventive maintenance by using quality gasoline, changing the oil regularly, and getting scheduled check-ups. Instituting these practices while the car is still new helps to extend its life and maintain peak performance, even as the car ages.

From 30,000 to 60,000 miles, the car generally runs well, but begins to have a few problems. Parts like tires, brakes, and shocks begin to wear out and usually have to be replaced. By 60,000 miles, problems occur more frequently and tend to be more serious. The car does not run as smoothly as it once did, and its pickup may be slower. Creaks and noises start appearing, valves may become blocked, and hoses and belts may become hardened and stiff. The car still runs, but not as well as it did at 20,000 miles. It is at this time that earlier abuse and neglect become apparent.

From 70,000 miles on, decline happens much more rapidly. In addition, when a car is not used for long periods of time, it begins to deteriorate to the point where it can no longer be driven. Tires get soft and flat, the frame rusts, and the battery dies. Although new technology has increased a car's life expectancy, without preventive maintenance, your car will have unnecessary problems as it ages and, ultimately, a shorter life span.

## Life Cycle of a Human Being

Babies, like new cars, need to be treated with special care and may have minor physical problems that need to be corrected. During their teens and twenties, most people are in their physical prime with few major health problems. After age thirty, problems begin to occur a little more often, and the body begins to function less efficiently. At age sixty, health problems occur still more frequently, and are often more severe. By age seventy and beyond, physical decline and deterioration are accelerated, eventually resulting in death.

Practicing preventive medicine is comparable to practicing preventive maintenance on your car. Failure to incorporate preventive health-care initially increases the likelihood that expensive replacement parts such as a new hip or heart will be required in the future. Less extreme, but perhaps more frustrating, will be your body's inability to function at its peak because of nagging pains or chronic degenerative problems.

Preventive healthcare can contribute to a longer, healthier life. Poor eating habits will increases the risk of developing blocked and rigid arteries that resemble the clogged fuel lines in an old car. Without regular exercise, the body becomes soft and flabby, like an unused tire. And, like the rusted moving parts of an abandoned car, joints that are not used often will lose flexibility, while unused muscles deteriorate and bones become brittle. The combined effects of poor diet and sedentary life style cause the heart to weaken and possibly be replaced like an unused battery. As with our cars, technology has helped extend the number of years we live, and preventive medicine can help improve the quality of those years.

Hopefully, this illustration will create a lasting mental image. From now on, when you take your car in for a tune-up, consider making an appointment for *your* annual physical or dental examination. When you put air in your tires or change the battery, think about getting more exercise. When you fill your car with gasoline, think about the food with which you have been filling your stomach. Is your body getting the nutrients it needs for healthy living, now and into the future?

**In the interest of good health and a long, active life, we should make a serious effort not to be like many Americans who take better care of their automobiles than they do of their bodies.**

# HOW TO USE THIS BOOK

Achieving optimal health is a multidimensional process with physical, emotional, environmental, and nutritional components. The multidisciplinary approach to holistic healthcare presented in this book targets the whole person by emphasizing both prevention and remediation of common health problems.

*Self-Care Anywhere* consists of two sections. The first, *Independently Healthy*, contains general guidelines for positive lifestyle changes. These provide a holistic framework that can help prevent many of today's health problems.

The second, *Common Health Problems*, provides natural remedies for a variety of medical problems. For each ailment or condition, underlying causes and physical and emotional symptoms, as well as traditional medical treatments, are briefly but comprehensively described.

Our self-care guidelines for both prevention and remediation of health-related problems provide a truly integrated approach. Each section features a range of modalities, which may include: mind/body medicine, aromatherapy, nutrition, exercise, vitamin and mineral supplementation, herbal medicine, and homeopathic medicine. In many instances, safer options that are less invasive, intrusive and toxic can be tried before resorting to prescription medication.

Read the *Independently Healthy* section carefully to assess your present level of compliance with each guideline, then select one or two areas for which positive changes would have the most profound impact on your health.

Do not attempt to make drastic revisions immediately; abruptly changing many aspects of behavior at once will be dooming your good intentions to failure. We suggest that you make changes gradually, at a comfortable pace. Use these guidelines as a point of reference to which you return frequently. The most important prescription for success is your commitment to practice preventive medicine and to become independently healthy.

Remedies in the *Common Health Problems* section are divided into two programs. The *EZ Care Program* may be the best place to begin, especially if you are new to the world of self-care. Included here are easy, basic treatment options that have been found to be most effective for the majority of people.

The second program, *Additional Recommendations,* is a supplement to the *EZ Care Program*. This program is for individuals who have had some experience with natural healing modalities, or for those who wish to go beyond the basic program. Remedies from each section may be combined or used individually

Unfortunately, people are not simple machines that can be fixed quickly and easily when they fail. Many symptoms have more than one cause, or are produced by a complex combination of factors. For example, an allergy sufferer may be allergic to something airborne, or something that has been eaten, *and* may have a stress-related problem that exacerbates the situation. Using the same protocol for a food allergy as for an environmental allergy may be ineffective. Finding the appropriate treatment can be compared to solving a complicated puzzle, which, as we all know, requires time, patience and experimentation.

Most of the supplements and supplies described in this book can be found in health food stores and health-oriented supermarkets. Items that are difficult to find locally can be purchased from a supplier listed in the Resource Guide, located in Appendix G.

*Self-Care Anywhere* is not meant to be a self-diagnostic program. Descriptions of disorders are provided for informational purposes only. Using this book may enable you to handle minor ailments or injuries, but is not intended to replace your physician. If medical intervention is indicated, this book can help you become knowledgeable about all treatment options, so that you and your physician can work as a team.

***Important words of caution:*** If you are currently being treated for a specific condition, consult your healthcare practitioner before trying any of the remedies in this book. Do *not* discontinue current prescription medications without first consulting your physician. While the remedies included here have been used safely and effectively, even natural remedies may cause reactions, especially in very sensitive or ill individuals, or when not used properly. In this case, conservative physician-supervised experimentation is key. And remember, more is not necessarily better with either conventional or alternative medicines.

### Getting The Most Out of *Self-Care Anywhere*

1. Read the ***Introduction*** and answer the questionnaires.
2. Read the ***Independently Healthy*** section to assess the health-promoting level of your current lifestyle.
3. Target one or two areas for change and begin slowly, but with determination.
4. Refer to the ***Common Health Problems*** section when confronted with a chronic or acute disorder.
5. Begin by implementing some, or all, of the **EZ Care Program.** Introduce each new remedy or technique slowly and, after a period of time, assess its effectiveness. Continue or discontinue its use accordingly, then add one or

two new options. Continue with this process until an effective, personalized treatment protocol has been established.

6. When ready to try new options, review the **Additional Recommendations** section and choose those remedies and techniques in which you are interested, and that can be applied relatively easily in your given situation.

7. Before beginning your program, review dosage guidelines and cautionary notes.

8. Always inform your healthcare practitioner about the modalities you are considering or using, especially if being treated for a specific illness.

*Self-Care Anywhere* can be a roadmap for an exciting journey because it provides directions for taking control of our health. Powerful, positive changes may occur when we begin to eat right, reduce stress, and assume a more natural, self-reliant approach towards our own health. Although at times the relief of chronic ailments and symptoms may seem miraculous, the power of this program is its ability to release the awesome potential for long-term health within each of us.

# SECTION I

## INDEPENDENTLY HEALTHY

The general guidelines presented in this section can be considered the foundation of a healthy lifestyle. Our program is complete, without being overwhelming. We suggest that changes be made gradually, and at your own pace. The most important thing is to make a commitment to yourself to break your medical dependency, and to take charge of your health. Go slowly, do what feels comfortable, and let each step be a building block for the next. In case of illness, always consult your healthcare practitioner before implementing any changes.

We tend to think of health as being a physical attribute; however, mental, emotional, and spiritual components of our lives also have an impact upon our physical well-being. If prevention is the cornerstone of our health program, nutrition, exercise, mental outlook, and stress reduction are the building blocks. In combination, these elements contribute to our overall health and wellness.

Following are a few easy steps for healthy living.
- Eat a diet high in water-content foods, such as fresh fruits and vegetables.
- Consider taking supplements, especially antioxidants.
- Avoid hydrogenated oils, found in things such as margarine and many baked goods.
- Avoid food coloring and artificial preservatives.
- Avoid refined sugar as much as possible.
- Eat more whole, unprocessed foods.
- Drink a liberal amount of pure water daily.
- Exercise daily.
- Get enough rest and sleep.
- Incorporate relaxation/stress management techniques into your daily routine.
- Develop a positive mental outlook.
- Learn to breathe fully.

Good health starts with respecting your body, and providing what it needs to resist disease and to thrive. The basic ingredients of a properly functioning body are good nutrition, exercise, and rest. The following guidelines form the basis of a healthy lifestyle:

## DIET AND NUTRITION

*Eat a diet high in water-rich foods*

A high-water-content diet consists predominantly of fresh fruits and vegetables, with smaller amounts of whole grains, legumes, nuts, seeds, fowl, fish and modest amounts of mono-unsaturated fats. Fresh fruits and vegetables are full of vitamins, minerals, and fiber. They also contain a class of beneficial natural compounds known as phytonutrients. Research has shown phytonutrients may lower cholesterol, prevent lung, breast, prostate, and colon cancers, prevent osteoporosis, and reduce menopausal symptoms. Select a colorful variety of fresh fruits and vegetables, avoiding white potatoes and iceberg lettuce, to obtain the most phytonutrients.

It is important to make dietary changes at a pace that is comfortable and natural for you. Radically changing your diet overnight could cause temporary problems, such as gas, bloating, constipation, cramping, fatigue, and often results in failure. If you currently eat little to no water-rich foods, you may want to start by including just one piece of fruit or one vegetable a day. Then increase by one fruit and one vegetable per day, and keep building.

The goal is five to nine servings of each per day. If possible, use organic fruits and vegetables, because they have fewer pesticides and are more nutritious. By replacing one of your regular snacks with a fruit or vegetable, you will soon develop good eating habits. The good news· the longer you do this, the easier it gets. Ideally, every meal should include some water-rich foods.

Coffee, milk, cereal, oatmeal mixed with water, soft drinks, and alcoholic beverages are not considered water-rich. The best way to increase your intake is to add a salad, fruit, or vegetable to every meal. If meat is usually the largest part of your meal, make it the smallest part and increase the proportion of fruits and vegetables. Be careful to add vegetables as well as fruit, because fruit has a much higher sugar-content.

Other eating tips include taking your time while eating, and chewing your food thoroughly. Inadequate chewing does not allow the digestive enzymes in the mouth to start breaking down the food, which often taxes the stomach to work harder to digest food. Also, be sure not to wash the food down with fluids, instead of chewing; once again, an important step in the digestion process is being skipped.

*Consider supplemental vitamins and minerals*

Vitamins and minerals are best when obtained from the food you eat, because they are proportionally correct and easily absorbed by the body.

Supplements are not a replacement for good nutrition, which is why they are called "supplements." Using supplements, however, can insure that you get enough of the right nutrients. The following are recommended:

♦ **Multivitamin/mineral combination** - one a day. Avoid those with talc, fillers, and artificial colorings. A multivitamin is recommended to supply nutrients that cannot always be obtained from diet alone.

♦ **Vitamin C** - may be used in doses of 500 to 1,000 mg., two to three times daily. The preferred form is mixed mineral ascorbates, such as calcium ascorbate, magnesium ascorbate, etc. Vitamin C is also available with bioflavonoids, which offer strong protection against free radical damage. Vitamin C can be beneficial in treating allergies, fighting colds, and healing wounds.

♦ **Vitamin E** - 400 international units (IU) if you are under age 40; consider 800 IU if you are over age 40. Make sure the vitamin E you choose is natural d-alpha tocopherol in a base of mixed tocopherols. If your multivitamin contains vitamin E, take additional vitamin E as needed to reach this recommended dosage. Higher doses of vitamin E may increase the risk of bleeding and bruising. Vitamin E is a powerful antioxidant that reduces your risk of a heart attack by up to 70% and may offer protection against Alzheimer's disease and colon cancer.

♦ **Selenium** - 200 micrograms (mcg.) daily, is best taken with vitamin E. If your multivitamin contains selenium, take as much additional selenium as needed to reach this recommended dosage. Research has shown that people with higher levels of this mineral have a lower incidence of cancer.

♦ **Omega-3 fatty acids** - (EPA) Dosage: 1,000 mg., 2 times daily, of preferably molecularly-distilled fish oil. They may also be obtained by eating a few servings of deep cold-water fish each week (e.g., mackerel, cod, halibut, salmon, herring, sardines), and by eating flaxseeds or adding flaxseed oil to salads. Omega-3 fatty acids reduce mediators of inflammation in our body, and can be useful to protect against asthma, eczema, allergies, colitis, premenstrual syndrome, depression, cancer, heart disease, hypertension, arthritis, hypercholesterolemia, autoimmune, and vascular diseases.

♦ **Calcium** - 1000 mg. for men and pre-menopausal women, 1500 mg. for post-menopausal, lactating, and pregnant women. This amount includes dietary consumption of calcium, which averages approximately 500 mg for individuals eating a healthy diet. Calcium is important in preserving bone health, and preventing osteoporosis and bone fractures. It is best taken in combination with 400 - 800 mg. of magnesium. Folic acid, vitamin D, vitamin K, boron, silica, copper, and zinc are also essential nutrients in the bone-building process.

In addition to these supplements, mixed carotenoids (preferably with lycopene), garlic, and coenzyme Q-10 are excellent additions to your daily regimen.

*Avoid any type of hydrogenated oil*

Hydrogenated oils contain trans-fatty acids. These man-made molecules fit unnaturally in the body due to their unusual molecular shape, which makes it difficult for the body to process the oil in a normal fashion, potentially causing many health problems. The increased use of hydrogenated and partially-hydrogenated oils parallels the increase of many degenerative diseases. These oils are prime suspects for heart disease, cancer, and many other twentieth-century health problems.

It is difficult to avoid hydrogenated oils, because they are in almost all baked goods. Another major culprit is margarine. Replace vegetable oils (e.g., corn, cottonseed, peanut oil) with cold-pressed oils high in mono-unsaturated fatty acids (e.g., olive oil, canola oil). It helps to read labels and shop in stores that carry healthier products. Most healthfood stores and a growing number of health-oriented supermarkets carry products baked without hydrogenated oils. These products are comparable in taste to unhealthy hydrogenated products.

*Avoid food coloring, preservatives and artificial sweeteners*

These have been linked to headaches, food allergies, hyperactivity, Attention Deficit Disorder (ADD), and a host of other health problems. These additives alter a food's natural state and can cause our brain neurotransmitters to malfunction. Before placing a child on a stimulant drug such as Ritalin, consider elimination of food colorings, preservatives, and artificial sweeteners from the diet.

*Avoid using refined sugar as much as possible*

As with hydrogenated oils, the increased use of refined sugar also parallels the increase in many degenerative diseases. Sugar is considered a stressor food. This means it supplies the body with no nutritional value, yet it taxes the body's metabolic processes in some way. Consumption of refined sugars is suspected of weakening the immune system, increasing obesity, promoting dental decay, increasing hyperactivity, and shortening attention spans. An excellent replacement for sugar and for artificial sweeteners is an herb called *stevia*. It is a non-caloric sweetener used widely around the world, and it does not affect blood-sugar metabolism. An extract of stevia is 100 to

300 times sweeter than table sugar; therefore, only a small amount is needed to replace an entire cup of sugar. Another alternative to sugar is natural fruit and fruit juice-sweetened items. Sucrose and corn syrup are *not* natural sweeteners, and should be avoided.

*Eat more whole foods*

Whole foods are those in their natural state. Foods that are processed, fried, or sweetened are not whole foods. Processing removes up to 90% of a food's minerals, vitamins, and fiber. The optimal diet is primarily composed of fresh fruits, vegetables, legumes, and whole grains. Examples of whole foods include brown rice rather than white rice, whole-grain cereals and flour rather than white flour, fresh whole pieces of fish rather than fish sticks, whole chicken rather than fried chicken or chicken nuggets, fresh fruits and vegetables.

*Drink an adequate amount of pure water daily*

Six to eight glasses of water a day help keep the body hydrated, help keep you regular, and remove toxins from the body. Pure water is absolutely the best thing you can put in your body. Pure water is either natural spring water from a reliable source, filtered water, or distilled water; depending on the source, drinking unfiltered tap water can be hazardous, because it often contains harmful chemicals.

## EXERCISE AND FITNESS

Exercise is critical to good health. There are three basic components to a well-rounded fitness program. These include aerobic exercise, strength-training exercise and stretching. Individually, each component has tremendous benefits. However, when done in combination, the benefits of the whole far outweigh that of each part individually.

Exercise is best performed daily. An easy way to accomplish this is to do strength training one day followed by aerobic training the next day, alternating on and off. After 6 days of this schedule, you may want to take a day off to give your body a rest; then resume your training program.

*Aerobic exercise*

The goal of aerobic exercise is to increase the heart rate and keep it elevated for a minimum of twenty minutes. Choose to walk, swim, jog, ride a bicycle, or do other aerobic exercises that are enjoyable, and that you will continue doing. You can even combine aerobic and strength training by doing a combination circuit.

Schedule a specific exercise time for each day (such as in the morning before work) and discipline yourself to adhere to it. On the days when you cannot do this, be creative: park further from the entrance; take steps instead of an elevator, escalator or ramp; go for a walk during lunch and/or during breaks. Any or all of these are effective, even if only for ten minutes.

*Strength training*

While most people understand the value of aerobic exercise to keep the heart in good condition as well as to burn calories, they usually discount the value of strength training. Not only does strength training improve our functional capacity, especially as we age, but it also enhances physical appearance, increases metabolic rate, reduces risk of injury, decreases resting blood pressure, increases bone density and protects against a variety of degenerative problems. In a study done at the YMCAs of America, Dr. Wayne Wescott found that people trying to lose weight lost three times the amount of body fat in an eight-week period when combining strength training with aerobic conditioning, as opposed to doing aerobic conditioning alone.

Strength training does not require going to a gym or lifting heavy weights. Much can be accomplished with twenty minutes of light dumbbell exercises, or by using an elastic stretch band, a medicine ball or even buckets of water or other weighted objects. Select a weight that will allow you to complete 12 – 15 repetitions of each exercise. Attempt to work each muscle group 2 - 3 times each week. Perform shoulder presses, bicep curls, chest presses, and bent-over rows for the upper body; squats, lunges, and calf raises to help tone the lower body.

*Stretching*

As we age, we lose elasticity in our muscles and joints. Regular stretching enables us to keep the body moving freely, while increasing range of motion, muscular balance, and coordination, as well as blood supply and nutrients to the joints. It also decreases the risk of injury, reduces low-back pain and stress. Yoga and Tai Chi are two very popular exercise programs that incorporate a great deal of stretching.

It is better to stretch a warm muscle (after you have done some moderate exercise) than a cold muscle. This enables you to increase the stretch and obtain more permanent results. It also reduces the risk of a stretching injury. The safest way to stretch is to perform slow, steady stretches. Also considered to be safe is a new stretching technique called "active isolation," which is done by contracting the opposing muscle from the muscle you intend to stretch. For example, you would tighten your thigh muscle when stretching your hamstring.

## STRESS REDUCTION

Good health relates to your thoughts and feelings. as well as your physical self. The mind is extremely powerful, and its role in health and wellness is just beginning to be understood. Studies have shown that people who handle stress well and have positive attitudes are healthier, happier, and more successful.

Most people lead stress-filled lives. Poorly managed stress is believed to cause or exacerbate a number of chronic and degenerative conditions, including back pain, heart disease, arthritis, and perhaps some forms of cancer. One way to relieve the physical symptoms of stress is through relaxation. The simplest way to relax is to take time for yourself to do something you enjoy, if only for a few minutes each day. Think of this not only as fun, but as good preventive medicine.

A more formal way to reduce stress is to learn a relaxation technique, such as meditation, deep breathing, yoga, or visualization, and to practice it daily. An excellent book on this subject is *The Relaxation & Stress Reduction Workbook* by New Harbinger Publications, Inc. Relaxation techniques put the mind into what is called an alpha state, in which the body can start to heal itself. Learning to control and relax your mind is one of the most important steps to your good health.

*Get enough sleep and rest*

Most people need at least 6 to 8 hour of sleep every night. Sleep is the time the body uses to repair itself. By depriving yourself of sleep, you weaken your immune system and decrease your ability to function; this increases your chance of becoming ill or being involved in an accident.  In addition to sleep, the body needs to rest, which means taking time to do nothing. Shopping, running errands and exercising are not rest.

*Develop a positive mental outlook*

Since the mind and body together play a role in the state of your health, your thoughts can have a major impact on maintaining good health. Having a positive mental outlook is more than just trying to think positive thoughts all the time. It relates to how you see the world; whether you see it as safe and loving, or dangerous and hostile; whether you see the glass as half full or half empty.

A positive attitude can be cultivated. With the desire to do so, a conscious effort, and an open mind, you can change the way you think. Following are a few techniques that can help you see your life in a more positive way:

♦ *Have at least one thing to look forward to everyday*

This can be something as simple as your favorite television show or as exciting as a weekend away. Perhaps you are expecting a package or a phone call. If you do not have anything to look forward to, you can create something. The important thing is to have something good that you can anticipate.

♦ *Find something everyday for which to be thankful*

Once again, it can be something very simple, such as a beautiful day, the rain, a good friend, or a warm room. Most people are unaware of how much they have until they've suffered an illness or loss.

Thankfulness often depends upon our perception of things. For example, to some parents, their children are burdens because they constantly need attention and restrict their freedom. Others, who consider their children a blessing, smile at the mere thought of them and look forward to seeing them. Many situations in our lives are mixed blessings. Seeing the good and being thankful for the events helps us develop a positive attitude.

♦ *Create a ritual to do each morning upon waking to start your day in a positive way*

You may want to take a few moments before getting out of bed to recognize all that you have to be thankful for and reflect on things you look forward to for the day. The first thing in the morning is the best time for this, because the brain has not yet started to process the day's activities and is relatively empty and ready to be programmed. *Begin with a smile;* then ask yourself, "What do I have to be thankful for?" and "What do I have to look forward to today?" By practicing this routine consistently, you will program your mind to think positively.

♦ *Practice smiling*

A smile is a powerful therapeutic tool. When you feel yourself beginning to get stressed or angry, *smile.* You will notice that your whole attitude begins to change quite rapidly. Smiling causes a tight jaw to release its tension and become relaxed. You also may notice a difference in your breathing, as it slows down and becomes more regular

Do not wait to smile until you actually feel angry or tense. In today's stress-filled environment, most people are not even aware of the tension in their bodies. Driving is a perfect example. Many of us drive every day without realizing that the constant process of starting, stopping, battling traffic, and watching out for other drivers is extremely stressful. Taking public transportation is not much better.

The next time you drive your car, become aware of your face. If you are like most people, you probably have a serious look and a tight jaw. *Now smile.* Notice how a simple smile can change your whole attitude, help you feel more relaxed, and even change some people's attitudes toward you.

◆ *Learn to breathe properly*

Most people breathe naturally and easily without having to think about what they are doing. Breath is life, and although we do it adequately enough to stay alive, many of us breathe incorrectly. We have been taught to hold in the stomach and breathe deeply by expanding the chest but, in fact, this is the opposite way we are meant to breathe.

A wonderful example of the correct breathing style is that of a baby. When you observe a baby breathing, you will notice that the breath goes down into the belly with each inhale and pushes out from the lungs with each exhale. By contrast, most adults breathe backwards by taking short breaths into the chest during the inhale and exhaling from the abdomen.

◆ *The stress response*

How you breathe affects your entire body. For example, when you are frightened, you automatically begin to take quick, shallow breaths as part of a natural response that also raises your blood pressure, heart rate, muscle tension, and metabolism. This stress response, also called "flight or flight" response, is a necessary survival mechanism. When faced with a threat — real or imagined, physical or mental — adrenaline and other powerful hormones are released into the body. These hormones enable us to quickly respond to danger and take appropriate action, such as to fight or run.

Unfortunately, the body cannot tell the difference between real physical danger, as in a speeding car coming at you, and the imagined danger of worry over problems at work. Worry, fear, anxiety, and tension keep the adrenaline flowing, which produces feelings of stress. Recent studies have shown that long-term effects of the fight-or-flight response can lead to permanent, harmful physiological changes.

♦ *The relaxation response*

One of the most effective ways to reduce feelings of stress and tension is through the relaxation response, which is the body's counterbalancing mechanism to the fight-or-flight response. A significant difference between the stress response and the relaxation response is that the stress response usually occurs involuntarily, but the relaxation response can be elicited at will.

Just as blood pressure, metabolism, muscle tension, heart rate, and breathing rate are raised by the fight-or-flight response, so they are lowered by controlled breathing. Consciously shifting to diaphragmatic breathing (belly breaths) helps to reduce the intensity of emotions and enables you to approach a difficult situation more effectively. Healthy breathing is the central focus of the exercise program, yoga, which is a five-thousand-year-old practice.

In addition to reducing feelings of stress, deep belly breathing also gets the lymph moving through the body, which helps carry out waste and bring fresh oxygen to the cells. This strengthens the immune system, increases available oxygen to the brain, and enables the entire body to function better.

♦ *Deep breathing techniques*

A simple test can tell whether you are breathing correctly. While standing, place one hand on your stomach and the other hand on your chest. Now inhale. If your chest moves up, and your stomach inward, you are breathing backwards. To breathe correctly, start with the exhale. Blow all the air out of your lungs by pressing in your abdomen and squeezing in your ribs. When you inhale, the air automatically will fill your lungs, causing the belly to expand. Try doing this several times a day. You can practice while driving, sitting at work, or watching TV. Soon you will be breathing correctly without any effort.

An excellent yoga breathing exercise is to inhale through your nose with a good belly breath, hold for a count of seven, then exhale through the mouth for a count of eight. Do this four times in the morning, and four times in the evening. The whole process takes only a few minutes, yet it produces powerful results. You also can do this anytime that you feel stressed or tense. With consistent practice, you will notice a much greater feeling of calmness, often leading to better sleep, less agitation, and overall improved health.

After becoming comfortable with this exercise, you can take it one step further to produce more profound relaxation. After finishing the four sets of inhales and exhales, take deep, long breaths, concentrating on nothing but the breath entering and leaving your body. To help control the pace of your breathing, inhale and exhale through the nose. While exhaling, with your lips lightly closed, try to make an *ahh* sound in your throat. With a little practice, you will begin to take much deeper, fuller breaths. Concentrate only on your breath, and the noise you are making. If your mind begins to wander, just say "Oh, well" and return to concentrating on the breath. You can come back to your other thoughts later.

This breathing technique not only helps expand lung capacity, it also can quiet what is referred to in yoga as the "monkey mind." Focusing on the breath helps calm the body as you enter a deep state of relaxation. When done before going to bed, this simple exercise can help you sleep better. When done first thing in the morning, it clears the mind for a productive and calm day.

## PRESCRIPTION FOR A HEALTHIER YOU

The guidelines in this section can help you stay healthy. If an illness strikes, they can help you deal with it more effectively. We all need to nurture ourselves, and to find a balance between work and play, independence and interdependence, caring for self and caring for others. This book can help you set your goals for being independently healthy. It is now up to you to begin.

# Acne

Acne occurs when the sebaceous glands in the skin excrete excessive amounts of sebum, causing the pores to become blocked, generally resulting in whiteheads, blackheads, and inflamed pustules. It is best not to touch or squeeze pustules, because this may result in permanent scarring.

Conventional therapies include manual extraction of comedomes and application of topical creams and lotions that may contain benzoyl peroxide, glycolic acid, antibiotics, and synthetic vitamin A derivatives. More severe cases may require oral antibiotics and synthetic vitamin A derivatives and steroid injection of large acne cysts.

| EZ Care Program | |
|---|---|
| Diet | **Avoid** sugar, soft drinks, alcohol, refined foods, fast foods, junk foods, high-fat foods, fried foods, excess salt intake, and high-sodium foods like potato chips, catsup, and French fries. |
| | **Eat a high-water-content diet** consisting of large quantities of fresh fruits and vegetables with comparatively smaller quantities of whole grains, legumes, seeds, nuts, fish, skinless chicken and turkey. |
| | **Identify personal food sensitivities**. Avoid all common allergenic foods (e.g., dairy, eggs, wheat, sugar, preservatives, corn). Rotate moderately allergic foods on a four-day schedule (see Appendix C). Food sensitivities are known to be a cause of acne. |
| Vitamins | **A** (natural, from fish liver oil) – Dosage: 10,000 to 25,000 IU daily with meals. May reduce sebum production and hyperkeratosis of oil glands. Topical application of a vitamin A cream or ointment also may help. *Note:* Vitamin A causes adverse reactions in some individuals. Reduce dosage or discontinue if you experience headaches, blurred vision, or skin rashes. The emulsified form is fat-soluble, and is better absorbed. Dosages above 10,000 IU are not recommended for pregnant women. |
| | **E** (natural d-alpha tocopherol in a base of mixed tocopherols) – Dosage: 800 IU daily with meals. Helps regulate the body's level of vitamin A, and may prevent acne scarring. |
| Minerals | **Selenium** – Dosage: 200 mcg. daily from l-selenomethionine. *Note:* Selenium and vitamin E are synergists; thus, they enhance each other's activity in the body. |
| | **Zinc** (take only if over 14 years of age) – Dosage: 50 mg. elemental zinc from amino acid chelate with meals. *Note:* Zinc is essential for local hormone activation, resolving inflammation, and supporting tissue regeneration. Also helps the body utilize and maintain the body's level of vitamin A. |
| Herbs | **Burdock Root** (Arctium lappa) – Dosage: 1 to 2 capsules, or 30-60 drops extract* in 4 oz. Water, three times daily. *Beneficial properties*: May help in bowel detoxification, and may be beneficial as a blood and skin purifier. |

| EZ Care Program | |
|---|---|
| Miscellaneous | **Lactobacillus Probiotic** (friendly intestinal bacteria that aid digestion, nutrient assimilation, and toxin elimination) (L. acidophilus, preferably with bifidobacterium and fructo-oligosaccharides) – Use according to directions on label, and keep refrigerated. |
| | **Gently wash the skin** two times daily, using an unscented herbal soap like calendula or rosemary. (Do not scrub the skin; this may irritate the condition.) Work a lather in with a gentle fingertip massage. Finish with a thorough cold-water rinse to remove soap residue. Herbal soaps are usually soothing to the skin and non-irritating, whereas some commercial soaps may exacerbate acne. |
| | **Reduce lifestyle stress** and implement a relaxation program. Harmonizing practices (e.g., biofeedback, meditation, yoga, Tai Chi exercise) may prove beneficial in cases of chronic acne. |

## Additional Recommendations

The EZ Care Program consists of basic remedies that are commonly used for acne, and have been found to work well in most cases. The remedies are most effective when combined, but can be used individually. The options stated below can supplement or replace EZ Care remedies, and may be combined when suggested doses are followed.

### Diet

♦ **Drink** 6 to 8 glasses of pure water per day. This is very important for tissue cleansing.

♦ In some cases, it may be important to **avoid high-iodine foods** such as shellfish, seaweed, and iodized table salt, because iodine may worsen acne.

### Vitamins

♦ **B3** (niacin) – Dosage: 100 mg. three times daily with meals.
*Note:* Niacin may cause a temporary skin flush, heat and itching; these generally subside after about half an hour.

♦ **B6** (pyridoxal 5-phosphate is preferred) – Dosage: 25-50 mg. daily. May be a specific for hormonal causative factors of acne, such as those associated with premenstrual aggravation.

♦ **B complex** – Dosage: 50-100 mg. balanced B complex capsule daily with meals.
*Note:* For highest assimilation, look for a multi-B vitamin in coenzyme form and avoid mega-potency B complex products. B vitamins are "anti-stress" nutrients. Stress is often a major factor in acne. Always use B3 and B6 in conjunction with a complete B complex formula, because high doses of one of the B vitamins may lead to imbalance in the body's pool of the other B vitamins.

♦ **C** (mixed mineral ascorbates mixed with bioflavonoids) – Dosage: 500 to 1,000 mg., three to four times daily with meals. May benefit healing the skin through its crucial role in producing and maintaining healthy collagen (the basis of the connective tissue that holds skin cells together).

## Minerals

◆ **Chromium** (polynicotinate is preferred form) – Dosage: 400 mcg. daily with meals.
   *Note:* Essential for blood-sugar regulation. High blood-sugar peaks may contribute to acne.

## Herbs

◆ **Tea** of **Burdock Root** (Arctium lappa) + **Echinacea Root** (Echinacea angustifolia or purpurea) + **Dandelion Root** (Taraxacum officinalis) + **Red Clover** (Trifolium pratense) + **Yellow Dock** (Rumex crispus) + **Sarsaparilla Root** (Smilax officinalis) – Prepare tea by decoction (see Appendix B) using 1 oz. of this herb mix to 3 cups pure water. Simmer 25 minutes. Dosage: Drink 8 oz. three times daily between meals.
   *Beneficial properties:* May help purify the blood and skin.

◆ **Chaste Tree Berries** (Vitex agnus castus) – Dosage: 2 capsules or 1 tsp. extract* upon arising, for at least 90 days.
   *Beneficial properties:* May assist hormonal harmonization in women; thus, may be specific for acne that is exacerbated by hormonal imbalance (e.g., premenstrual flare-up).

◆ **Goldenseal Root** (Hydrastis canadensis)    Dosage: 1 to 2 capsules or 30-60 drops extract* in 4 oz. water three times daily.
   *Beneficial properties*: Detoxifying and antibacterial.

◆ **Gentian Root** (Gentiana lutea) – Dosage: 1 to 2 capsules or 30-60 drops extract* in 4 oz. water, three times daily.
   *Beneficial properties:* Tonic bitter; traditionally used to aid digestion and elimination, and as a liver cleanser.
   *Note:* Extract may be preferable in this case, because actual perception of its bitter taste will enhance the body's response.

◆ **Milk Thistle Seed Extract** (Silybum marianum) – Dosage: 250 mg. daily of standardized extract or 30-60 drops liquid extract* in 4 oz. water three times daily with meals.
   *Beneficial properties:* May help protect the liver, which is the body's major detoxification organ, from toxins, thus supporting the blood-cleansing processes required for clear skin.

◆ **Oregon Grape Root** (Berberis aquifolium) – Dosage: 1 to 2 capsules or 30-60 drops extract* in 4 oz. water, three times daily.
   *Beneficial properties:* Contains antibacterial components that may inhibit harmful bacterial growth in the large intestine and on the skin. Also may help as a blood purifier.

## Aromatherapy

Choose one or more of these oils: **Grapefruit** (Citru paradisi), **Geranium** (Pelargonium graveolens) or **Tea Tree** (Melaleuca alternifolia).

Prepare a **Head Vapor** (see Appendix D), adding a total of 6 to 8 drops of one of the above essential oils *or* a combination of two or three of the oils. Steam face for several minutes until face sweats freely. Rinse or spray face with cold water for 30 to 60 seconds. *While skin is still wet,* massage in 2 drops of any one of the essential oils mixed with 1 tbsp. lemon juice plus 1 tbsp. water. Continue this massage until face is dry.

<u>Homeopathy</u>

See Appendix E for proper use and handling instruction prior to administering remedies described below.

♦   **Belladonna 6C** – Very severe acne, with red lesions deep in the skin and no pus showing through. Dosage: 5 pellets under the tongue, one to two times daily.

♦   **Hepar Sulph 6C** – Pimples heal slowly, and easily suppurate white pus. Dosage: 5 pellets under the tongue, one to two times daily.

♦   **Sulphur 6C** – General homeopathic remedy for acne on nose, dandruff of scalp and eyebrows, eruptions worse with washing and with heat. Dosage: 5 pellets under the tongue, one to two times daily.
    Also, often alternated with the specific indicated remedy. For example, use the indicated remedy two to three weeks, then sulphur 6C for one week, then the indicated remedy for two weeks, etc., until the condition clears.

♦   **Thuja 6C** – Severe or even scarring acne of the face and nose, with inflammation of skin; face greasy or oily; history of repeated or failed vaccinations. Dosage: 5 pellets under the tongue, one to two times daily.

<u>Miscellaneous</u>

♦   **Avoid** synthetic cosmetics, lotions and creams, as these may aggravate or even cause acne.

♦   **Carrot** or **Cucumber Mask** – Apply a mask of steamed and pureed carrots, *or* raw, pureed cucumbers. May soothe, cleanse, and nourish the facial skin. Leave in place up to 1 hour; rinse with cold water. Follow with either the essential oil/lemon juice rub *or* the essential oil/aloe vera application (see Aromatherapy above).

♦   **Clay Mask** – May soothe inflamed and irritated skin, as well as draw out impurities.
    *Preparation:* (1) Mix green or rose clay with water to form a paste. (2) Spread over affected area or entire face. (3) Allow to remain on skin for 1 to 2 hours. (4) Rinse with clear, warm water. (5) Rinse with cold water. If any clay adheres to skin, dab area with aloe vera juice to help remove.

♦   **Epsom Salt Bath** (see Appendix D) – Dosage: To encourage perspiration, before entering tub and while in tub, drink several cups of yarrow (Achillea millefolium) tea prepared by infusion (see Appendix B). Do not dry. Wrap in a cotton sheet, go to bed, and cover for at least 1 hour.

Take a second round of sweating in another bath (sweating helps the body reduce the elevated toxic load that may be contributing to skin eruptions). Then take a tepid shower. Follow with a brisk towel rub. Rest at least 1 hour.

♦ **Expose** face to **fresh air** as much as possible, as well as small amounts of **sunlight** (before nine a.m. or after 4 p.m. for 10-15 minutes). Do not overdo sunlight. Avoid sunburn and excessive exposure. Sunlight may increase the peeling of surface keratin and prevent blockage of skin glands.

♦ **Fiber Supplement** – Dosage: 1 to 3 tsp. psyllium husk fiber in 8 oz. pure water, one to two times daily between meals.
*Note:* Carefully read label; some brands require additional water. Constipation is often a contributing factor of acne.

♦ **Keep hands away from face**. Do not prop face on hands.

♦ **Regularly exercise** to support blood circulation, tissue oxygenation, and lymphatic drainage, which are crucial for healthy skin. Exercise also encourages sweating, which is a primary avenue of skin detoxification.
*Note:* Cleanse skin immediately after exercising, to prevent further clogging of the pores.

♦ **Shampoo regularly**. Cut hair short and keep off face.

* Most herbal extracts contain alcohol. Avoid use if alcohol sensitive or if there is a history of alcohol abuse. *Note:* Alcohol content can be reduced through evaporation by adding extract to very hot water (just below boiling point) and allowing to stand 5 to 7 minutes before drinking.

# Angina

Angina is a potentially serious condition that should never be cared for without the assistance of a licensed healthcare professional. The information in this book is intended to help you be aware of options available to you.

Angina occurs when there is an inadequate supply of blood to the heart due to clogging or constriction of the arteries. This low supply of blood reduces the amount of oxygen available to the heart muscle when demand for the muscle is high. A pressure or heaviness is often felt in the center of the chest, sometimes radiating to the arms, back, neck, or jaw. It may occur at rest or with exertion. In some individuals, angina presents itself as shortness of breath.

Conventional treatments include drugs that dilate arteries or those that reduce the heart's workload, such as nitrates, beta-blockers or calcium-channel blockers. When medical therapy is not enough, or the narrowing becomes significant, angioplasty may be used. More severe vessel disease with heart dysfunction is treated with coronary-bypass surgery.

*Special Note:* An alternative medical treatment to angioplasty or bypass surgery is **chelation therapy**. For more information on chelation therapy, see Appendix F.

| EZ Care Program | |
|---|---|
| Diet | **Avoid** intake of **red meats, fried foods,** and **partially hydrogenated oils (e.g., margarine).** |
| | **Eat a high water-content diet** consisting of large quantities of fresh fruits and vegetables, with comparatively smaller quantities of whole grains, legumes, seeds, nuts, and cold-water fish. |
| | **Eliminate** all **caffeine, sugar, and alcohol.** |
| Vitamins | **E** (natural d-alpha tocopherol in a base of mixed tocopherols) – Dosage: Begin with 200 IU daily. Increase intake each week by 200 IU daily to attain a level of 800 IU daily in divided doses with meals. Vitamin E is a crucial antioxidant that may benefit cardiovascular function. |
| Minerals | **Magnesium** (elemental magnesium from amino acid chelate) – Dosage: 250 mg., two to four times daily. If loose stools occur, reduce the dosage to bowel tolerance. Magnesium aids in heart contractions, maintaining dilation of the coronary arteries, and preventing arrythmia. |
| Herbs | **Cayenne Pepper** (Capsicum annuum) – Dosage: 1 to 2 capsules or ¼ tsp. per meal. May be beneficial during acute angina episodes, as an adjunct to medication. In this case, add 1 tsp. cayenne to 8 oz. Warm water and sip slowly. <br> *Beneficial properties*: May improve blood circulation, reduce blood vessel spasm, and assist the action of other herbs. |
| | **Garlic** (Allium sativa) – Dosage: 1 to 2 capsules per meal of standardized allicin garlic or aged garlic extract. Fresh, raw garlic—a whole, living food—is preferable (4-6 cloves daily with meals); however, capsules should be considered if use of raw garlic is inconsistent. <br> *Note:* Fresh parsley taken with raw garlic helps prevent "garlic breath" and enhances garlic's blood-cleansing effects. <br> *Beneficial properties*: May improve circulation, purify blood, lower cholesterol, and lower blood pressure. |
| | **Ginkgo Biloba** – Dosage: 1 to 2 capsules (40-80 mg.) of 24% standardized extract or 30-60 drops of extract* in 4 oz. water three times daily. <br> *Beneficial properties*: May improve general circulation and blood flow to the heart. |
| | **Hawthorn Leaves** (Crataegus oxycantha) – Dosage: 250 mg. three times daily of a standardized extract or 35 to 50 drops liquid extract* in 4 oz. of warm water, two to three times daily between meals. Hawthorn leaves are preferred to berries because of their potency. <br> *Beneficial properties*: May help strengthen the heart and decrease severity of angina. |
| Homeopathy | **Mag Phos 6X** – Antispasmodic cell salt and **principal cell salt remedy for angina**. Dosage: Dissolve 5 pellets under the tongue, three times daily between meals. During acute episodes, repeat dosage every 5 to 10 minutes, or as required. |
| Miscellaneous | **Coenzyme Q-10** – A nutrient required for full oxygenation of heart cells that is often deficient in patients with heart disease. Dosage: 100 mg., two to four times daily. For greatest assimilation of this fat-soluble nutrient, use an emulsified form of coenzyme Q-10. <br> *Note:* HMG-CoA reductase inhibitors (statin drugs), used to treat high |

| EZ Care Program |
|---|
| cholesterol, will deplete coenzyme Q-10 stores in the body. |
| **Eliminate** use of **tobacco,** a major factor in cardiovascular disease. |
| **Institute a physician-approved program of exercise**. Gradually increase intensity in accordance with tolerance. If symptoms appear, slow down or stop until the pain subsides, then resume. Exercise is a crucial element in cardiovascular health. |
| **L-Carnitine** – 500 mg. three times a day. A nutrient involved in producing energy in cardiac muscle. Supplementation may help increase efficient oxygen utilization by heart cells. |
| **L –Arginine** – 1000 –2000 mg. three times daily away from food. L-arginine is an amino acid, which causes coronary vessel dilation by the release of nitric oxide. It is also beneficial in aiding heart function. *Note:* L-Arginine works in a mechanism similar to nitroglycerine, so consult your physician before using. Any nitrate supplement can lower blood pressure, causing a fainting episode. |
| **Reduce** lifestyle **stress** and implement a relaxation program. Harmonizing practices, such as biofeedback, meditation, yoga, and Tai Chi exercise, may prove beneficial. |

# Additional Recommendations

The EZ Care Program consists of basic remedies commonly used for angina and has been found to work well in most cases. The remedies are most effective when combined, but can be used individually. The options stated below can supplement or replace EZ Care remedies and may be combined when suggested doses are followed.

## Diet

♦ **Avoid frying and sautéing. Add cold-pressed vegetable oils**, especially extra-virgin olive oil, after steaming to lend a sautéed texture to vegetables. Keep vegetable oils refrigerated after opening.

♦ **Avoid artificial sweeteners** and **food preservatives** because these may cause spasm of arterioles (small arterial branches) and impede blood circulation to the heart.

♦ **Drink** adequate amount of pure water daily as recommended by physician.

♦ **Eat fish** such as mackerel, herring, trout, and salmon, as these contain rich amounts of omega-3 fatty acids.

♦ **Eat generous** amounts of raw **garlic** and **onions**; they contain antioxidants important for heart and blood vessel health.

♦ **Eat high fiber foods** such as grains, legumes, broccoli, raw cabbage, and dark green, leafy vegetables

◆ **Include flaxseed oil**: 1 to 2 tbsp. daily. Flaxseed oil contains anti-inflammatory omega-3 fatty acids that help protect arteries and decrease resistance to blood flow.

◆ **Limit salt** intake; salt may increase blood pressure in salt-sensitive individuals. If salt is tolerated, use only an unrefined sea salt that contains an abundance of beneficial trace minerals.

## Vitamins

◆ **C** (mixed mineral ascorbates mixed with bioflavonoids) – Dosage: 500 to 1,000 mg two to three times daily with each meal. Vitamin C is essential for structural integrity of the heart and blood vessels, and for maintaining normal serum cholesterol and triglyceride levels.

◆ **B complex** – Dosage: 50 mg. balanced B complex capsule with morning meal.
*Notes:* (1) For highest assimilation, use a B vitamin in the coenzyme form which contains the vitamins in their coenzyme form and avoid mega-potency B complex products. (2) B vitamins are "anti-stress" nutrients. Stress is often a major factor in cardiovascular symptoms.

◆ **Tocotrienols** – Dosage 200 – 800 IU divided twice daily. Tocotrienols are members of the vitamin E family and are found in rice bran oil. Tocotrienols inhibit the cholesterol forming enzyme HMG-CoA reductase, and may aid in plaque removal from arteries.

## Aromatherapy

In a small, amber glass bottle, make a blend of 1 part each of **essential oils of Ginger** (Zingiber officinalis) **and Ylang-Ylang** (Cananga odorata). During angina attacks, tap 4 drops of this blend onto the palm of one hand, then rub palms together vigorously. Inhale deeply several times from cupped palms, exhaling to the side. Repeat every few minutes, or as required.

## Homeopathy

See Appendix E for proper use and handling instruction prior to administering remedies described below.

◆ **Carbo Veg 6C** – Angina due to excessive flatulence generally accompanied by great chilliness. Dosage: Dissolve 5 pellets under the tongue, two to three times daily between meals. During acute episodes, repeat dose every 15 to 30 minutes, or as required.

◆ **Glonoinum 6C** – Violent beating as if heart will burst through chest; labored breathing and pain radiating in all directions, particularly radiating down; weakness of left arm. Dosage: Dissolve 5 pellets under the tongue, two to three times daily between meals. During acute episodes, repeat dose every 15 to 30 minutes, or as required.

- **Naja 6C** – Constriction of the chest; pain as if heart is gripped in a vise. In the absence of a clear and specific indication, Naja may prove beneficial. Dosage: Dissolve 5 pellets under the tongue, two to three times daily between meals. During acute episodes, repeat dose every 30 minutes, or as required.

## Miscellaneous

- **Elevating the head of the bed** may help angina that occurs only at night.

- **Avoid becoming chilled.** Always dress warmly in cold weather, and avoid exposing face to cold wind.

- **Avoid cold drinks**.

- **Bromelain** – 500 mg. three times daily between meals. The enzyme derived from pineapple may help reduce inflammation and reduce atherosclerotic plaque formation in blood vessels.

# Anxiety

The most common psychiatric symptom—anxiety—is the sense of fear or impending doom. In the acute form, it is known as a "panic attack." Anxiety is a component of many psychiatric disorders, but also may be a part of everyday life. Physical symptoms of anxiety include heart palpitations, a feeling of shortness of breath, sweating, and dizziness.

Conventional treatments include psychotherapy and short-term use of sedatives, antidepressants, beta-blockers, and serotonin reuptake inhibitors.

| EZ Care Program | |
|---|---|
| Diet | **Avoid** all refined sugar, juice concentrates, and high fructose corn syrup. Use raw honey in moderation or stevia as a sweetener. |
| | **Avoid** all stimulants, especially those with caffeine, including coffee and decaf, black tea, soda, and chocolate. |
| Vitamins | **B complex** – B vitamins are major nerve and "anti-stress" nutrients. Dosage: 50 to 100mg. balanced B complex capsule with morning meal. *Note:* For highest assimilation, use a multi B complex which contains the vitamins in their coenzyme form and avoid mega-potency B complex products. |
| | **Inositol** – Dosage 4 – 8 g. daily. Inositol is a B vitamin shown in studies to reduce symptoms of anxiety, depression, and obsessive-compulsive disorder. It has a calming effect on the central nervous system. |

| EZ Care Program | |
|---|---|
| Herbs | **Chamomile flowers** (Matricaria recutita) – Dosage: 2 to 3 capsules or 4-8 oz of tea, three times daily.<br>*Beneficial properties*: Antispasmodic and soothing to the nerves. Especially indicated for anxiety in children. (See Appendix B) At bedtime, ½ tsp. of raw, unrefined honey can be added to warm tea to enhance sleep. |
| | **Kava Kava** (piper methysticum) – Dosage: 2 capsules of a standardized extract or 30 drops liquid extract* in 4 oz. water three times daily.<br>*Beneficial properties*: Significant relaxant properties.<br>*Note:* Do not mix with any other herbs that affect mental functioning without consulting your healthcare professional. |
| Homeopathy | **Kali Phos 6x** – The principal cell salt remedy for calming and strengthening nerves. Specific for nervousness, sleeplessness, lowered vitality, weariness, grumpiness, and anxiety with nervous exhaustion. Dosage: Dissolve 5 pellets under the tongue, two to four times daily between meals, and at bedtime. During acute episodes, dissolve 5 pellets every 15 to 30 minutes, until acute anxiety subsides. |
| Miscellaneous | **Breathing exercise** – Thousands of years ago in India, it was written that when breathing is rushed and incomplete, the mind acts like a "chariot driven by wild horses." Mental poise derives in large part from practicing deep, rhythmic breathing; this can be developed through regular practice of breathing exercises. Following is a yoga breathing exercise for calming the mind: Inhale through the nose with a deep belly breath for a count of 4, hold for a count of 7, exhale through the mouth for a count of 8. Practice two times per day, four to eight sets each time. |
| | **L-5HTP** (5-hydroxytryptophan) – Dosage: 100 mg. twice daily. This derivative of the amino acid tryptophan has sedative and anti-depressive effects. L-5HTP helps the natural production of the neurotransmitter serotonin, which is responsible for mood balance.<br>*Note:* The effects of L-5HTP are not immediate, and therefore not recommended for acute bouts of anxiety. Consult your healthcare practitioner if you are taking prescription antidepressants. |

# Additional Recommendations

The EZ Care Program consists of basic remedies that are commonly used for anxiety and have been found to work best in most cases. The remedies are most effective when combined, but can be used individually. The options listed below can supplement or replace EZ Care remedies and may be combined when suggested doses are followed.

## Diet

◆   **Identify personal food sensitivities**. Avoid all common allergenic foods (e.g. dairy, eggs, wheat, sugar, preservatives, corn). Rotate moderately allergic foods on a four-day schedule (see Appendix C).

◆ **Eat small meals** frequently throughout the day. This may help balance blood sugar, and may have positive effects on anxiety.

## Minerals

◆ **Calcium** (elemental calcium from amino acid chelate) – Dosage: 125 to 250 mg. daily with each meal and at bedtime. Essential for relaxing the nervous system. Considered a "lullaby" mineral.

◆ **Chromium** (polynicotinate is preferred form) – Dosage: 200 mcg. one to two times daily with meals. May help balance blood sugar fluctuations. The body's ability to maintain optimal blood sugar levels is crucial for sustaining emotional equilibrium and energy levels.

◆ **Magnesium** (elemental magnesium from amino acid chelate) – Dosage: 125 to 250 mg. daily with each meal and at bedtime. Essential for relaxing the nervous system. Considered a "lullaby" mineral.

## Herbs

◆ **Lemon Balm** (Melissa officinalis) and **Hops** (Humulus luplulus) and **Scullcap** (Scutellaria lateriflora) **combination tea** – Prepare by infusion, using 1 tsp. of each herb to 2 cups pure water. Steep for 25 minutes, let cool, then strain. Drink 6 oz. warm tea two to four times daily. All three herbs are prominent relaxants; when taken in combination, they elicit a more dynamic calming response.

◆ **St. John's Wort** (Hypericum perforatum) – 1 to 3 capsules of standardized extract (0.3% hypericin ) or 8 oz. of tea three times daily.
*Beneficial properties*: Antianxiety, antidepressant, and sedative. (See Appendix B)
*Note:* Consult your healthcare practitioner if you are taking prescription antidepressants. Avoid exposure to strong sunlight and tanning beds because skin can become photosensitive.

◆ **Valerian Root** (Valeriana officinalis) – Dosage: 2 capsules or 30-60 drops liquid extract* in 4 oz. water two to three times daily.
*Beneficial properties*: Sedative and calming to the nerves. Traditionally used for insomnia, excitability, and nervous exhaustion. May be combined with **Passion Flower (Passiflora incarnata)** which has similar properties, or with **Oat Seed Extract (Avena sativa)** which is a nerve nourisher. Administer in equal amounts when using in combination.

## Aromatherapy

Combine equal amounts of 2 or 3 of the following essential oils: **Blue Chamomile** (Matricaria chamomilla), **Lavender** (Lavendula vera), **Neroli** (Citrus aurantium var. amara) and **Ylang- Ylang**. During acute episodes, tap 4 drops of the blend onto the palm of one hand, then rub the palms together vigorously. Inhale deeply from the cupped palms several times, exhaling to the side. Repeat every few minutes or as required. This application may be used between acute episodes, to reduce proneness to anxiety.

## Homeopathy

See Appendix E for proper use and handling instruction prior to administering remedies described below.

- **Aconitum 6C** – Sense of panic and frantic impatience; fearful that something terrible is going to occur; easily startled; anxiety that you will die from an illness. Dosage: Dissolve 5 pellets under the tongue, two to three times daily. During acute episodes, dissolve 5 pellets every 30-60 minutes, until acute anxiety subsides.

- **Argentum Nit. 12C** – Performance anxiety (e.g., prior to an exam); stage-fright; very anxious that something will go wrong. Dosage: Dissolve 5 pellets under the tongue, one to two times daily or weekly. During acute cases, 5 pellets every hour until acute anxiety subsides.

- **Arsencium 12C or 30C** – Fastidious, fussy, perfectionist; worry about everything, especially when something is expected of you; exaggerate severity of an illness or stress challenge; very chilly; thirsty for small sips of cold water. Dosage: Dissolve 5 pellets under the tongue, one to two times daily or weekly. During acute episodes, 5 pellets every hour, until acute anxiety subsides.

- **Phosphorus 12C or 30C** – Highly impressionable; pick up on other people's worries and anxieties; desire company, affection, and sympathy; fear of the dark, being alone, thunderstorms, and spiders; fear felt in pit of stomach; restless and fidgety. Dosage: Dissolve 5 pellets under the tongue, one to two times daily or weekly between meals and at bedtime. During acute episodes, 5 pellets every hour, until acute anxiety subsides.

## Miscellaneous

- **Neutral Bath** – Fill tub with water that is comfortably warm, not too hot or too cold. Dim lighting and quiet atmosphere. Enter tub. Cover exposed parts, such as knees, with a towel; or cover the top surface of the tub with a sheet. Add warm water as required to maintain a neutral temperature. Remain relaxed and quiet. Do not scrub. Move about as little as possible. Remain in water 20 minutes to 2 hours. If in tub longer than 30 minutes, be careful when standing up; ask for assistance, if necessary. After getting out of tub, pat dry (do not rub; friction is stimulating and offsets the calming effect of the neutral bath). Lie down and rest for at least one hour.

- **Reduce** lifestyle **stress** and implement a relaxation program. Harmonizing practices (e.g., biofeedback, meditation, yoga, Tai Chi exercise) may prove beneficial.

- **Rescue Remedy** – a Bach flower remedy that may be helpful for emotional disturbances. Dosage: 5 drops sublingually, three times daily. Hold the drops in the mouth for one minute before swallowing. During acute cases, take every 15 to 30 minutes, until acute anxiety subsides.

- \*   Most herbal extracts contain alcohol. Avoid use if alcohol sensitive or if there is a history of alcohol abuse. *Note:* Alcohol content can be reduced through evaporation by adding the extract to very hot water (just below boiling point) and letting it stand 5 to 7 minutes before drinking.

# Arthritis (Osteoarthritis)

Osteoarthritis, also known as degenerative joint disease, is the most common form of arthritis. It afflicts an estimated 80% of the population over age 50. In osteoarthritis, the cartilage covering the ends of the bones begins to wear away, causing the rough surfaces of bones to rub together at the joint, bringing on symptoms of stiff and painful joints as well as loss of mobility.

Conventional medicine treats this condition with pain relievers, such as acetaminophen and anti-inflammatory drugs (NSAIDs) like ibuprofen, naproxen, and aspirin as the first line of treatment. Cold packs, warm compresses and baths, along with a regular low impact exercise program, are also recommended. For intense pain, corticosteroid injections or even surgery are used. Corticosteroid injections should be used with extreme caution. Side-effects include tendon weakness, tendon rupture, atrophy, and flaring of pain.

*Special Note:* **Prolotherapy** is an alternative therapy to treat arthritis. This reconstructive injection therapy can be highly successful in relieving symptoms of arthritis pain. Prolotherapy injections stimulate tissue regrowth, allowing for normal joint function. Contact a physician skilled in prolotherapy for treatment. See Appendix F for more information.

| EZ Care Program | |
| --- | --- |
| Diet | Eat a **high-water content diet** consisting of large quantities of fresh fruits and vegetables with comparatively smaller quantities of whole grains, legumes, seeds, nuts, fish, skinless chicken and turkey. |
| | **Include flaxseed oil** – 1 to 2 tbsp. daily. Flaxseed oil contains anti-inflammatory omega-3 fatty acids that help maintain joint function, and reduce joint pain. |
| Vitamins | **C** (from mixed mineral ascorbates) – Dosage: 500 to 1,000 mg. three times a daily with meals. May protect against erosion of cartilage tissue and stimulate repair of connective tissue. |
| Herbs | **Capsaicin cream** (made from cayenne pepper) – Dosage: Use according to directions on label. Inhibits the pain-producing chemical known as Substance P. *Beneficial properties*: May help to relieve pain. *Note:* A Localized burning sensation may occur during initial period of use. Wash hands thoroughly after application. |
| Miscellaneous | **Chondroitin Sulfate** – Dosage: 500 mg. three times a day for two months. May help rebuild damaged joints. |

## EZ Care Program

| |
|---|
| **Glucosamine Sulfate** – Dosage: 500 mg. three times daily for at least three months. May help regenerate joint cartilage as well as decrease the pain of osteoarthritis. Glucosamine sulfate can also prevent the onset of cartilage degeneration.<br>*Note:* Heavier individuals should speak to a physician about increasing dosage. |
| **Methyl sulfonyl methane** (MSM) – Dosage 1000 mg. twice daily. Provides a source of natural sulfur, which aids in the structure of ligaments and tendons. MSM also has analgesic properties, and can boost the immune system, aid in liver detoxification, and relieve allergies. Most effective in oral forms; less effective in creams. |
| **Exercise** at least a half an hour every day. May be beneficial in promoting blood circulation to and from the joints as well as weight loss. Exercises such as swimming, walking, Tai Chi exercise, and yoga are gentle and less likely to aggravate joint inflammation. |

## Additional Recommendations

The EZ Care Program consists of basic remedies commonly used for osteoarthritis and has been found to work well in most cases. The remedies are most effective when combined, but can be used individually. The options stated below can supplement or replace EZ Care remedies and may be combined when suggested doses are followed.

### Diet

♦ **Avoid excessive intake of protein,** especially from animal sources, because this worsens swelling and restriction of joint movement.

♦ **Avoid** nightshade family vegetables, including tomatoes, eggplant, red and black peppers, and potatoes. These aggravate arthritis in many cases; however, please note: this is not a universal rule.

♦ **Drink** 8 glasses of pure, room-temperature **water** daily.

♦ **Eliminate** coffee and decaf, black tea, chocolate, soda, alcohol, and sugar.

♦ **Identify personal food sensitivities**. Avoid all common allergenic foods (e.g., dairy, eggs, wheat, sugar, preservatives, and corn). Rotate moderately allergic foods on a four-day schedule (see Appendix C).

### Vitamins

♦ **B3** (niacinimide) – Dosage: 500 mg., four times daily with meals and at bedtime. May help decrease pain and increase joint mobility.

♦ **B5** (pantothenic acid) – Dosage: 100 mg., two to four times daily with meals and at bedtime. In some cases of osteoarthritis, low tissue levels of vitamin B5 may be an important developmental factor.

♦ **B complex** – Dosage: 50 – 100 mg. daily with meals. *Note:* For highest assimilation, use a multi B complex which contains the vitamins in their coenzyme form and avoid mega-potency B complex products.

♦ **D** (from fish liver oil) – Dosage: 400 to 1000 IU daily. Necessary for absorbing calcium. Emulsified forms of vitamin D, a fat-soluble nutrient, are better absorbed, and are preferred for older individuals whose digestive powers have diminished.

♦ **E** (natural d-alpha tocopherol in a base of mixed tocopherols) – Dosage: 800 to 1200 IU daily with meals. May protect against the breakdown, and stimulate regeneration of, cartilage tissue.

## Minerals

♦ **Calcium** (elemental calcium from amino-acid chelate) – Dosage: 150 to 250 mg., three to four times daily with meals and at bedtime. Required for developing and maintaining muscle and bone tissue.

♦ **Magnesium** (elemental calcium from amino acid chelate) – Dosage: 150 to 250 mg., three to four times daily with meals and at bedtime. Helps promote the absorption and metabolism of other minerals, including calcium, phosphorus, and potassium. Required for bone rebuilding. Helps in utilization of B complex vitamins, vitamin C, and vitamin E.

♦ **Potassium** (from potassium citrate) – Dosage:100 to 300 mg., daily. May help dissolve toxic accumulation in the joints, and flush from the body. Some authorities attribute apple cider vinegar's healing power to its high potassium content.

## Herbs

♦ **Alfalfa** (Medicago sativa) tablets – Dosage: 10 to 20 tablets daily.
*Beneficial properties*: An excellent restorative tonic that rejuvenates the whole system and provides rich nutrition for muscle and joint tissue.

♦ **Boswellia** – Dosage: 1 capsule of standardized extract twice to three times daily. Boswellia is an Indian Ayurvedic herb, which inhibits inflammatory pathways, leading to increased joint mobility and decreased morning stiffness.

♦ **Cat's Claw** (Uncaria tomentosa) – Dosage: 200 mg. standardized to contain 3% alkaloids, 1 capsule three times daily with meals.
*Beneficial properties*: May reduce inflammation in affected areas.

♦ **Ginger Root** (Zingiber officinalis) – Dosage: 2 capsules or 6 - 8 oz. of dried ginger root tea three times daily. For enhanced effect, add a pinch of cayenne to each serving (see Appendix B).
*Beneficial properties*: May aid circulation and reduce joint inflammation.

♦ **Grape Seed Extract** or **Pine Bark Extract** (Pycnogenol) – Dosage: 50 mg., three times daily.

*Beneficial properties*: May reduce inflammation in affected areas.

♦   **Kelp** tablets – Dosage: 3 to 6 tablets daily with meals.
*Beneficial properties*: Kelp is a rich source of vital vitamins and minerals that long have been used in treating musculo-skeletal disorders.

♦   **Licorice Root** (Glycyrrhiza uralensis) – Dosage: 1 to 2 capsules or 40-50 drops liquid extract * two times daily.
*Beneficial properties*: May reduce inflammation as well as support the adrenal glands that produce natural cortisone.
*Note:* If you have high blood pressure, consult a physician before using this herb, because it may increase blood pressure via increased water retention. It may also lower serum-potassium levels, leading to irregular heart rhythms. Chinese licorice root is less problematic in this regard than the western variety (Glycyrrhiza glabra).

## Aromatherapy

Use the following essential-oil combination. Blend and store the combination in amber glass bottles.

**Reduce Inflammation and Pain Relief** – 2 parts **Blue Chamomile** (Chamomilla matricaria) + 2 parts **Lavender** (Lavendula vera) + 1 part **Rosemary** (Rosmarinus officinalis)

**Prepare massage oil** using the following proportion: 25 drops of the blend for each 1 oz. jojoba or emu oil. Shake well before each use. Rub massage blend into affected joints two to three times daily.

## Homeopathy

See Appendix E for proper use and handling instruction prior to administering remedies described below.

♦   **Apis 30C or 200C** – Hot, red, swollen, tender joints with stinging pain; better with cold applications and cold air; worse in a warm room when touched or when pressure is applied. Dosage: Dissolve 5 pellets under the tongue, one to two times weekly or monthly or as required.

♦   **Bryonia 6C** – Pain aggravated by the slightest motion and relieved by moderate pressure and warmth; inflamed joints hot and swollen but feel chilly. Dosage: Dissolve 5 pellets under the tongue, one to two times daily or as required.

♦   **Rhus Tox 6C or 30C** – Hot, swollen, painful joints; pain of a tearing character; symptoms better with warmth, rubbing, and change of position; worse in damp weather and damp climate; pain worse on first motion, better with continued motion, worse with excessive motion. Dosage: Dissolve 5 pellets under the tongue, one to two times daily or weekly or as required.

## Miscellaneous

♦ **Apple Cider Vinegar** – Choose one or more of the following options:

(1) Each morning on rising, drink ½ tsp. unfiltered apple cider vinegar in 6 oz. fresh apple juice. Immediately afterward, eat an apple.

(2) Add 1 tbsp. unfiltered apple cider vinegar to a raw salad, two times daily.

(3) Take 2 tsp. unfiltered apple cider vinegar + 1 to 2 tsp. raw honey in 8 oz. water, two times daily between meals.

In conjunction with apple cider vinegar intake, eat a raw apple two times daily between meals. Unfiltered apple cider vinegar is an excellent source of potassium and other important nutritional factors and may help improve joint mobility and reduce musculo-skeletal stiffness and pain.

♦ **Betaine HCL and Pepsin** – Dosage: One to two 700 mg., capsules at beginning of every meal with protein. Provides hydrochloric acid and pepsin (required for normal mineral metabolism); aids stomach phase of digestion. Many older individuals no longer produce adequate amounts of these two digestive substances.
*Note:* Avoid if suffering from stomach or duodenal ulcers. Discontinue use if experience a burning sensation in the stomach.

♦ **Clay Poultice** (see Appendix B) – Leave in place for several hours, or overnight. After removing the poultice, wash and dry skin, then rub into the affected area one of the aromatherapy massage blends described above. Repeat three or more times weekly or as required.

♦ **Eliminate** use of all **tobacco** products.

♦ **Hot and Cold Contrast Baths** – **two to three times weekly** (*not on days when taking warm bath with hayflowers tea*). Begin by immersing the affected part (e.g., hand) in a basin of hot (110°-115°F) water for up to 4 minutes. Then immerse it in a basin of cold (55°-60°) water for 45 seconds. Alternate back and forth for 20-40 minutes. Add hot and cold water to the respective basins or as required to maintain the temperatures.

♦ **Proteolytic Enzyme Formula** (protein-digesting enzyme that includes protease, bromelain, papain) – Dosage: 3 or more capsules, three times a day *between* meals, to decrease inflammation and speed healing of tissues. When taken with meals, the enzymes are used up in the digestive process.
*Note:* Avoid if there are stomach or duodenal ulcers; proteolytic enzymes may aggravate ulcers and induce bleeding.

♦ **S-adenosylmethionine** (SAMe) Dosage: 400 mg per day of enteric coated tablets in the butanedisulfonate form on an empty stomach. May help alleviate pain and inflammation.

◆ **Weight loss** – Excessive body weight places abnormal stress on the skeletal system, including the joints. Body tissues can truly heal only when the stress on them is reduced to within their threshold of tolerance.

\* Most herbal extracts contain alcohol. Avoid use if alcohol sensitive or if there is a history of alcohol abuse. *Note:* Alcohol content can be reduced through evaporation by adding extract to very hot water (just below boiling point) and allowing to stand 5 to 7 minutes before drinking.

# Arthritis (Rheumatoid)

Rheumatoid arthritis is classified as an autoimmune disease in which the body attacks its own tissues. The disease causes inflammation of the joints and, over time, degeneration and disfiguration. It often begins with the small joints in the hands, which become swollen, tender, and often deformed; it also affects the wrists, elbows, feet, shoulders, knees, hips, and neck. Symptoms tend to occur symmetrically; joints on both sides of the body are affected at the same time. Other symptoms include fever, fatigue, stiffness, and loss of appetite.

Conventional treatments during early stages may include using aspirin or anti-inflammatory drugs, such as ibuprofen or naproxen sodium for fever, inflammation, and pain. For more severe symptoms, treatment may include gold injections, and prednisone. Drugs used to fight malaria or immunosuppressants such as methotrexate also may be prescribed. However, their side-effect profiles are less favorable. Splints are used to immobilize the joints. Surgery is a last resort, and removes and replaces diseased joints. Physician-supervised regular exercise is recommended.

| EZ Care Program | |
|---|---|
| Diet | **Eat a high water-content foods diet** consisting predominantly of fresh fruits and vegetables with smaller amounts of whole grains, legumes, nuts, seeds, fowl, and fish. |
| | **Eliminate** sugar, soda, coffee, alcohol, and stimulants. |
| | **Identify personal food sensitivities**. Avoid all common allergenic foods (e.g., dairy, eggs, wheat, sugar, preservatives, corn). Rotate moderately allergic foods on a four-day schedule (see Appendix C). These are often a major cause of rheumatoid arthritis. |
| | **Avoid** nightshade family vegetables, including tomatoes, eggplant, red and black peppers, and potatoes; in many cases, they aggravate arthritis. |
| | **Include flaxseed oil** – contains anti-inflammatory omega-3 fatty acids that help to reduce joint swelling. Dosage: 1 to 2 tbsp. daily. |

| | EZ Care Program |
|---|---|
| | **Eat fish** such as mackerel, herring, trout and salmon as these contain high quantities of omega-3 fatty acids. |
| Minerals | **Calcium** (elemental calcium from amino acid chelate) – 150 to 250 mg., three to four times daily with meals and at bedtime. Required for developing and maintaining muscle and bone tissue. |
| | **Magnesium** (elemental magnesium from amino acid chelate) – 150 to 250 mg., three to four times daily with meals and at bedtime. Helps promote absorption and metabolism of other minerals, including calcium, phosphorus, and potassium. Helps in utilization of B complex vitamins, vitamin C, and vitamin E. |
| Herbs | **Devils Claw** (Harpagophytum procumbens) – Dosage: 2 capsules three times a day. *Beneficial properties*: Traditionally used to relieve inflammation, joint, tendon and muscle pain. |
| | **Curcumin** – Dosage: 400 mg. three times daily with meals. Curcumin is a flavonoid that gives tumeric its yellow color. Has anti-inflammatory properties that can reduce joint pain, swelling, and stiffness. |
| | **Evening Primrose Oil** (Oenothera biennis) – Dosage: 1300 mg., two times daily with meals. *Beneficial properties*: Contains gamma-linoleic acid (GLA) that may inhibit inflammatory processes. |
| Miscellaneous | **Exercise** at least half an hour daily. This is a crucial part of the physical therapy program for rheumatoid arthritis. May be beneficial in promoting blood circulation to and from the joints, as well as lymphatic drainage of joint toxins. Swimming, walking, Tai Chi exercise, and yoga are gentle exercises that are less likely to aggravate joint inflammation. Of particular benefit: **gentle stretching and deep-breathing exercises**. |
| | **Lactobacillus Probiotic** (friendly intestinal bacteria that aid digestion, nutrient assimilation, and toxin elimination) (L. acidophilus, preferably with bifidobacterium and fructo-oligosaccharides) – Use according to directions on label and keep refrigerated. |
| | **Methyl sulfonyl methane** (MSM) – Dosage: 1000 mg. twice daily. Provides a source of natural sulfur, which aids in the structure of ligaments and tendons. MSM also has analgesic properties, and can boost the immune system, aid in liver detoxification, and relieve allergies. Most effective in oral forms; less effective in creams. |
| | **Omega-3 Fatty Acids** (Max EPA) – Dosage 1000 – 4000 mg. twice daily with meals. *Beneficial properties:* Contains eicosapentaenoic acid (EPA) and docosahexanoic acid (DHA) which inhibit inflammatory processes. |
| | **Reduce** lifestyle **stress** and implement a relaxation program. Harmonizing practices (e.g., biofeedback, meditation, yoga, Tai Chi exercise) may prove beneficial. |

## Additional Recommendations

The EZ Care Program consists of basic remedies commonly used for rheumatoid arthritis and has been found to work well in most cases. The remedies are most effective when combined, but can be used individually. The options stated below can supplement or replace EZ Care remedies and may be combined when suggested doses are followed.

## Diet

♦ **Avoid** intake of **red meats, fried foods,** and **partially hydrogenated oils** (e.g., margarine).

♦ **Eat flavonoid-rich foods** such as apricots, cherries, blackberries, blueberries, grapes, grapefruits, and lemons. Flavonoids exert antioxidant and anti-inflammatory effects.

♦ **Short two-to-three day fasts** (consult physician before undertaking). Maximum frequency: once every other week. It is best to consume only pure distilled water during a fast; if this is not feasible, include in the fast, fresh salt-free vegetable broths and fresh vegetable juices.

## Vitamins

♦ **B3** (niacinimide) – Dosage: 500 mg., three times daily. May help decrease pain and increase joint mobility.

♦ **B5** (pantothenic acid) – Dosage: 100 mg., three to four times daily with meals and at bedtime. Supports the adrenal glands (which produce natural cortisone) and may benefit arthritis.

♦ **B6** (pyridoxal 5-phosphate is preferred) – Dosage: 50 mg., two times daily taken with meals. Required for synthesizing collagen and maintaining healthy cartilage tissue.

♦ **B complex** – Dosage: 50 mg. Always use recommended B3, B5 and B6, in addition to a complete B complex formula, because high doses of one of the B vitamins can lead to imbalance in the body's pool of the other B vitamins. *Note:* For highest assimilation, use a multi B complex which contains the vitamins in their coenzyme form and avoid mega-potency B complex products.

♦ **C** (as mineral ascorbates with bioflavonoids) – Dosage: 1000 mg., three to four times daily. May be very helpful as an anti-inflammatory and detoxicant.

♦ **E** (natural d-alpha tocopherol in a base of mixed tocopherols) – Dosage: total of 800 IU daily taken with meals.

♦ **K** – Dosage: 5 to 10 mg., three times a day. May help stabilize joint linings.

## Minerals

♦ **Copper** – Dosage: 2 mg., (glycinate or salicylate) one to two times daily with meals. Associated with the antioxidant enzyme *superoxide dismutase* (SOD), that may be deficient in rheumatoid arthritis.
*Note:* (1) Zinc and copper compete for absorption; therefore, when high doses of zinc are taken, over time a copper deficiency can develop. (2) Although copper is required for forming SOD and other essential substances, it is potentially toxic, so before taking it,

consult a physician who applies a hair-analysis test to assess the body's stores of copper and to determine if a shortfall exists (see Resource Guide). (3) Given the fact that some areas have high water or soil content of copper, professional assessment and guidance should be utilized before using a copper supplement.

♦ **Manganese** – Dosage: 5 to 10 mg., (aspartate or citrate) one to three times daily with meals. Associated with the antioxidant enzyme *superoxide dismutase* (SOD) which may be deficient in rheumatoid arthritis.

♦ **Selenium** – Dosage: 200 mcg. daily from l-selenomethionine. May help reduce production of inflammatory prostaglandins.
*Note:* Selenium and vitamin E are synergists and should be taken together.

♦ **Zinc** (take only if over 14 years of age) – Dosage: 25 mg., elemental from amino acid chelate two times daily. Associated with the antioxidant enzyme *superoxide dismutase* (SOD) that may be deficient in rheumatoid arthritis.

## Herbs

♦ **Burdock Root** (Arctium lappa) – Dosage: 1 to 2 capsules or 30-60 drops of extract* in 4 oz. water three times daily.
*Beneficial properties*: May help detoxify bowels; may be beneficial as a blood purifier.

♦ **Boswellia** – 1 capsule of standardized extract twice to three times daily. Boswellia is an Indian Ayurvedic herb that inhibits inflammatory pathways leading to increased joint mobility and decreased morning stiffness.

♦ **Cayenne Pepper** (Capsicum annuum) – 1 to 2 capsules three times daily with meals.
*Beneficial properties*: May invigorate circulation, promote tissue repair, and reduce pain.
*Note:* Begin with a low dosage, because this herb may worsen preexisting gastrointestinal irritation and inflammation, or may initiate irritation if used to excess. Due to the herb's powerful effects on circulation, avoid use during pregnancy.
*Also available:* Capsicum (cayenne) cream for topical application may relieve pain. Apply locally as directed. Localized burning sensation may occur during initial use. Apply with gloves to help avoid local irritation. Avoid contact with broken or irritated skin.

♦ **Licorice Root** (Glycyrrhiza uralensis or glabra) – 1 to 2 capsules or 40-50 drops liquid extract * two times daily.
*Beneficial properties*: May reduce inflammation, as well as support the adrenal glands (which produce natural cortisone).
*Note:* Avoid use if you have kidney or heart disease. If you have high blood pressure, consult a physician before using this herb, because it may increase blood pressure via increased water retention. Chinese licorice root (uralensis) is less problematic in this regard than the western variety (glabra).

## Aromatherapy

Use following essential oil combination:

2 parts **Helichrysm** (Helichrysm italicum) + 2 parts **Yarrow** (Achillea millefolium) + 1 part **Pine** (Pinus sylvestris). Blend and store in amber glass bottle.

*Prepare massage oil using the following proportion:* 25 drops of a given blend for each 1 oz. jojoba or emu oil. Shake well before each use. Rub massage blend into affected joints, two to three times daily.

## Homeopathy

See Appendix E for proper use and handling instruction prior to administering remedies described below.

♦ **Apis 30C or 200C** – Hot, red, swollen, tender joints with stinging pain; better with cold applications and cold air; worse in a warm room and when touched or pressure applied. Dosage: Dissolve 5 pellets under the tongue, one to two times weekly or monthly or as required.

♦ **Bryonia 6C** – Pain aggravated by the slightest motion; relieved by moderate pressure and warmth; inflamed joints hot and swollen but patient chilly. Dosage: Dissolve 5 pellets under the tongue, one to two times daily or as required.

♦ **Causticum 12C or 30C** – Symptoms worse with overuse, strain, bathing, dry weather, and when cold; better in damp and warm weather; contractures of muscles and tendons; affected joints stiff, and tendons shortened; deformity of the joints; more comfortable when it rains; rheumatoid arthritis, affecting primarily hands and fingers. Dosage: Dissolve 5 pellets under the tongue, one to two times daily, weekly, or monthly or as required.

♦ **Rhus Tox 6C or 30C** – Hot, swollen, painful joints; pain of a tearing character; symptoms better with warmth, rubbing and change of position; worse in damp weather and damp climate; pain worse on first motion, better with continued motion, worse with excessive motion. Dosage: Dissolve 5 pellets under the tongue, one to two times daily or weekly or as required.

## Miscellaneous

♦ **Alternating Hot and Cold Contrast Baths** to affected joints. Begin by immersing the affected part (e.g., hand) in a basin of hot (110°-115°F) water for up to 6 minutes. Then immerse it in a basin of cold (55° - 60°) for 1 to 3 minutes. Alternate back and forth for 20-40 minutes. Add hot and cold water to the respective basins as required to maintain the temperatures.

♦ **Bromelain capsules** – Dosage: 6 to 8 capsules daily in divided doses between meals. This enzyme, derived from pineapple, may help reduce swelling and inflammation of soft tissue.

♦ **Boswellia caspules** – Dosage: 1 capsule, 3 times daily. This Aryvudeic herb from India acts as a natural analgesic and anti-inflammatory.

- **Clay poultice** (see Appendix B) – Leave in place for several hours or overnight. After removing the poultice, wash and dry the skin, then rub in both above and below the affected area one of the aromatherapy massage blends. Repeat three or more times weekly or as required.

- **Crushed ice in a plastic bag** – Applied topically may provide significant relief when joint is acutely inflamed with redness and swelling.

- **Gentle spinal manipulation** from a qualified practitioner may be beneficial.

- **Moist heat application** for 15 to 30 minutes. Just prior to exercise, a warm shower may reduce muscle spasm and stiffness.

- **Proteolytic Enzyme Formula** (protein digesting enzyme that includes protease, bromelain, and papain) – Dosage: 3 or more capsules three times a day between meals. May decrease inflammation and speed healing of tissues when taken between meals; if taken with meals, the enzymes are used up in the digestive process.
  *Note:* Avoid with active stomach or duodenal ulcers; proteolytic enzymes may aggravate ulcers and induce bleeding.

\* Most herbal extracts contain alcohol. Avoid use if alcohol sensitive or if there is a history of alcohol abuse. *Note:* Alcohol content can be reduced through evaporation by adding extract to very hot water (just below boiling point) and allowing to stand 5 to 7 minutes before drinking.

# Asthma

Asthma is a potentially serious condition, and should never be cared for without the assistance of a licensed healthcare professional. The following information is intended to help you be aware of the options available to you.

Asthma is caused by chronically hyperreactive and inflamed airways. An asthma attack can cause muscles in the airways to constrict, lung tissue to swell, and mucus to accumulate, all of which make breathing difficult. An allergic reaction, infection, emotional reaction, or even exercise can induce asthma. Patients with asthma may have symptoms such as a dry cough, wheezing, stridor, or shortness of breath. Severe asthma can be life-threatening and requires immediate emergency medical attention.

Conventional treatments include using an inhaler with prescribed corticosteroids, bronchodilators, and a peak flow meter to measure airflow. Corticosteroid pills, theophilline preparations, and leucotriene inhibitors for more severe asthma.

*Special Note:* Alternative medicine physicians can perform an injection into the infraspinatus muscle. This injection point, known as the infraspinatus respiratory reflex (IRR), is an acupuncture site that controls breathing. Patients with asthma may notice increased airflow, less chest tightness, and diminished coughing after receiving an IRR injection.

| EZ Care Program | |
|---|---|
| Diet | Eat a **high-water-content** diet consisting of large quantities of fresh fruits and vegetables, and comparatively smaller quantities of whole grains, legumes, seeds, nuts, fish, skinless chicken and turkey. |
| | **Identify personal food sensitivities**. Avoid all common allergenic foods that may aggravate asthma (e.g., dairy, which increases mucus production; artificial preservatives, nuts, wheat, sugar, corn and white flour). Rotate moderately allergic foods on a four-day schedule (see Appendix C). |
| Vitamins | **B complex** – Dosage: 50 mg. of a balanced B complex. *Note:* For highest assimilation, use a multi B complex which contains the vitamins in their coenzyme form, and avoid mega-potency B complex products. |
| | **C with bioflavanoids** – Dosage 1000 mg. twice daily. May increase for acute asthma attacks and viral infections. Acts as a natural anti-histamine, boosts the immune system, and eases bronchial hyperreactivity. |
| Minerals | **Magnesium** (elemental magnesium from amino acid chelate) – Dosage: 250 mg., four times daily with meals and at bedtime. Relaxes the smooth muscles of the bronchial tubes, thus may ease breathing and increase uptake of air by asthmatic patients. |
| Herbs | **Licorice Root** (Glycyrrhiza uralensis or glabra) – 1 to 2 capsules or 40-50 drops liquid extract * two times daily. <br> *Beneficial properties*: May reduce inflammation and support adrenal glands (which produce natural cortisone). <br> *Note:* Avoid use if you have kidney or heart disease. If you have high blood pressure, consult a physician before using this herb, because it may increase blood pressure via increased water retention. Chinese licorice root (uralensis) is less problematic in this regard than the western variety (glabra). |
| | **Lobelia** (Lobelia inflata) mixed with **Cayenne** (Capsicum annuum) – Dosage: mix 3 parts lobelia liquid extract* with 1 part cayenne liquid extract.* Put 20 drops of mixture in 4 oz. warm water at onset of asthmatic attack. Repeat every 30 minutes or as required. <br> *Beneficial properties*: Powerfully antispasmodic. |
| Miscellaneous | **Breathing exercises** – Following is a yoga breathing exercise: Inhale through the nose with a deep belly breath for a count of 4. Hold for a count of 7. Exhale through the mouth for a count of 8. Practice two times per day, four to eight sets each time. <br> *Note:* To enhance concentration and be certain the exercise is performed properly, you might lie down, place a lightweight book on your abdomen, then peacefully observe the book's rise-and-fall motion as you breathe deeply. |

| EZ Care Program | |
|---|---|
| | **Omega-3 Fatty Acids** (Max EPA) – Dosage 1000 – 4000 mg. twice daily with meals. <br> *Beneficial properties:* Contains eicosapentaenoic acid (EPA) and docosahexanoic acid (DHA), which inhibit inflammatory processes. |
| | **Quercitin** – 250 mg., two to four times daily in divided doses between meals. One of the most pharmacologically active flavonoids, quercitin inhibits the release of histamine, which is a substance that stimulates tissue inflammation. |
| | **Reduce** lifestyle **stress** and implement a relaxation program. Harmonizing practices (e.g., biofeedback, meditation, yoga, Tai Chi exercise) may prove beneficial. |

# Additional Recommendations

The EZ Care Program consists of basic remedies commonly used for asthma and has been found to work well in most cases. The remedies are most effective when combined, but can be used individually. The options stated below can supplement or replace EZ Care remedies and may be combined when suggested doses are followed.

## Diet

♦ **Eat fish** such as mackerel, herring, trout and salmon as these contain anti-inflammatory omega-3 fatty acids.

♦ **Drink** 6 to 8 glasses of pure water daily.

♦ **Eliminate** all junk foods, fast foods, sugar, high-fat foods, refined and denatured foods, highly-seasoned foods, alcohol, caffeine, excess salt, and foods containing artificial sweeteners, preservatives and colorings.

## Vitamins

♦ **A** (Natural, from fish liver oil) – Dosage: 10,000 to 25,000 IU once daily with meals. vitamin A is required to maintain the integrity of the epithelial lining of the respiratory tract.
*Note:* Consult a physician before using higher doses of vitamin A. Avoid use if pregnant. Discontinue use if experience nausea, dry skin, sore lips, blurred vision, or other signs of vitamin A toxicity.

♦ **B6** (pyridoxal 5-phosphate is preferred form) – Dosage: 50 mg., one to two times daily with meals. May decrease frequency, duration, and severity of wheezing and asthmatic attacks.
*Note:* Always use recommended B6 and B12 in addition to a complete B complex formula, because high doses of one of the B vitamins can lead to imbalance in the body's pool of the other B vitamins. For highest assimilation, use a multi B complex that contains the vitamins in their coenzyme form and avoid mega-potency B complex products.

♦ **B12** – Dosage: 500 to 1,000 mcg. daily for thirty days. Then every other day for two months.
*Note:* In cases of B12 deficiency, intramuscular B12 injections administered by a physician are the primary and most effective option. Always use recommended B12 in addition to a complete B complex formula, because high doses of one of the B vitamins can lead to imbalance in the body's pool of the other B vitamins.

♦ **E** (natural d-alpha tocopherol in a base of mixed tocopherols) – Dosage: 800 IU daily with meals. Exerts antioxidant, anti-inflammatory actions that may help prevent asthmatic attacks.

## Minerals

♦ **Calcium** (elemental calcium from amino acid chelate) – Dosage: 100 mg., four times daily with meals and at bedtime. Calcium calms the nerves and decreases nerve irritability.

♦ **Manganese** (elemental manganese from amino acid chelate) – Dosage: 5mg., two to three times weekly for three months. Manganese may function as a protective antioxidant in lung tissue as part of the enzyme *superoxide dismutase* (SOD), thus protecting these tissues from degeneration.

## Herbs

♦ **Anise Seed** (Pimpinella anisum) – Dosage: serve 6 to 8oz. of tea prepared by infusion (see Appendix B) two to three times daily between meals. Use 2 tsp. anise seed : cup pure water when preparing infusion.
*Beneficial properties*: A mild expectorant recommended by Hippocrates that may prove useful for asthmatic children.

♦ **Garlic** (Allium sativa) – Dosage: blend 1 large garlic clove with 8 oz. hot water. Sip slowly. Take one to two times daily between meals or as required.
*Beneficial properties*: May help loosen bronchial secretions.

♦ **Mullein (**Verbascum thapsiforme) – Dosage: two to four capsules or 40-50 drops liquid extract* four times daily. Option: mullein tea. Serve 6 to 8 oz. of tea prepared by infusion (see Appendix B) two to three times daily between meals. Use 2 tsp. mullein leaf per cup pure water when preparing infusion.
*Beneficial properties*: May soothe respiratory tract in case of acute or chronic asthma.

♦ **Thyme** (Thymus vulgaris) **tea** – Dosage: serve 6 to 8 oz. of tea prepared by infusion (see Appendix B) two to three times daily between meals. Use 2 tsp. dried thyme per cup pure water when preparing infusion. To enhance effect of the tea, to each serving add 10-15 drops **Lobelia liquid extract**.
    Also consider **Thyme syrup** prepared as follows: Prepare an infusion using 3 tbsp. dried thyme **or** 6 tbsp. fresh thyme: 2 cups pure water. Steep 35 minutes. Strain and add 16 oz. raw honey. Bottle in glass and refrigerate. Dosage: 1 to 2 tbsp. two to four times daily or as required. In treating asthma, valued for antispasmodic and expectorant (i.e., loosens and brings up phlegm) properties.

## Aromatherapy

Blend and store the oil combination in an amber glass bottle. Use as a massage oil. Also, several times daily tap 3 to 4 drops of one of these blends onto the palm. Rub the palms together, then take 10-15 deep breaths from the cupped palms, turning the head to the side when exhaling.

1 part **Blue Chamomile** (Chamomilla matricaria) + 1 part **Lavender** (Lavendula vera) + 2 parts **Eucalyptus** (Eucalyptus globulus)

Prepare massage oil using the following proportion: 25 drops of the blend for each 1 oz. jojoba or sweet almond oil. Shake well before each use. Rub massage blend into upper chest and throat, two to three times daily.

## Homeopathy

See Appendix E for proper use and handling instruction prior to administering remedies described below.

♦ **Arsenicum Album 12C or 30C** – Asthmatic attacks generally occur just after midnight until about 2 a.m.; chilly but better with warmth; anguish, restlessness, and fear of suffocation; dry burning cough and soreness in chest; worse in damp weather and near the seashore. Dosage: Dissolve 5 pellets under the tongue, two to three times daily or weekly or as required. During acute episodes, administer dose every 30-60 minutes until symptoms subside.

♦ **Carbo Veg 6C or 30C** – Asthmatic attacks generally occur in the evening and are associated with long coughing attacks with soreness and burning in the chest; asthma from accumulation of gas in the stomach; worse in open air and after eating or talking; desire to be fanned. Dosage: Dissolve 5 pellets under the tongue, two to three times daily or weekly or as required. During acute episodes, administer dose every 30-60minutes until symptoms subside.

♦ **Kali Carbonicum 6C or 30C** – Wheezing worse between 2 a.m. and 4 a.m. or at 5 a.m.; anxiety, weakness with chest tightness and oppression; cannot lie flat, rests on knees with head buried in pillow. Dosage: Dissolve 5 pellets under the tongue, two to three times daily or weekly or as required. During acute episodes, administer dose every 30-60minutes until symptoms subside.

♦ **Nux Vomica 12C or 30C** – Asthma of digestive origin, generally caused by overeating with bloating of the stomach; nighttime attacks with suffocating tightness of the chest preceded by anxious, disturbing dreams; better with belching, loosening clothing, lying on back, changing sides, or sitting up; irritable temperament. Dosage: Dissolve 5 pellets under the tongue, two to three times daily or weekly or as required. During acute episodes, administer dose every 30-60minutes until symptoms subside.

♦ **Pulsatilla 6C or 30C** – Asthma in timid individuals who are subject to rapid changes in mood; worse in warm, stuffy rooms, warm weather, or after eating rich fatty foods; crisis often occurs around 10 p.m. or late evening; yellowish green mucus easily brought up; desires open air. Dosage: Dissolve 5 pellets under the tongue, two to three times daily or weekly or as required. During acute episodes, administer dose every 30 to 60minutes until symptoms subside.

## Miscellaneous

♦ **Avoid environmental pollutants** and allergens as much as possible. Consider an air purifier or filter such as a HEPA filter.

♦ **Betaine HCL and Pepsin** – Dosage: 1 to 2 capsules (700 mg. each) at beginning of any meal containing protein. Provides hydrochloric acid and pepsin (required for normal mineral metabolism) to aid stomach phase of digestion. Many older individuals no longer produce adequate amounts of these two digestive substances.
*Note:* Avoid if suffering from stomach or duodenal ulcers. Discontinue use if experience a burning sensation in the stomach. Asthma patients often secrete subnormal amount of stomach acids, thus increasing their propensity to allergic reactions to food.

♦ **Branched-Chain Amino Acids** – Dosage: 500 – 1000 mg. twice daily. The branched-chain amino acids, leucine, isoleucine, and valine help ease bronchial hyperreactivity and open the breathing passageways.

♦ Consider **manipulative work** such as deep tissue massage, chiropractic, and manual lymphatic drainage.

♦ **Head Vapor** (see Appendix D for details) – Add 10 drops of the undiluted essential oil combination blend described above.

♦ **Hot Compress to Chest and Neck** – During an acute attack, the following technique may prove of good service: Apply a hot wet compress to back of neck plus thoracic region of back and chest; simultaneously, keep the feet in a hot foot bath. Keep the head cool by sponging it with cool water. Continue application until the attack subsides (generally 15 to 30 minutes). Follow with a warm shower. Then rest in bed, remaining covered until the sweating ceases.

♦ **Lime juice** – 1 tsp. undiluted three times a day between meals.

♦ **N-Acetyl Cysteine (NAC)** – Dosage: 600 mg. three times daily. NAC, a precursor to the antioxidant glutathione, is important for liver detoxification. This amino acid serves as a natural mucolytic, aiding in the thinning and expelling of mucus secretions.

♦ **Proteolytic Enzyme Formula** (protein digesting enzyme that includes protease, bromelain, papain) – Dosage: 3 or more capsules three times a day between meals. Can decrease inflammation and speed healing of tissues if taken between meals; if taken with meals, the enzymes are used up in the digestive process.
*Note:* Avoid with active stomach or duodenal ulcers; proteolytic enzymes may aggravate ulcers and induce bleeding.

♦ **Short two-to-three day fasts** (consult physician before undertaking fast) – Maximum frequency: once every other week. Pure distilled water is best; if this is not feasible, include in the fast, fresh salt-free vegetable broths and fresh vegetable juices.

♦ **Wet Chest Pack** – Dip a towel in cold water and wring it out to slightly dripping. Place over chest and throat and cover with a dry towel of equal dimension. Then tuck in tightly with a blanket from feet to chin. Leave in place for 30 to 60 minutes.

\* Most herbal extracts contain alcohol. Avoid use if alcohol sensitive or if there is a history of alcohol abuse. *Note:* Alcohol content can be reduced through evaporation by adding extract to very hot water (just below boiling point) and allowing to stand 5 to 7 minutes before drinking.

# Athlete's Foot

Athlete's foot, also known as tinea pedis, is a fungal growth on the skin of the foot and occasionally the toenails. Symptoms include scaling, itching, burning, and cracking of the skin.

Conventional treatments include keeping the foot dry and clean, as well as using antifungal powders. Treatment must continue five to six weeks, which is the time it takes for new skin to grow and replace the old infected skin.

Fungal infection of the toenails requires oral antifungal treatment. This form of treatment requires a liver function test every three to four months. Infected toenails may not show signs of clearing for 6-12 months, which is the time it takes for new nails to grow.

| EZ Care Program | |
|---|---|
| Aromatherapy | **Tea Tree Oil (Melaleuca alternifolia)** – Mix 30 drops of tea tree oil in 1 oz. **Apple cider vinegar**. Apply for several days until the area has dried. Then switch to a 5% olive oil dilution (i.e., 5 drops tea tree oil for every 95 drops olive oil) which is emollient and soothing. tea tree oil has powerful antifungal properties. *Note:* (1) Tea tree oil may be used alone as an effective treatment. (2) It is important to continue treatment for six weeks, even if infection seems cleared. tea tree oil also may be used for toenail fungus, with treatment continuing for six months (i.e., the time it takes for toenails to completely regrow). |
| Miscellaneous | **Wash feet daily** for six weeks, before putting on fresh socks. Scrub with washcloth and clean well between toes to assist sloughing off dead skin cells. To prevent recurrence, continue this hygienic practice even after fungal infection has cleared. |
| | **Change socks** daily. It is best to wear cotton socks, because synthetic socks do not "breathe." *Note:* Athletes foot powder may be sprayed in the socks to assist in keeping the foot dry and prevent spreading the fungus. |

| EZ Care Program | |
|---|---|
| | **Keep your feet very dry**, especially after getting out of a shower. Towel-dry well between the toes. Whenever possible, remove shoes and socks and expose feet to light and air. Sunlight is especially helpful. Continue this hygienic practice even after the fungal infection has cleared. |

## Additional Recommendations

The EZ Care Program consists of basic remedies commonly used for athlete's foot and has been found to work well in most cases. The remedies are most effective when combined, but can be used individually. The options stated below can supplement or replace EZ Care remedies and may be combined when suggested doses are followed.

### Vitamins

♦ **A** (Natural, from fish liver oil) – 10,000 to 25,000 IU one to two times daily until the infection clears. Then reduce dosage to 10,000 IU once daily. Helps protect skin tissue from infection.
*Note:* Consult a physician before using higher doses of vitamin A. Avoid use if pregnant. Discontinue use if you experience nausea, dry skin, sore lips, blurred vision, or other signs of vitamin A toxicity.

♦ **C** (mixed mineral ascorbates) – Dosage: 500 to 1000 mg., two to three times daily with meals. vitamin C helps fight infection and is required for forming and maintaining collagen, which is the basis of connective tissue found in skin.

♦ **E** (natural d-alpha tocopherol in a base of mixed tocopherols) – Dosage: 800 IU once daily with a meal. vitamin E exerts antioxidant activity that protects skin tissue, helping limit extent of damage incurred by infections.

### Herbs

♦ **Calendula** (Calendula officinalis) cream or oil – Dosage: Apply two to three times daily. For a more dynamic effect, make 5% tea tree oil dilution in a base of calendula oil (5 drops tea tree oil in 95 drops calendula oil).
*Beneficial properties*: May relieve itching and promote the healing of affected tissue.

♦ **Echinacea Root** (Echinacea angustifolia or purpurea) – Dosage: 50 drops of liquid extract* in 4 oz. water two to three times daily between meals. Echinacea has potent antifungal properties.

♦ **Garlic Foot Bath** followed by dusting with **Goldenseal Root** (Hydrastis canadensis) **powder** – Dosage: 2 cloves of garlic blended with 1 qt. hot water (110°-120°F). Place in a shallow basin. For an enhanced effect, add 2 drops each of essential oils of tea tree, lavender, and myrrh (see below). Soak feet for 20 minutes. Dry well. Dust with powdered goldenseal root.

♦ **Garlic** (Allium sativum) – 1 to 2 capsules per meal of standardized allicin garlic or aged garlic extract. Fresh, raw garlic (a whole, living food) is preferable; however, capsules should be considered if raw garlic is not taken consistently.
*Beneficial properties:* Powerful antifungal.
*Note:* Raw parsley taken with raw garlic helps prevent "garlic breath", and enhances garlic's blood-cleansing effects.

♦ **Garlic Oil** – Mince 8 oz. peeled garlic cloves. Place in a large jar, cover completely with olive oil, and shake well. Place in a dark, moderately warm spot for three to four days. Then strain through unbleached cotton or cheesecloth. Bottle and store in a cool place. Wash the feet with hot, soapy water. Then rinse and dry well. Rub garlic oil into affected areas. Perform this procedure two-to-three times daily. After infection disappears, continue application of garlic oil for another seven days, to help prevent recurrence.
*Beneficial properties:* Powerful antifungal.

### Miscellaneous

♦ **Alternating Hot and Cold Foot Bath** (see Appendix D for details) – Soak feet in hot water for 6 minutes, then in cold water for 1 minute. Alternate three times, finishing with cold.

♦ **Lactobacillus Probiotic** (friendly intestinal bacteria that aid digestion, nutrient assimilation, and toxin elimination) (L. acidophilus, preferably with bifidobacterium and fructo-oligosaccharides) – Use according to directions on label and keep refrigerated.

# Atherosclerosis

Atherosclerosis is a potentially serious condition, and should never be cared for without the assistance of a licensed healthcare professional. The following information is intended to help you be aware of the options available to you.

Atherosclerosis is a gradual clogging or hardening of the arteries. It is the predecessor to other problems such as heart attacks, strokes, and high blood pressure. Most Americans will develop athersclerosis in their early twenties but usually do not develop symptoms for years. Early symptoms often include chest pressure or tightness (angina) with exertion, fatigue, and leg cramps. More advanced symptoms include shortness of breath, angina at rest, cold extremities, and ulcerated skin.

Conventional treatments include low fat, low salt diets; weight reduction if necessary; normalization of cholesterol through diet and exercise, as well as pharmacological agents such as statin drugs (e.g. Lipitor, Zocor, and Pravachol if necessary. Aspirin is also used to reduce the incidence of heart attack and stroke. More severe cases of atherosclerosis may require angioplasty or bypass procedures.

High cholesterol is only one factor in the development of atherosclerosis. Only approximately 40% percent of patients with vascular disease suffer from hypercholesteremia. The converse also holds true; many patients with elevated cholesterol may never encounter the disease. New research suggests other markers of vascular disease may be more predictive of future heart attacks and strokes than just cholesterol. These markers include homocysteine, lipoprotein (a), fibrinogen, apoproteins A and B, and cardiac C-reactive protein.

*Special Note:* An alternative medical treatment for atherosclerosis **chelation therapy**. For more details on chelation therapy, see Appendix F.

| EZ Care Program | |
| --- | --- |
| Diet | **Avoid** intake of **red meats**, **fried foods,** and **partially hydrogenated oils** (e.g., margarine). |
| | Eat a **high-water-content** diet consisting of large quantities of fresh fruits and vegetables, with comparatively smaller quantities of whole grains, legumes, seeds, nuts, fish, skinless chicken and turkey. |
| | **Eliminate** all caffeine, sugar, and alcohol. |
| Vitamins | **E** (natural d-alpha tocopherol in a base of mixed tocopherols) – Dosage: 800 IU daily taken with meals. vitamin E is an antioxidant that may protect the arterial walls, strengthen the heart, and help inhibit abnormal clotting in blood vessels. |
| | **Tocotrienols** – Dosage: 200 – 800 IU divided twice daily. Tocotrienols are members of the vitamin E family and are found in rice bran oil. Tocotrienols inhibit the cholesterol-forming enzyme HMG-CoA reductase and may aid in plaque removal from arteries. |
| Minerals | **Calcium** (elemental calcium from amino acid chelate) – Dosage: 150 mg., two to three times daily. Calcium, along with magnesium, regulates heart contraction and relaxation. Calcium supplementation also may help decrease serum cholesterol and triglyceride levels. |
| | **Magnesium** (elemental magnesium) – Dosage: 150 mg., two to three times daily. Magnesium is antispasmodic and essential for normal cardiac muscle relaxation. |
| Herbs | **Garlic** (Allium sativum) – Dosage: 1 to 2 capsules per meal of standardized allicin garlic or aged garlic extract. Fresh, raw garlic (a whole, living food) is preferable; however, capsules should be considered if raw garlic is not taken consistently. <br> *Beneficial properties*: May improve circulation, purify blood, help reduce build-up in the arteries and reduce high blood pressure. <br> *Note:* Raw parsley taken with raw garlic helps prevent "garlic breath" and enhances garlic's blood-cleansing effects. |

| | EZ Care Program | | |
|---|---|
| | **Ginkgo Biloba** – Dosage: 1 to 2 capsules (40-80 mg.) of 24% standardized extract or 30-60 drops of extract* in 4 oz. water three times daily. <br> *Beneficial properties*: May improve general circulation and blood flow to the heart. |
| | **Hawthorn Leaves** (Crataegus oxycantha) – Dosage: 250 mg., three times daily of a standardized extract. <br> *Beneficial properties*: May strengthen the heart and help decrease angina. |
| Miscellaneous | **Coenzyme Q-1O** (a fat-soluble nutrient) – Dosage: 100 mg., two to four times daily. The emulsified forms are preferred, because they have a much higher level of assimilation. Helps in oxygenation of heart cells. <br> *Note:* HMG-CoA reductase inhibitors (statin drugs), used to treat high cholesterol will deplete coenzyme Q-10 stores in the body. |
| | **Eliminate use of tobacco,** which is a major factor in cardiovascular disease. |
| | **L-Carnitine** – Dosage: 500 mg., three times a day. An amino acid used for cardiac muscle energy production. Supplementation may help increase efficiency of oxygen utilization by heart cells. |
| | **Reduce** lifestyle stress and implement a relaxation program. Harmonizing practices (e.g., biofeedback, meditation, yoga, Tai Chi exercise) may prove beneficial. |

# Additional Recommendations

The EZ Care Program consists of basic remedies commonly used for atherosclerosis and has been found to work well in most cases. The remedies are most effective when combined, but can be used individually. The options stated below can supplement or replace EZ Care remedies and may be combined when suggested doses are followed.

### Diet

- **Avoid frying or sautéing. Add cold-pressed vegetable oils**, especially extra-virgin olive oil, after steaming to lend a sautéed texture to vegetables. Be sure to keep vegetable oils refrigerated after opening.

- **Avoid artificial sweeteners** and **food preservatives**; they may cause spasm of arterioles (small arterial branches) and impede blood circulation to the heart.

- **Drink** pure water at the level recommended by your healthcare practitioner.

- **Eat fish** such as mackerel, herring, trout, and salmon as these contain anti-inflammatory omega-3 fatty acids that help protect arteries and decrease resistance to blood flow.

- **Eat generous amounts of raw garlic and onions**; these are considered blood and artery cleansers.

♦ **Eat high fiber foods** such as grains, legumes, broccoli, raw cabbage, and dark green, leafy vegetables.

♦ **Include flaxseed oil**: 1 to 2 tbsp. daily. Contains anti-inflammatory omega-3 fatty acids.

♦ **Limit** or **eliminate salt** intake; salt may increase blood pressure in salt-sensitive individuals. If salt is tolerated, use only unrefined sea salt that contains an abundance of beneficial trace minerals.

## Vitamins

♦ **B3** (Flush free niacin or niacin with inositol) – Dosage: 500 mg., three to four times daily with meals and at bedtime. May help lower total serum cholesterol level and raise HDL, the protective cholesterol. Niacin can also lower lipoprotein (a) levels.
*Note:* Avoid niacin products that do not contain insoitol. They may produce a hot, itchy reddening of the skin called "niacin flush". Patients taking niacin, especially long-acting prescription forms require periodic monitoring of blood liver enzymes. If you experience abdominal pain, nausea, muscle pain, or itching while using this product, consult your physician.

♦ **B6** (pyridoxal 5-phosphate is preferred) – Dosage: 50 mg., one to two times daily with meals. May help prevent accumulation of an artery damaging-agent known as homocysteine and may inhibit clot formation in bloodstream.
*Note:* B vitamins are "anti-stress" nutrients. Stress is often a major factor in cardiovascular symptoms. B vitamins also may improve the unsaturated to saturated fatty acid profile in the blood.

♦ **B complex** – Dosage 50 - 100 mg. Always use recommended B3, B6, and folic acid, in addition to a complete B complex formula, because high doses of one B vitamin may lead to imbalance in the body's pool of the other B vitamins. *Note:* For highest assimilation, use a multi B complex which contains the vitamins in their coenzyme form, and avoid mega-potency B complex products.

♦ **C** (mineral ascorbates mixed with bioflavonoids) – Dosage: 500 to 1000 mg., two to three times daily with meals. vitamin C is required to maintain integrity of arterial walls and normal serum cholesterol levels.
*Note:* If these dosages cause loose stools or excessive flatulence, reduce dosage to within bowel tolerance.

♦ **Folic Acid** – Dosage: 800 mcg. one to two times daily with meals. A coenzyme in the conversion of homocysteine to methionine, which is an essential amino acid.

## Minerals

♦ **Chromium** (chromium polynicotinate) – Dosage: 200 mcg. one to two times daily with meals. May help decrease serum cholesterol and triglyceride levels and retard development of, or encourage regression of, atherosclerotic plaques.

◆ **Potassium** (elemental potassium from potassium aspartate) – Dosage: 99 mg., one to three times daily. Potassium deficiency is associated with cardiac arrhythmia, hypertension, and decreased tolerance to certain heart medications.

◆ **Selenium** (from l-selenomethionine) – Dosage: 200 mcg. once daily with a meal. Selenium is a vitamin E synergist that may help prevent damage to arterial linings and formation of abnormal clots in blood vessels.

## Herbs

◆ **Alfalfa** (Medicago sativa) – Dosage: 10 to 20 tablets daily. An excellent restorative tonic that rejuvenates the whole system and may help reduce serum cholesterol levels and shrink atherosclerotic plaques.

◆ **Cayenne Pepper** (Capsicum annuum) – Dosage: 1 to 2 capsules or ¼ tsp. per meal. *Beneficial properties*: May improve blood circulation, reduce blood vessel spasm, and assist action of other herbs. May be of good service during acute anginal episode as an adjunct to medication. In this case, add 1 tsp. cayenne to 8 oz. warm water and sip slowly.

## Miscellaneous

◆ **Bromelain** – Dosage: 500 mg., three times daily between meals. Enzyme derived from pineapple that may help reduce inflammation and reduce atherosclerotic plaque formation in blood vessels.

◆ **Lecithin granules** – Dosage: 1 tbsp. two to three times daily with meals. May help in removing cholesterol deposited in blood vessels.

◆ **Omega-3 Fatty Acids** – Dosage: 300 mg. of EPA and DHA from marine lipid concentrate one to four times daily with meals. May help raise HDL ("good cholesterol") levels and reduce risk of cardiovascular disease.

◆ **Unfiltered Apple Cider Vinegar** – Dosage: 5 drops of apple cider vinegar in 4 oz. water three times daily between meals. A rich source of potassium, and may act as a heart tonic.

\* Most herbal extracts contain alcohol. Avoid use if alcohol sensitive or if there is a history of alcohol abuse. *Note:* Alcohol content can be reduced through evaporation by adding extract to very hot water (just below boiling point) and allowing to stand 5 to 7 minutes before drinking.

# Back Pain

Back pain in the United States has reached nearly epidemic proportions. Eighty percent of the population will suffer from back pain, making this the number one cause of employee absenteeism, and the second most common cause for doctor visits. Causes include improper lifting techniques, falls and accidents, poor posture, lack of exercise, weight gain and stress. Back pain can be divided into two types: acute and chronic. Acute pain comes on suddenly, lasts for a period of time, sometimes hours, days or weeks, then goes away, often to return at a later time. Chronic back pain is pain that persists for more than three months, often increasing in severity over time.

Although 90% of back problems resolve without treatment within a month of onset, some can be more serious. Self-care remedies, in many cases, reduce the duration of injury and help prevent future problems. There are, however, "red flags" of back pain that may indicate a more serious condition. If you have trouble urinating or have loss of control of bowel or bladder; numbness, tingling, or shooting pain in your leg or buttocks, weakness in the legs, accompanying fever, weight loss or night sweats, immediate physician attention is recommended.

Conventional treatments for acute back pain include ice along with analgesics and anti-inflammatory drugs such as aspirin or ibuprofen. For unremitting, intense pain, stronger muscle relaxants and anti-inflammatory agents are prescribed. Treatments also may include physical therapy and back exercises to stretch and strengthen the appropriate muscles. Surgery is used to treat patients with acute neurological compromise from a herniated disc.

However, many patients do not have pain originating from a herniated disc. A review of healthy 60-year-old people revealed 60% of those without back pain had at least one herniated disc on MRI-scanning. Other studies have shown that patients who do not have an acute surgical emergency have similar outcomes after treatment with physical therapy or surgery. In fact, in measuring pain levels three years after treatment, either group had similar outcomes to those who received no treatment whatsoever.

*Special Note:* **Prolotherapy** is an alternative therapy to treat back pain and the only treatment that gave the former Surgeon General, C. Everett Koop relief. This reconstructive-injection therapy can be highly successful in relieving symptoms of back pain. Prolotherapy injections stimulate tissue regrowth, allowing for normal joint function. Contact a physician skilled in prolotherapy for treatment. See Appendix F for more information

| EZ Care Program (Acute Pain) | |
|---|---|
| Homeopathy | **Arnica montana** – 6c or 30c: Backache from injury or overuse of muscles. May help reduce swelling, and pain and speed healing in cases of injury, especially if accompanied by bruising. For best results, use immediately after injury. Dosage: Dissolve 5 pellets under the tongue, every 30 minutes to 4 hours following back injury, in accord with severity of injury. Adjust dosage as symptoms subside. |
| | **Arnica oil or gel** – Use externally by rubbing small amount onto affected area. *Note: Toxic when taken internally.* Avoid mouth, eyes, and any open cuts. Apply every one to four hours in accord with severity of back injury. |
| Herbs | **Capsaicin cream** (made from cayenne pepper) – Dosage: Use according to directions on label. Inhibits the pain-producing chemical known as Substance P. *Beneficial properties*: May help to relieve pain. *Note:* A Localized burning sensation may occur during initial period of use. Wash hands thoroughly after application. |
| Miscellaneous | **Methyl sulfonyl methane** (MSM) – Dosage: 1000 mg. twice daily. Provides a source of natural sulfur, which aids in the structure of ligaments and tendons. MSM also has analgesic properties, and can boost the immune system, aid in liver detoxification, and relieve allergies. Most effective in oral forms; less effective in creams. |
| | **Take it easy** and give your back a chance to rest, because time is the best healer. If possible, avoid complete bedrest, because studies show that it prolongs back injuries. |
| | **Ice** the area of pain the first 48 hours. Ice may help reduce swelling and effectively relieve pain. *Method of application:* (**1**) Fill a paper cup with water and freeze it. (**2**) Peel back the paper and expose approximately one-half inch of ice. (**3**) Ice the painful area, using a circular motion. Keep the ice moving 5 to 10 minutes, until the skin turns pinkish. (**4**) If direct ice-to-skin contact is too painful, ice through a thin towel placed over the affected area; in this case, continue icing for 15-20 minutes. (**5**) With either method, repeat icing every 1 to 2 hours. (**6**) If lying on stomach is uncomfortable during icing, the following alternative method may be preferable: Wrap a plastic bag filled with crushed ice in a wet towel. While lying on back, with knees flexed, slide ice pack under affected area of back. |
| | **Apply heat** to injured area after the first 48 hours. Both wet and dry heat increases blood flow, increases circulation, promotes healing and relaxes muscle spasms. |

## Additional Recommendations

The EZ Care Program consists of basic remedies commonly used for acute back pain and has been found to work well in most cases. The remedies are most effective when combined, but can be used individually. The options stated below can supplement or replace EZ Care remedies and may be combined when suggested doses are followed.

# Acute Back Pain

Try to make yourself as comfortable as possible, giving the aggravated muscle a chance to relax. Often the most comfortable position is lying flat on the back with legs bent at a 90-degree angle and the calves resting on the cushion of a chair or couch. This helps relieve some of the pressure on the back. Once a little more comfortable, you may want to try to relieve your pain.

### Minerals

♦   **Magnesium** (elemental magnesium from amino acid chelate) – Dosage: 200 mg., four times daily with meals and at bedtime. Magnesium plays an important role in neuromuscular contractions and can act as a muscle relaxant. It is also required for absorbing and metabolizing calcium.

### Herbs

♦   **Antispasmodic Extract** (see below for instructions on preparation) – Dosage: 40-50 drops of extract* in 4 oz. warm water every 30 minutes until pain subsides, then reduce dosage accordingly.
    *Beneficial properties:* See antispasmodic extract description under "Chronic Back Pain".

♦   **St. John's Wort** (Hypericum perforatum) – Dosage: 40-50 drops of the liquid extract* or 6 oz. of tea prepared by infusion every 15-30 minutes until pain subsides (see Appendix B); use 2 tsp. dried flowering tops per 1 cup pure water.
    *Beneficial properties:* specific for muscular bruises, deep soreness, soreness and tenderness of the spine, and concussion shock or injury to the spine accompanied by great pain.

♦   **White Willow Bark** (Salix alba) – Dosage: 4 oz. of tea prepared by decoction every 15 to 30 minutes until pain subsides, then reduce dosage accordingly (see Appendix B); use 2 tsp. bark per cup pure water. For a more dynamic effect, add 25 drops of antispasmodic extract* to each 4 oz. dose of white willow tea.
    *Beneficial properties:* traditionally used to relieve pain; original source for active ingredient in aspirin.
    *Note:* Avoid use with history of a gastric or duodenal ulcer; may aggravate bleeding.

### Homeopathy

See detailed **homeopathy** section below under Chronic Back Pain.

### Miscellaneous

♦   **Proteolytic Enzyme Formula** (protein digesting enzyme that includes protease, bromelain, papain) – Dosage: 3 or more capsules three times daily between meals. May decrease inflammation and speed healing of tissues if taken between meals; if taken with meals, the enzymes are used in the digestive process.

*Note:* Avoid with active stomach or duodenal ulcers; proteolytic enzymes may aggravate ulcers and induce bleeding.

♦ **Spinal manipulation or acupuncture** by a qualified professional may help start the healing process and also bring significant relief.

# Chronic Back Pain

## Vitamins

♦ **B complex** – Dosage: 50 - 100mg. balanced B complex capsule daily with meals. B complex vitamins support the strength and health of nerve tissue. *Note:* For highest assimilation, use a multi B complex which contains the vitamins in their coenzyme form and avoid mega-potency B complex products.

♦ **C** (from mixed mineral ascorbates) – Dosage: 500 to 1000 mg., three to five times daily with meals. May protect against erosion of cartilage tissue and stimulate repair of connective, bone, and nerve tissue.
*Note:* If these dosages cause loose stools or excessive flatulence, reduce dosage to within bowel tolerance.

## Minerals

♦ **Calcium** (elemental calcium from amino acid chelate) – Dosage: 200 mg., four times daily with meals and at bedtime. Calcium plays an important role in muscle growth and contraction, nerve transmission and maintenance of healthy bones. May be very important for strengthening weak back muscles.

♦ **Magnesium** (elemental magnesium from amino acid chelate) – Dosage: 200 mg., four times daily with meals and at bedtime. Magnesium plays an important role in neuromuscular contractions and can act as a muscle relaxant. It is also required for absorbing and metabolizing calcium.

## Herbs

♦ **Antispasmodic Extract** – For chronic, recurring back pain, it is worth the effort to prepare and keep on hand. This standard medication of American herbalism traditionally has been used for centuries to relieve spasm and associated pain. Muscle spasm is frequently a prominent factor in back pain. *Prepare as follows:* Add the following herbs (preferably organically-grown or wildcrafted) to a glass jar: 1 part **Lobelia Seed** (Lobelias inflata), 1 part **Scullcap** (Scutellaria lateriflora), 1 part **Skunk Cabbage Root** (Symplocarpus foetida), 1 part **Gum Myrrh** (Commiphora myrrha), 1 part **Black Cohosh Root** (Cimicifuga racemosa), 1/2 part **Cayenne** (Capsicum annuum). Pour vodka over herbs until alcohol level is 1-1/2 inches higher than top level of the herbs. Close lid tightly and shake well. Store in warm, dark place. Shake well daily for two to three weeks. Then strain through folded cheesecloth or undyed linen. Squeeze or press remaining herb mass. Discard herbs. For immediate use, pour some of the extract into an amber glass dropper bottle. Store remainder in a mason jar in a cool, dark place. Dosage: 40 to 5 drops of extract* in 4 oz. warm water two to three times daily or as required.

*Note*: For added benefit, take **Mag Phos 6X** (see below under Homeopathy) with every dose of antispasmodic extract.

♦ **St. John's Wort** (Hypericum perforatum) – Dosage: 40-50 drops liquid extract* or 6 oz. of tea, two to three times daily.
*Beneficial properties*: considered specific for muscular bruises, deep soreness, soreness and tenderness of the spine, and concussion shock or injury to the spine accompanied by great pain. Consider its use in any case of back pain accompanied by sciatica.
*Note:* Wait at least two hours after taking St. John's wort before exposure of skin to sunlight, because this herb may increase photosensitivity.

♦ **White Willow Bark** capsules (Salix alba) – Dosage: 2,000 mg., two to three times daily with meals or 4 oz. of tea two to three times daily between meals.
*Beneficial properties:* traditionally used to relieve pain; original source for active ingredient in aspirin.
*Note:* Avoid use with history of a gastric or duodenal ulcer; may aggravate bleeding.

## Aromatherapy

Blend and store the combination in an amber glass bottle. Use it as hydrotherapy adjunct as described below, as well as massage oil. **Prepare massage oil** using the following proportion: 25 drops of blend for each 1 oz. jojoba or sweet almond oil. Shake well before each use. Rub massage blends into areas of back pain two to three times daily.

**Lavender** (Lavendula vera) + **Marjoram** (Origanum marjorana) + **Sweet Birch** (Betula lenta)

## Homeopathy

See Appendix E for proper use and handling instruction prior to administering remedies described below.

♦ **Bryonia 6C or 30C** – Aching or stitching pain from the slightest motion; muscles sensitive to touch; bruised feeling in back when lying on it; worse when dry and cold; better when lying down and at rest; firm pressure gives some relief. Dosage: Dissolve 5 pellets under the tongue, two to three times daily, weekly or as required. During acute pain, use every 15 minutes, three times daily or as required. Adjust dosage as symptoms subside.

♦ **Colocynthis 6C** – Pain in back extends down upper part of thigh and buttock; pain concentrates in a small area causing limping; may become so severe that cannot stand or walk; severe burning in lower part of back and upper buttock. Dosage: Dissolve 5 pellets under the tongue, every 30 minutes to 4 hours in accord with severity of pain. Adjust dosage as symptoms subside.

♦ **Hypericum 6C or 30C** – Sharp or shooting back pain caused by either a fall or blow to the back; lifting arms aggravates the pain; severe nerve pain extends through the hip joint (e.g., sciatica). Dosage: Dissolve 5 pellets under the tongue, every 30 minutes to 4 hours after the back injury in accord with severity of injury. Adjust dosage as symptoms subside.

♦ **Rhus Tox 6C or 30C** – Pain worse on first motion but lessens as motion continues; pain returns if motion continues for too long; stiff neck, pain between shoulder blades (sacroiliac pain); pain and stiffness worse at night and first thing in the morning; bruised or burning pain; worse when cold; better when warm; back pain or strain caused by overexertion or lifting heavy objects. Dosage: Dissolve 5 pellets under the tongue, every one to two hours or two to three times daily or weekly or as required.

## Miscellaneous

♦ **Avoid standing** in the same position for extended periods of time.

♦ **Prolotherapy** for ligament and tendon rebuilding. See Appendix F for more information.

♦ **Check for flat feet**. Use arch support if necessary. Flat feet affect spinal alignment.

♦ Concentrate on **maintaining good posture** while sitting, standing, and walking.

♦ **Exercise daily.** Gentle stretching exercises and walking are best. Sedentary habits worsen a bad back and prevent it from healing.

♦ **Feldenkreiss Method** – A very gentle therapy that corrects body movements, thus aiding the body's own effort to rid itself of back pain.

♦ **Hot and Cold Hydrotherapy for Low Back Pain** – Apply hot moist compress to lower back region. Continue hot applications every 15 minutes. Follow with an alternating hot (2 minutes) and cold (20-30 seconds) strong shower spray directed at area of pain. Alternate between hot and cold two to three times. Then dry the treated area and rub in the aromatherapy massage blend described above several times daily or weekly or as required. Alternate this therapy several times weekly with the **Neutral Bath** described below.

♦ **Lift with legs, not back.**

♦ **Neutral Bath** – Fill tub with water between comfortably warm and tepid. Keep lighting dim and atmosphere quiet. Enter tub. Cover exposed parts, such as knees, with a towel, or cover the top surface of the bathtub with a sheet. Add warm water or as required to maintain neutral temperature. Remain relaxed and quiet. Do not scrub, and move about as little as possible. Remain in water 20 minutes to 2 hours. If in tub longer than 30 minutes, be careful when standing up; ask for assistance if necessary. Drain water from tub and rub briskly with a wash cloth dipped in cold water. Thoroughly massage entire body with cold, damp wash cloth. Dip cloth in cold water whenever it begins to warm. Then dry using a brisk towel rub. Finish by rubbing into the area of back pain the aromatherapy massage blend described above. Lie down and rest for at least one hour. Alternate this therapy several times weekly with the **Hot and Cold Hydrotherapy for Low Back Pain** described above.

♦ **Reduce** lifestyle **stress** and implement a relaxation program. Harmonizing practices (e.g., biofeedback, meditation, yoga, Tai Chi exercise) may prove beneficial in cases of chronic back pain. Very often, tension is internalized and manifests as a form of back pain termed TMS (Tension Myositis Syndrome).

♦ **Relieve constipation.** Habitual straining at the stool and chronic gas pressure may cause or worsen back pain.

♦ **Rolfing** – A type of therapeutic bodywork. May help correct faulty posture through soft tissue manipulation. Similar to a very strong and deep massage (see Resource Guide).

♦ **Rolling on two tennis balls placed inside a sock** – Position balls below back with spine between the two balls. Roll back and forth, and rock side to side, for 10 seconds on descending areas of the spine. Begin at base of skull; work all the way downward to base of sacrum. This may offer pain relief via trigger point or acupressure point reflex action. *Note:* Check with your doctor first to make sure you do not have unstable bone spurs that may break off due to applied pressure and worsen back pain.

♦ **Spinal manipulation** by a chiropractor or osteopathic physician may help start the healing process and may bring significant relief.

♦ **Stop smoking**. Studies link smoking to chronic low back pain.

♦ **Unfiltered apple cider vinegar** – Dosage: 2 tsp. of unfiltered, apple cider vinegar + 1 tsp. raw honey in 8 oz. warm water one to two times daily between meals. Traditional therapy for rheumatic pain.

♦ When sitting, **use a straight chair** with a firm back, or **support** the lower back with a firm cushion.

♦ **When driving, push the car seat forward** to raise the knees higher and reduce strain on the back and shoulder muscles. Also, support the lower back with a firm cushion.

# Bites and Stings

Bites and stings occur when a person comes into contact with an insect or animal. The bite or sting often causes some form of reaction, including pain, swelling, and general discomfort. Many bites and sting symptoms may be easily and safely alleviated with home care. However, it is best that a professional evaluates all bites from humans, animals, and poisonous reptiles. Individuals who have severe reactions—such as fever, difficulty breathing, dizziness, extreme redness, pus or streaking at the site of the bite, or shock should also see their healthcare professional immediately.

Conventional treatments include careful removal of the stinger if possible, ice applications to reduce swelling, antihistamines, and analgesics like Tylenol or ibuprofen to reduce pain. A topical paste of meat tenderizer mixed with water is commonly used for stings of many common insects, because it breaks down the protein left by the sting. If a ringlike rash with a central clearing appears, the bite may be from a tick; this may be the first sign of Lyme disease, which requires treatment with antibiotics.

| EZ Care Program | |
|---|---|
| Miscellaneous | **Bromelain or papaya enzyme tablets** – May help break down harmful proteins found in venom. Mix a thick paste of water and mashed tablets; apply directly to the sting. If these are not available, use a slice of fresh pineapple core (the source of bromelain) or green papaya. |
| | **Apply ice** to injured area **immediately** to reduce inflammation and pain. Keep ice pack in place for five minutes; remove for one to two minutes and repeat. Continue this alternation as required. |
| | **Charcoal poultice** – may help absorb venom. Make a paste by mixing a small amount of water with the contents of two activated charcoal capsules. For a more dynamic effect, add essential oils as discussed below under Aromatherapy. Spread paste evenly on a paper towel or small square of linen. Cover affected area with the poultice, fasten with bandage, and keep in place for several hours. Then remove, wash area well, and apply aloe vera gel or Calendula cream. |
| | Review **homeopathy** section below for appropriate remedy. |

## Additional Recommendations

The EZ Care Program consists of basic remedies that are commonly used for bites and stings and have been found to work well in most cases. The remedies are most effective when combined, but can be used individually. The options stated below can supplement or replace EZ Care remedies and may be combined when suggested doses are followed.

### Vitamins

♦ **C** (mineral ascorbates mixed with bioflavonoids) – Dosage: 1000 mg., three to four times daily with meals. May decrease reactivity to stings as well as reduce swelling and pain.

### Herbs

♦ **Aloe vera gel** – Apply externally four to six times daily.
*Beneficial properties:* May promote healing of tissue and prevent infections.

♦ **Calendula** (Calendula officinalis) oil or cream – Apply externally four to six times daily.
*Beneficial properties:* May promote healing of tissue and prevent infections.

♦ **Echinacea Root** (Echinacea angustifolia or purpurea) – Dosage: 50 drops liquid extract* in 4 oz. warm water or as required. A poultice of dry or fresh root may be applied externally as well.
*Beneficial properties*: Traditionally used for treating animal bites, including snake bites.

♦ **Plantain** (Plantago major or lanceolata) poultice – Common herb found growing on roadsides and in backyards. Chop fresh herb and place in blender with a little water. Puree to make a thick paste. Spread on gauze and apply to bite or sting. Keep moist.

Repeat as required. When hiking or camping and blender is not available, chew fresh plantain and apply mash to affected area.
*Beneficial properties*: Traditionally used for treating insect bites or stings.

♦  **White Oak Bark** (Quercus alba) – Prepare a poultice using powdered bark blended with sufficient water to create a thick paste. Spread on gauze and apply to bite or sting. Keep moist. Repeat as required.
*Beneficial properties* Traditionally used for antivenomous properties.

## Aromatherapy

Mix 3 to 5 drops of essential oil of **Lavender** (Lavendula vera) in a small amount of aloe vera gel. Apply directly to bite or sting. Repeat as required.

## Homeopathy

See Appendix E for proper use and handling instruction prior to administering remedies described below.

♦  **Acetic Acid 6C** – Cat bite produces a lacerated wound; swelling of entire limb when bite is on limb. Dosage: Dissolve 5 pellets under the tongue, every 15 to 60 minutes until symptoms stop increasing. Then 5 pellets two to four times daily until symptoms subside. Moisten skin, dissolve pellets in water and apply directly to wound.

♦  **Apis 12C or 30C** – Red, inflamed insect bites or stings that cause burning or stinging pain; worse from heat and warm applications; relieved by cold and cold applications. Dosage: Dissolve 5 pellets under tongue every 15 to 60 minutes until symptoms stop increasing. Then 5 pellets two to four times daily until symptoms subside.

♦  **Hypericum 30C** – Sharp or shooting pains from a bite or sting; dog bites or other animal bites when the wound does not heal, has shiny red edges, and produces a burning and stinging pain. Dosage: Dissolve 5 pellets under the tongue, every 15 to 60 minutes until symptoms stop increasing. Then 5 pellets two to four times daily until the symptoms subside.

♦  **Lachesis 6C** – Bites of tarantula, dog, or leeches. Dosage: Dissolve 5 pellets under the tongue, every 15 to 60 minutes until symptoms stop increasing. Then 5 pellets two to four times daily until the symptoms subside.

♦  **Ledum 30C** – Relieves symptoms associated with bites or stings of mosquitoes, bees, wasps, scorpions, spiders, and rats; bites of angry animals; symptoms sensitive to touch and relieved by cold applications. Dosage: Dissolve 5 pellets under the tongue, every 15 to 60 minutes until symptoms stop increasing. Then 5 pellets two to four times daily until symptoms subside. Moisten skin, dissolve pellets in water, and apply directly to wound.

♦  **Stapysagria 12C** – Mosquito or other insect bites that are extremely itchy and raise large welts. Dosage: Dissolve 5 pellets under tongue every 15 to 60 minutes until symptoms stop increasing. Then 5 pellets two to four times daily until symptoms subside.

**Miscellaneous**

♦ **Clay poultice** – Prepare a clay poultice (see Appendix B) by mixing clay with 1 part cider vinegar to 1 part pure water.

\* Most herbal extracts contain alcohol. Avoid use if alcohol sensitive or if there is a history of alcohol abuse. *Note:* Alcohol content can be reduced through evaporation by adding extract to very hot water (just below boiling point) and allowing to stand 5 to 7 minutes before drinking.

# Black Eye

Trauma to tissue around the eye results in broken blood vessels, inflammation, and discoloration. While usually a benign injury, any internal eye damage, bony deformities, or vision loss should immediately be treated by a medical professional. Conventional treatments include ice, along with anti-inflammatory analgesics such as ibuprofen.

| EZ Care Program | |
|---|---|
| Homeopathy | **Arnica montana 30C** – Homeopathic medicine. Dosage: Dissolve 5 pellets sublingually one to three times daily during the first one to two days after injury. May help reduce swelling and speed healing. For best results, use immediately after injury. |
| | **Arnica oil or gel** – Use externally by rubbing small amount onto affected area. May reduce swelling and pain and speed healing. *Note: Toxic when taken internally. Avoid mouth, eyes, and any open cuts.* |
| Miscellaneous | **Apply ice** to injured area **immediately** to reduce inflammation and pain. Keep ice pack in place for five minutes. Remove for one to two minutes and repeat. Continue this alternation as required. |
| | **Alternate hot and cold** compresses to the eye - **Begin 24 hours after injury** to encourage vigorous blood circulation and reduce tissue edema. Alternate two minutes hot with one minute cold; several times; always end with cold. If swelling continues, opt for one minute hot and one minute cold in alternation. |
| | **Bromelain** – Dosage: 500 mg., three times daily between meals. Enzyme derived from pineapple. May help reduce inflammation and speed healing. |

## Additional Recommendations

The EZ Care Program consists of basic remedies that are commonly used for black eyes and have been found to work well in most cases. The remedies are most effective when combined, but can be used individually. The options stated below can supplement or replace EZ Care remedies and may be combined when suggested doses are followed.

## Diet

♦ **Eat** large quantities of fresh fruits and vegetables daily to supply bioflavonoids required for maintaining capillary integrity.

## Vitamins

♦ **C** (mineral ascorbates mixed with bioflavonoids) – Dosage: 1000 mg., three to four times daily with meals. May be beneficial for healing damaged blood vessels and tissues.

## Herbs

♦ **Prepare a poultice** for application to the black eye, using one of the following herbs: **Comfrey Root** (Sympthytum officinalis), **Hyssop** (Hyssop officinalis), **St. John's Wort** (Hypericum perforatum) or **Witch Hazel Bark** (Hamamelis virginiana).

*Prepare poultice as follows:* **(1)** Blend a sufficient quantity of pure water with the powdered herb to form a paste. Spread on gauze and apply over black eye. Keep moist. Repeat or as required. **(2)** Whenever possible, it is preferable to use fresh comfrey, hyssop, or St. John's wort for this poultice. In this case, blend the fresh herb with as little water as possible.

*Note:* Wait at least two hours after applying St. John's wort before exposure of treated area to sunlight, because this herb may increase photosensitivity.

## Aromatherapy

Mix 2 drops of **Hyssop** (Hyssop officinalis) essential oil with a small amount of aloe vera gel. Apply to skin around the eye. Repeat as required.
*Note: Be very careful to avoid direct contact of eyes with essential oil.*

## Homeopathy

See Appendix E for proper use and handling instruction prior to administering remedies described below.

♦ **Ledum 6C – Primary homeopathic remedy for a black eye**. Helps relieve pain and clear up discoloration. A keynote of ledum is "relief obtained from cold applications." Dosage: Dissolve 5 pellets under tongue two to four times daily.
*Note:* Use either in place of arnica or after treatment when arnica has been discontinued; do not use simultaneously.

♦ **Symphytum 6C** – Black eye with pain in eyeball. Dosage: Dissolve 5 pellets under tongue two to four times daily as required.

# Boils

Boils are painful, red and hot infected inflammatory lesions of the hair follicle. The infection may be accompanied by fever. Because the lesion can spread, several are often found in a group that may form an area known as a carbuncle. Pus usually accumulates, comes to a head, then opens and drains. Infected boils often require medical attention, and may require drainage.

Conventional treatments include warm compresses, whirlpool therapy, and antibiotics. If severe, spreading, or unrelenting, a surgical incision, drainage and intravenous antibiotic therapy may be used to avoid systemic spread, especially in diabetics and immuno-compromised persons (those with AIDS or cancer).

| EZ Care Program | |
|---|---|
| Herbs | **Goldenseal** – (Hydrastis canadensis ) Dosage: 2 to 4 capsules or 40-50 drops liquid extract* three times daily for up to 14 days. In addition, apply extract topically with cotton swab.<br>*Beneficial properties*: Traditionally used as an antibacterial.<br>*Note:* Decrease dosage if you experience nausea, loose stools, or other gastrointestinal symptoms. |
| | **Echinacea** (Echinacea purpurea) – Dosage: 2 to 4 capsules or 50 drops liquid extract* three times daily for two weeks.<br>*Beneficial properties*: Traditionally used to help fight infections. Boosts the immune system. |
| Miscellaneous | **Charcoal poultice** – may help draw and bring boil to a head. Make a paste by mixing a small amount of water with contents of two activated charcoal capsules. Spread paste evenly on a paper towel or small square of linen. Cover affected area with the poultice, fasten with a bandage, and keep in place for several hours. Also consider papaya pulp poultices and the topical application of raw, unfiltered honey described in the Miscellaneous section below.<br>*Note:* Also see poultice note under Miscellaneous. |
| | **Moist heat** – Apply tolerably hot, wet towels to the boil to bring it to a head and let the pus drain. Seek medical attention if the infection worsens or persists. If hot towels do not improve the boil, try alternating hot with cold using two minutes of hot, followed by one minute of cold. Repeat this procedure five to six times in a row. Repeat the entire process three times a day. The pumping action of the hot and cold often resolves a boil. |

# Additional Recommendations

The EZ Care Program consists of basic remedies that are commonly used for boils and have been found to work well in most cases. The remedies are most effective when combined, but can be used individually. The options stated below can supplement or replace EZ Care remedies and may be combined when suggested doses are followed.

## Diet

♦ **Eat oranges** – Traditional naturopaths consider the orange a specific for boils.

♦ **Short two-to-three day fast** (consult physician before undertaking fast) – Maximum frequency: once every other week. Drink pure distilled water during fast; if this is not feasible, include in the fast fresh, salt-free vegetable broths and fresh vegetable juices.

♦ **Identify personal food sensitivities**. Avoid all common allergenic foods (e.g., dairy, eggs, wheat, corn, sugar, preservatives). Rotate moderately allergic foods on a four-day schedule (see Appendix C).

## Vitamins

♦ **A** (natural, from fish liver oil) – Dosage: 10,000 to 25,000 IU one to two times daily with meals until affected area improves. May help protect skin tissue from infection.
*Note:* Consult a physician before using higher doses of vitamin A. Avoid use if pregnant. Discontinue use if you experience nausea, dry skin, sore lips, blurred vision, or other signs of vitamin A toxicity.

♦ **C** (from mixed mineral ascorbates) – Dosage: 500 to 1000 mg., three to four times daily with meals and at bedtime. May help protect skin against infection and support skin integrity through formation and maintenance of collagen, which is the basis of connective tissue found in skin.

♦ **E** (natural d-alpha tocopherol in a base of mixed tocopherols) – Dosage: 800 IU daily with a meal. Exerts an antioxidant action that may help protect damaged tissue from oxidative damage and reduce possibility of scarring.

## Minerals

♦ **Zinc** (take only if over 14 years of age) – Dosage: 25 to 50 mg., elemental zinc from amino acid chelate taken with a meal. Zinc is required for the utilization of vitamin A. It may help maintain healthy skin cells and generate new skin after injury or infection.

## Herbs

♦ **Burdock Root** (Arctium lappa) and **Yellow Dock Root** (Rumex crispus) **tea and wash** – Prepare a decoction (see Appendix B) using 2 tsp. of each herb to 3 cups pure water. Drink 4 oz. of tea three to four times daily between meals. Also, wash affected area with the tea three to four times daily. Consider using as a wash after removing poultices and compresses described below.

♦ **Comfrey Root** (Symphytum officinalis) **poultice** – Blend fresh chopped Comfrey root with a quantity of water sufficient to form a thick paste. Spread on gauze and apply over affected area. Cover with a cabbage leaf. Cover all with cheesecloth and secure with surgical tape. Keep in place for two hours. Repeat one to four times daily or as required.

♦ **Hops poultice** (Humulus lupulus) – Mix powdered hops leaves with a quantity of water sufficient to form a thick paste. Spread on gauze and apply over affected area. Cover with a cabbage leaf. Cover all with cheesecloth and secure with surgical tape. Keep in place for two hours. Repeat one to four times daily or as required.

## Aromatherapy

Dab 1 drop of one of the following oils on boil three to four times daily or as required: **Lemon** (Citrus limonum) or **Tea Tree** (Melaleuca alternifolia). Consider applying essential oils after removing poultice or compress and subsequent washing of treated area described in herbal section above.

## Homeopathy

See Appendix E for proper use and handling instruction prior to administering remedies described below.

♦ **Belladonna 6C** – Hot, shiny, red, inflamed boils with throbbing pain; more effective when given before the formation of pus. Dosage: Dissolve 5 pellets under tongue two to four times daily or as required.

♦ **Hepar Sulph 6C** – When taken in early stages, aborts the formation of pus. If pus has already formed and boil is draining, Hepar. Sulph is indicated; pus is thick and yellow, boil is extremely sensitive to touch and produces sharp, sticking pains; patient chilly but better in wet weather. Dosage: Dissolve 5 pellets under the tongue, two to four times daily until suppuration stops.

♦ **Sulphur 6C** – Small red, hot boils constantly occurring in crops; boils return soon after previous ones disappear; red or purplish circle around the eruption; boils frequently form on buttocks. Dosage: Dissolve 5 pellets under tongue two to four times daily or as required.

## Miscellaneous

♦ **Alternate Hot and Cold Shower Spray** – Use a hand-held shower attachment. Concentrate hot shower spray on the area for 2 minutes. Then switch to a cold spray for 30 seconds. Alternate back and forth three to four times. Dry the area. Follow with one of the poultices described below.

*Note:* After completing each application of the poultices or compresses described below, wash the treated area with salt water (1 handful sea salt : 1 quart water) or burdock root/yellow dock decoction described above under Herbs.

♦   **Clay poultice** – Apply clay poultices (see Appendix B) on affected area, renewing every one to four hours or as required. Clay poultices help draw out pus. Continue clay poultices until shooting pains are experienced in the treated area. Then switch to a raw cabbage poultice (puree chopped cabbage with just enough water to form a thick paste). Once the boil ripens, reintroduce clay poultices during the day. At night, cover affected area with a cheesecloth soaked in clay water solution. Place a cabbage leaf on top to keep area moist, cover with a dry cheesecloth, and secure all with surgical tape.

♦   **Papaya pulp poultices** – Puree a green or semi-ripe papaya with a sufficient quantity of water to make a thick, non-runny mash. If necessary, add ground flaxseed as a thickener. Spread on a piece of gauze and place over affected area. Cover with a piece of cheesecloth and secure all with surgical tape. Keep in place over night.

♦   **Raw, unfiltered honey compress** – Spread honey over affected area and cover with gauze. Keep in place for several hours. Repeat several times daily.

*   Most herbal extracts contain alcohol. Avoid use if alcohol sensitive or if there is a history of alcohol abuse. *Note:* Alcohol content can be reduced through evaporation by adding extract to very hot water (just below boiling point) and allowing to stand 5 to 7 minutes before drinking.

# Brittle Nails

Brittle nails are weak nails that chip and break easily. This condition could be a signal of poor nutrition or mineral deficiency, as well as different forms of arthritis. In smokers, this can be a sign of poor oxygen delivery. It is advisable to mention this to your healthcare professional.

Conventional therapy may include diagnosis for the underlying cause and improvement in diet, along with mineral supplementation, exercise, and adequate fluid intake.

| EZ Care Program | |
|---|---|
| Diet | **Increase** consumption of digestible **protein**. |
| | **Increase** foods high in the B vitamin **biotin**: unsulphured blackstrap molasses, cauliflower, legumes, nuts, and egg yolks. |
| Herbs | **Black Currant Seed oil** (Ribies nigrum) – Dosage: 500 mg., two times daily for at least two months. *Beneficial properties*: Traditionally used for skin conditions, including nails. |

## Diet

♦ **Include in the diet** some of the following **high-silicon** foods: cabbage, cucumber, dandelion, leaf lettuce, onion, dark leafy greens, kelp, nettles, and sunflower seeds.

## Vitamins

♦ **A** (Natural, from fish liver oil) – Dosage: 10, 000 to 25,000 IU daily with meals. A shortfall of vitamin A in the diet may cause dryness and brittleness of nails.
*Note:* Consult a physician before using higher doses of vitamin A. Avoid use if pregnant. Discontinue use if you experience nausea, dry skin, sore lips, blurred vision, or other signs of vitamin A toxicity.

♦ **B complex** – Dosage: 25 to 50 mg. balanced B complex capsule taken with a meal. Insufficient B-vitamins causes nails to become fragile with horizontal or vertical ridges appearing.
*Note:* For highest assimilation, use a multi B complex which contains the vitamins in their coenzyme form and avoid mega-potency B complex products.

♦ **C** (from mixed mineral ascorbates) – Dosage: 500 to 1000 mg., two to three times daily with meals. vitamin C plays a major role in forming collagen, which is the protein that forms the basis of connective tissue.

♦ **D** (from fish liver oil) – Dosage: 400 to 1000 IU daily with a meal. Aids in absorption of calcium from intestinal tract.

## Minerals

♦ **Calcium** (elemental calcium from amino acid chelate) – Dosage: 200 mg., three to four times daily taken with meals. Required for normal cell division and essential to integrity of intracellular cement.

## Herbs

♦ **Horsetail (Equisetum arvense)** – Dosage: 2 to 3 capsules of standardized extract three times daily with meals.
*Beneficial properties*: A rich source of silica, a trace element required for structural strength and rigidity of tissues.

## Homeopathy

See Appendix E for proper use and handling instruction prior to administering remedies described below.

♦ **Silicea 6X.** – Homeopathic form of silicon. The cell salt specific for brittle nails. Nails rough, yellow, brittle, and powdery when cut. Dosage: Dissolve 5 pellets under the tongue, two to three times daily.

### Miscellaneous

♦ **Betaine HCL and Pepsin** – Dosage: one to two 700 mg. capsules at beginning of every meal with protein. Provides hydrochloric acid and pepsin that are required for normal mineral metabolism and digestion of protein. Many older individuals no longer produce adequate amounts of these two digestive substances.
*Note:* Avoid if suffering from stomach or duodenal ulcers. Discontinue use if burning sensation in stomach is experienced.

♦ **Methyl sulfonyl methane (MSM)** – Dosage: 1000 mg. twice daily. Provides a source of natural sulfur, which is essential in nail matrix strength.

♦ **Proteolytic Enzyme Formula** (protein digesting enzyme that includes protease, bromelain, papain) – Dosage: 1 to 2 capsules three times daily with meals.
*Note:* Avoid if there are stomach or duodenal ulcers; proteolytic enzymes may aggravate ulcers and induce bleeding.

# Bronchitis

Bronchitis is a viral or bacterial infection or irritation of the lining of the bronchial tubes, resulting in inflammation and swelling of the air passages. The most common characteristic is a deep, raspy, painful cough that may be accompanied by fever, shortness of breath, and an increase in phlegm. Bronchitis can lead to pneumonia if not treated promptly. See your health care professional if your cough lasts longer than one week.

Conventional treatments include acetaminophen or ibuprofen to reduce fever and pain, as well as expectorants and cough suppressants. Steam inhalation and adequate water consumption are also recommended. Antibiotics are generally over-prescribed for bronchitis, as the majority of infections are viral in origin.

| EZ Care Program | |
|---|---|
| Diet | **Avoid all processed sugar**, because this may suppress immunity and increase mucus production. |
| | **Avoid milk** and all milk products, because they increase mucus formation. Consider dairy alternatives such as soy, nut milks, and cheeses. |
| Vitamins | **C** (mineral ascorbates with bioflavonoids) – Dosage: 1,000 – 2000 mg., three to four times daily with meals. May help control infection and reduce severity and duration of symptoms. Reduce dosage if loose stools occur. |

| | EZ Care Program |
|---|---|
| Herbs | **Echinacea** (Echinacea purpurea) – Dosage: 50 drops liquid extract or two capsules, every two to three hours for acute bronchitis. *Beneficial properties:* Traditionally used as an immune stimulant to help fight infections. |
| | **Goldenseal Root** (Hydrastis canadensis) – Dosage: 1 to 2 capsules or 30 to 50 drops liquid extract* every four hours for acute infections. *Beneficial properties:* Traditionally used to fight infections. |
| | **Wild Cherry Bark** (Prunus serotina) – Dosage: 2 capsules or 4 oz. of tea every 2 to 3 hours for acute infections (see Appendix B). Serve warm with a pinch of cayenne pepper. *Beneficial properties:* May resolve coughs, especially in the bronchi. |
| Hydrotherapy | **Head Vapor** (i.e., steam inhalation) (See Appendix D for complete instructions) – Add essential oil blend described below under Aromatherapy. Where the formula for the blend calls for "1 part" of a given essential oil, use 1 drop; for "2 parts," use 2 drops. If a stronger treatment is desired, double the number of drops (i.e., 12 drops total instead of 6 per formula described); one to two times daily to soothe irritated bronchial lining, enhance oxygenation, destroy pathogenic bacteria, and dislodge phlegm. |
| Miscellaneous | **N-Acetyl Cysteine** (NAC) – Dosage 600 mg. three times daily. NAC, a precursor to the antioxidant glutathione, is a natural mucolytic, aiding in the thinning and expelling of mucus secretions. |
| | **Avoid** all tobacco and second-hand smoke. |

# Additional Recommendations

The EZ Care Program consists of basic remedies commonly used for bronchitis and have been found to work well in most cases. The remedies are most effective when combined, but can be used individually. The options stated below can supplement or replace EZ Care remedies and may be combined when suggested doses are followed.

## Diet

♦ **Identify personal food sensitivities** for chronic bronchitis. Avoid all common allergenic foods (e.g., dairy, eggs, wheat, corn, sugar, preservatives). Rotate moderately allergic foods on a four-day schedule (Appendix C).

## Vitamins

♦ **A** (natural, from fish liver oil) – Dosage: 10,000 to 25,000 IU daily taken with a meal. Required for maintaining structural integrity and lubrication of epithelial tissues lining lungs, nose, and throat.
*Note:* Consult a physician before using higher doses of vitamin A. Avoid use if pregnant. Discontinue usage if you experience nausea, dry skin, sore lips, blurred vision, or other signs of vitamin A toxicity.

♦ **Beta-carotene** – Dosage: 25.000 to 50,000 IU three times daily with meals. A potent antioxidant that protects lung tissue; converts to vitamin A in the body.

## Minerals

♦ **Zinc** (take only if over 14 years of age) – Dosage: 25 to 50 mg. elemental zinc from amino acid chelate one to two times daily with meals for one week; or one 25 mg. zinc lozenge four times daily for one week. Zinc supports immune function , and requirements increase during acute or chronic infection.
*Note:* Zinc helps utilize and maintain the body's level of vitamin A; these two vitamins work well together in this context.

## Herbs

♦ **Garlic** (Allium sativum) – Dosage: 1 to 2 capsules per meal of standardized allicin garlic or aged garlic extract. Fresh, raw garlic (a whole, living food) is preferable, but capsules should be considered if use of raw garlic is problematic.

♦ **Garlic juice** mixed at a ratio of 1 to 2 with raw honey, or several garlic cloves (or a similar quantity of raw onion) pureed and mixed with a sufficient quantity of raw honey to make a thick syrup; also may prove of good service for bronchitis. Take 1 tbsp. of either syrup every one to two hours or as required.
*Beneficial properties:* Garlic exerts a powerful antibiotic action. It has a special affinity for the respiratory tract where it helps limit infection, act as an expectorant, and positively influence bronchial secretions.
*Note:* Raw parsley taken with raw garlic helps prevent "garlic breath" and enhances garlic's blood-cleansing effects.

♦ **Marshmallow Root** (Althea officinalis) – Dosage: 6 oz. tea prepared by decoction (see Appendix B) every two to three hours for acute bronchitis; for chronic bronchitis, two to three times daily between meals. Serve warm with a pinch of ginger root powder.
*Beneficial properties:* May soothe the pain and cough of bronchitis.

♦ **Mullein tea** (Verbascum thapsus) – Dosage: 6 oz. warm tea prepared by infusion (see Appendix B) three to four times daily between meals. Traditionally used to treat bronchial irritation and asthmatic bronchitis.

♦ **Slippery Elm Bark tea** (Ulmus fulva) – Dosage: 6 oz. tea prepared by decoction (see Appendix B) every two to three hours for acute bronchitis; for chronic bronchitis, two to three times daily between meals. Serve warm with a pinch of ginger root powder.
*Beneficial properties*: Contains an abundant mucilage that may soothe and quiet inflamed bronchial linings.

♦ **Thyme tea** (Thymus vulgaris) – Dosage: 6 oz. tea prepared by infusion (see Appendix B) three to four times daily between meals. May exert a healing, antiseptic action in the respiratory tract. Thyme forms the basis of the Listerine antiseptic compound.

## Aromatherapy

Use the following undiluted essential oil combination. Blend and store in amber glass bottle. This also may be used as an adjunct to suggested hydrotherapies, as well as local massage oil.

2 part **Eucalyptus** (Eucalyptus globulus) + 2 parts **Lavender** (Lavendula vera) + 2 parts **Pine** (Pinus sylvestrus)

Tap 3 to 4 drops of the blend onto a palm several times daily. Rub the palms together, then take 10 to 15 deep breaths from the cupped palms, turning the head to the side when exhaling.

**Massage oils preparation**: 25 drops of a given blend for each 1 oz. jojoba or sweet almond oil. Shake well before each use. Rub massage blend into upper chest, upper back, neck and throat two to three times daily.

## Homeopathy

See Appendix E for proper use and handling instruction prior to administering remedies described below.

♦ **Aconitum 6C** – Administer during the first stages of acute bronchitis when there are high fever and lung congestion preceded by a chill due to suppressed perspiration or exposure to cold drafts, anxiety and great restlessness. Dosage: Dissolve 5 pellets under the tongue, every one to two hours or as required.

♦ **Antimonium Tart 6C** – Chest feels heavy, as if a weight has been placed on it, plus mental depression and hoarseness; wheezing and rattling, loose cough but unable to raise mucus; labored breathing; white, creamy coating on tongue; aversion to food; worse about four a.m. Dosage: Dissolve 5 pellets under the tongue, every two to three hours or as required.

♦ **Carbo Veg 6C** – Chronic bronchitis in the elderly; evening hoarseness and rawness in the throat; profuse yellow, foul mucus, sometimes mixed with blood from bronchial hemorrhage; difficulty raising mucus; coldness of extremities and blueness of fingernails. Dosage: Dissolve 5 pellets under the tongue, every two to four times daily or as required.

♦ **Drosera 6C** – Chronic bronchitis with a spasmodic, tickling, choking cough that is worse after midnight, especially around two a.m.; cough is dry, loud, barking, deep sounding, and painful; hold chest while coughing to control pain; feel chilly yet perspire profusely.Dosage: Dissolve 5 pellets under the tongue, every two hours or two to four times daily or as required.

♦ **Rumex 6C** – Bronchitis with spasmodic cough; tickling in throat; difficulty raising phlegm; feeling of soreness all the way down the trachea and underneath the breastbone; extremely sensitive to cold air; place blanket over head to avoid breathing cold air; worse at night and with motion. Dosage: Dissolve 5 pellets under the tongue, every two to three hours or as required.

♦ **Spongia 6C** – Dry, barking, croupy cough; dry air passages and no phlegm; worse with cold air, cold fluids, sweets, tobacco, smoke, warm room, lying with the head low and talking; better with warm food and drinks, sitting up and leaning forward. Dosage: Dissolve 5 pellets under the tongue, every two to three hours or as required.

### Miscellaneous

♦ **Epsom Salt Baths** (see Appendix D) – Treatment: nightly during acute stage, to help break up congestion and detoxify the system. Drink hot lemon water (juice of 1 lemon in 16 oz. hot water) while in tub, to encourage free perspiration. This procedure activates the skin, which, like the lungs, is a respiratory organ.

♦ **Steam Pack over Throat and Chest** (see Appendix D for details) – Traditionally used to relieve congestion.

\* Most herbal extracts contain alcohol. Avoid use if alcohol sensitive or if there is a history of alcohol abuse. *Note:* Alcohol content can be reduced through evaporation by adding extract to very hot water (just below boiling point) and allowing to stand 5 to 7 minutes before drinking.

# Bruises

Trauma to tissues causes blood to leak out of capillaries and collect just beneath the skin, resulting in a black and blue mark on the surface of the skin. Bruising is a normal function of the body when there is trauma. However, if you bruise easily or spontaneously, without any history of trauma, you should see your physician.

Conventional treatments include ice along with anti-inflammatory analgesics, such as ibuprofen.

| EZ Care Program | |
|---|---|
| Vitamins | **C** (mineral ascorbates mixed with bioflavonoids) – Dosage: 1,000 mg., three to four times daily with meals. May help heal damaged blood vessels and tissues. |
| Homeopathy | **Arnica 6C or 30C** – Dosage: Dissolve 5 pellets under the tongue, one to three times daily for the first day or two after injury. May help reduce swelling and speed absorption of blood from under the skin. For best results, use immediately after injury. |
| | **Arnica oil or gel** – Use externally by rubbing small amount into affected area. <br> *Note: Arnica gel is toxic when taken internally. Avoid mouth, eyes, and any open cuts.* |
| Miscellaneous | **Apply ice** to injured area **immediately** to reduce inflammation and pain. Place a piece of cotton cloth over the bruised area. Secure an ice bag in place over cloth with an elastic bandage to create a small amount of compression. Keep in place for no longer than 30 minutes. Repeat one to three more times throughout the day. |

| | |
|---|---|
| **EZ Care Program** | |
| | **Alternate hot and cold** compresses to the bruise – **Begin _24-48 hours after_ the injury** to encourage vigorous blood circulation and reduce tissue edema. Alternate 2 minutes heat with 1 minute ice several times. Always end with ice. If swelling continues, alternate 1 minute heat and 1 minute ice. <br> _Note: Never use heat on a bruise before_ 24 to 48 hours have passed, because heat may restart the subcutaneous bleeding and worsen the inflammation. |
| | **Bromelain** – Dosage: 500 mg., three times daily between meals. Enzyme derived from pineapple that may help reduce inflammation and reduce healing time. |

# Additional Recommendations

The EZ Care Program consists of basic remedies that are commonly used for bruises and have been found to work well in most cases. The remedies are most effective when combined, but can be used individually. The options stated below can supplement or replace EZ Care remedies and may be combined when suggested doses are followed.

## Diet

♦   **Eat** large quantities of fresh fruits and vegetables daily, to supply vitamin C and bioflavonoids that are required to maintain capillary integrity. Dark leafy green vegetables are a good source of vitamin K, which is a blood clotting, anti bruising agent.

♦   **Eat** lima beans and other legumes, dark leafy green vegetables, dried prunes, black mission figs, blackstrap molasses, and other iron-rich foods.

♦   **Eat** whole grains, nuts, legumes, brewer's yeast, and other foods rich in B vitamins.

## Vitamins

♦   **Bioflavonoids** (full potency bioflavonoids) – Dosage: 500 mg., two to three times daily with vitamin C. Bioflavonoid deficiency results in weakening and easy breakage of small blood vessels, and subsequently subcutaneous bleeding and bruising.

♦   **B complex** – Dosage: 25 to 50 mg. of balanced B complex capsule one to two times daily with meals. B complex vitamins are essential for healthy tissues in the circulatory system and to prevent anemia. <br> _Note:_ For highest assimilation, use a multi B complex which contains the vitamins in their coenzyme form and avoid mega-potency B complex products.

♦   **D** (from fish liver oil) – Dosage: 400 IU one to two times daily with meals. Excessive bruising may be a sign of deficiency in vitamin D that is a natural blood-clotting agent.

## Herbs

♦ **Comfrey Root** (Symphytum officinalis), **Hyssop** (Hyssop officinalis), or **Witch Hazel Bark** (Hamaelis virginiana) **poultice** – Prepare a poultice for application to the bruise using either comfrey root or hyssop or witch hazel bark. **(1)** Blend a sufficient quantity of pure water with the powdered herb to form a paste. Spread on gauze and apply over bruise. Keep moist. Repeat or as required. **(2)** Whenever possible, it is preferable to use fresh comfrey root or hyssop for a poultice. In this case, blend the fresh herb with as little water as possible.

♦ **Marshmallow Root** (Althea officinalis) **and Chamomile flowers** (Matricaria chamomilla) **compress** – Prepare infusion (see Appendix B) of these two herbs using 4 tbsp. of each herb : 2 quarts pure water. Steep 35 minutes. Saturate a cotton or linen cloth with the infusion and apply to bruised area. Whenever the cloth begins to dry, dip it back into the infusion. Continue the compress for one hour. Repeat two to three times daily or as required.

Other herbs that may be useful as a compress for bruising: **Calendula flowers** (Calendula officinalis) and **Yarrow** (Achillea millefolium). Substitute either of these herbs for marshmallow root and chamomile flowers in the formula given above and apply in like manner.

## Aromatherapy

Mix 2 to 4 drops of one of the following essential oils with a small amount of aloe vera gel and apply to bruised skin: **Hyssop** (Hyssop officinalis) or **Lavender** (Lavendula vera). Repeat as required.

## Homeopathy

See Appendix E for proper use and handling instruction prior to administering remedies described below.

♦ **Hypericum 6C** – Bruises of body parts rich in nerves, such as fingers, toes, nail beds. Dosage: Dissolve 5 pellets under the tongue, two to four times daily or as required.

♦ **Ledum 6C** – Consider this remedy when Arnica fails to initiate significant improvement. Primary homeopathic remedy for a black eye. Helps relieve pain and clear discoloration. Keynote: "relief obtained from cold applications." Dosage: 5 pellets under the tongue, two to four times daily or as required. *Use either in place of arnica or after treatment when arnica has been discontinued Do not use simultaneously.*

♦ **Ruta 6C** – Bruises of the periosteum (i.e., bone bruises), especially when hard nodules form under the skin. Dosage: Dissolve 5 pellets under the tongue, two to four times daily or as required.

### Miscellaneous

♦ **Desiccated liver or liver extract capsules** (from Argentinean or New Zealand range-fed cattle) – Dosage: 2 to 8 capsules daily in divided doses with meals. A good source of highly assimilable iron.

♦ **Horse Chestnut Extract** – Dosage: 1 capsule, three times daily. Helps to maintain the integrity of the circulatory system. It is especially effective in patients with varicose veins.

# Burns

Burns occur when our skin comes in contact with anything over 120°F. Burns are categorized by degrees of injury. First-degree burns are the least severe and cause local skin redness that may peel. Second-degree can be differentiated from first-degree burns by the onset of blistering. Third-degree burns are the most severe. The affected area has reduced sensation and looks charred, white, or waxy. Burns of any level can become infected and should be evaluated by a physician. Never break any blisters, because this can cause infection and scarring.

Conventional treatments include applying cold water and wet wraps at the first onset of a burn. This aids in the removal of heat from the area and may lessen the severity of the burn. Follow with application of burn ointments, such as silvadene cream. Burns that involve a large area of the body require hospitalization, and are treated with intravenous fluids and antibiotics.

| EZ Care Program | |
|---|---|
| Diet | **Eat protein-rich foods** such as fish, chicken, turkey, legumes, and cultured dairy products if not sensitive to dairy. Protein is used to heal skin tissue. |
| Vitamins | **A** (natural, from fish liver oil) — Dosage: 10,000 to 25,000 IU daily with meals. Important for skin health. May help repair tissues and prevent infection after injury.<br>*Note:* Consult a physician before using higher doses of vitamin A. Avoid use if pregnant. Discontinue use if you experience nausea, dry skin, sore lips, blurred vision, or other signs of vitamin A toxicity. |
|  | **Beta Carotene** — Dosage: 25,000 to 50,000 IU three times daily with meals. Non-toxic precursor of vitamin A. |

| EZ Care Program | | |
|---|---|---|
| | **C** (mineral ascorbates mixed with bioflavonoids) — Dosage: 1,000 mg., three to four times daily with meals. May enhance immune system response to burns and discourage infection. Important in tissue rebuilding and collagen formation. | |
| | **E** (natural d-alpha tocopherol in base of mixed tocopherols) — Dosage: 800 IU daily with meals. May relieve pain and promote healing in burns. *Note:* Pure vitamin E (squeezed from a capsule) applied externally may promote healing. However, do not use on open wounds or cuts. | |
| Minerals | **Zinc** (take only if over 14 years of age) — Dosage: 50 mg. elemental zinc from amino acid chelate taken with meals. *Note:* Zinc and vitamin A are synergists and work well together in this context. Zinc supports the immune system's response and promotes wound healing. | |
| Herbs | **Aloe vera gel** (from whole leaf) — Apply externally three to four times daily. *Beneficial properties:* May promote healing of tissue and prevent infections. | |
| | **Calendula** (Calendula officinalis) oil or cream or St. John's wort (Hypericum perforatum) oil or lotion — Apply externally three to four times daily, alternating with aloe gel. *Beneficial properties:* May promote healing of tissue and prevent infections. | |
| Miscellaneous | **Immediately run cold water over burned area**, or submerge in ice water for 5 to 10 minutes with brief breaks. *It is critical to do this within the first twenty minutes.* *Note:* Do not put the ice directly on the burn. | |

# Additional Recommendations

The EZ Care Program consists of basic remedies that are commonly used for burns and have been found to work well in most cases. The remedies are most effective when combined, but can be used individually. The options stated below can supplement or replace EZ Care remedies and may be combined when suggested doses are followed.

### Diet

♦ **Eat** generous servings of **raw fruits** and **vegetables**.

### Minerals

♦ **Potassium** (aspartate or citrate) – Dosage: 18 to 36 mg., one to two times daily to support fluid and pH balance.

### Aromatherapy

♦ Essential oil of **Lavender** (Lavendula vera) – Mix 1 part essential oil to 10 parts aloe vera gel. Apply to burn often. Repeat every few hours or as required. In some cases, pouring undiluted Lavender oil onto a sterile gauze and applying to the burn may prove of good service. Repeat every few hours or as required.

## Homeopathy

See Appendix E for proper use and handling instruction prior to administering remedies described below.

♦ **Arnica 6C or 30C** – Dosage: Dissolve 5 pellets under the tongue, immediately after occurrence to relieve pain. Repeat every 30 to 60 minutes or as required until the pain subsides, then switch to one of the following remedies:

♦ **Cantharis 12C** – Pain of second and third degree burns and sunburns. Dosage: Dissolve 5 pellets under the tongue, three to four times daily or as required.

♦ **Causticum 12C** – For chronic burns that do not heal, and second degree burns. Dosage: Dissolve 5 pellets under the tongue, two to three times daily or as required.

♦ **Phosphorus 6C** – Electrical burns. Dosage: Dissolve 5 pellets under the tongue, two to four times daily or as required.

## Miscellaneous

♦ **Apply honey** to the burn for its soothing effects and healing properties.
*Note:* Raw honey contains live enzymes and is the preferable form.

♦ **Fresh cucumber juice or ginger juice** – Apply to affected area. Repeat as required throughout the day. These are traditional burn remedies.

♦ **Clay poultice** – Apply thick, cold clay poultices on top of the gauze that has been placed over the burn; remove the poultice after one hour. If the gauze sticks to the burn, leave it in place until it falls off or washes off by itself. Apply a fresh clay poultice as soon as the old one is removed. Change poultices in this fashion every hour throughout the day. At night, use some of the other topical applications discussed above, such as Lavender oil.

After new tissue has begun to form, reduce the frequency of applications of clay poultices to three to four times daily, leaving each in place for two hours. For burns of hands and feet, consider dipping the affected part directly into the clay paste. Immerse the part for one hour. Repeat as required.

Clay helps burns heal more rapidly and cleanly, especially if applied immediately after the burn.

# Bursitis

Bursitis is inflammation of the bursa – a small fluid filled sac located near joints throughout the body. The bursa cushions large joints such as the shoulder, hip, and knee. Overuse, irritation, or injury can inflame the bursa, causing bursitis. Shoulders, elbows, knees, wrists, hands, hips, heels, and the big toe are the areas most commonly affected. A short period of rest for the particular joint is often advisable so it has time to heal.

Conventional treatments include resting and icing the affected joint, and anti-inflammatory analgesics such as aspirin and ibuprofen. For more severe cases, corticosteroid injections or fluid removal from the bursa with a syringe may be performed. Corticosteroid injections should be used with extreme caution. Side effects include tendon weakness, tendon rupture, atrophy, and flaring of pain. As a last resort, the bursa may be surgically removed.

| EZ Care Program | |
|---|---|
| Diet | **Eliminate** coffee and decaf, black tea, chocolate, soda, alcohol, and sugar. |
| Vitamins | **Beta Carotene** – Dosage: 25,000 IU three times daily. May exert beneficial anti-inflammatory action. |
| | **B12** (sublingual) – Dosage: 2000 mcg. for seven to ten days, then three times weekly for three weeks; then one to two times weekly thereafter or as required. May help reduce pain and reduce abnormal calcium deposits. |
| | **Bioflavonoids** (full potency) – Dosage: 500 mg., two to three times daily taken with vitamin C. May help reduce inflammation and limit tissue destruction. |
| | **C** (mineral ascorbates mixed with bioflavonoids) – Dosage: 1,000 mg., three to four times daily with meals. vitamin C plays a crucial role in producing and maintaining collagen, which is the intercellular ground substance required for forming tendons and bursal tissues. |
| Herbs | **Devils Claw** (Harpagophytum procumbens) – Dosage: 1 to 2 capsules or 30 - 50 drops of extract* in 4 oz. water three times daily. *Beneficial properties:* Traditionally used to relieve inflammation and pain associated with joints, tendons, and muscles. |
| | **Bromelain** (enzyme derived from pineapple) – Dosage: two 500 mg. capsules three times daily between meals. May help reduce inflammation and decrease healing time. |
| | **White Willow Bark** (Salix alba) – Dosage: 1 to 2 capsules or 30 - 50 drops of extract* in 4 oz. water two times daily. *Beneficial properties:* Traditionally used to relieve pain. |

# Additional Recommendations

The EZ Care Program consists of basic remedies that are commonly used for bursitis and have been found to work well in most cases. The remedies are most effective when combined, but can be used individually. The options stated below can supplement or replace EZ Care remedies and may be combined when suggested doses are followed.

## Diet

◆ Eat a **high-water-content** diet consisting of large quantities of fresh fruits and vegetables and comparatively smaller quantities of whole grains, legumes, seeds, nuts, fish, skinless chicken and turkey.

◆ **Identify personal food sensitivities**. Avoid all common allergenic foods (e.g., dairy, eggs, wheat, corn, sugar, preservatives). Rotate moderately allergic foods on a four-day schedule (see Appendix C). In addition, eliminate nightshade family foods (e.g., potatoes, tomatoes, peppers, eggplant).

◆ **Short two-to-three day fasts** (consult physician before undertaking fast) – Maximum frequency: once every other week. Drink pure, distilled water if possible; if this is not feasible, include in the fast, fresh salt-free vegetable broths and fresh vegetable juices.

◆ Use only **cold-pressed oils**, such as olive, flax, or sesame; or use butter.

## Vitamins

◆ **E** (natural d-alpha tocopherol in a base of mixed tocopherols) – Dosage: 800 IU daily with meals. May help reduce inflammation and reduce healing time.

## Minerals

◆ **Selenium** – Dosage: 200 mcg. daily from l-selenomethionine. May help decrease inflammation by inhibiting free radical damage.
   *Note:* Selenium and vitamin E are synergists, in that they enhance each other's activity in the body.

◆ **Zinc** (picolinate or lysinate) – Dosage: 25 mg., two times daily with breakfast and dinner. May support tissue repair and reduce healing time.

## Herbs

◆ **Burdock Root** (Arcium lappa) – Dosage: 1 to 2 capsules or 30 - 50 drops of extract* in 4 oz. water three times daily.
   *Beneficial properties:* May help ameliorate bursitis via blood purification and reduction of lymphatic congestion.

◆ **Cayenne Pepper** (Capsicum annuum) – Dosage: 1 to 2 capsules three times daily with meals.
   *Beneficial properties:* May stimulate circulation, promote tissue repair, and reduce pain.

*Note:* Begin with a low dosage, because this herb may worsen preexisting gastrointestinal irritation and inflammation or initiate irritation when used to excess. Due to its powerful effects on circulation, cayenne pepper should be avoided during pregnancy.
*Also available:* Capsicum (cayenne) cream for topical application. May reduce pain. Apply locally as directed. Localized burning sensation may occur during initial use.

♦ **Curcumin** (extracted from tumeric) – Dosage: 300 mg., two to three times daily between meals.
*Beneficial properties:* Traditionally used to relieve inflammation and pain associated with joints, tendons, and muscles.

## Aromatherapy

Choose one of the following essential oils or use them in combination: **Blue Chamomile** (Matricaria chamomilla) or **Lavender** (Lavendula vera). Prepare a massage oil by mixing in an amber glass bottle 10 drops of one of these essential oils, *or* 5 drops of each of the two per 100 drops of olive oil or emu oil. Shake well. Gently rub into the affected area two to four times daily or as required. For a synergistic effect, apply the prepared blend after completing application of ice pack as described below.

## Homeopathy

See Appendix E for proper use and handling instruction prior to administering remedies described below.

♦ **Apis 6C or 30C** – Inflamed, hot, swollen, tender joint; stinging pain; worse when touched and with applied pressure; better with cold applications. Dosage: Dissolve 5 pellets under the tongue, two to three times daily or weekly or as required.

♦ **Bryonia 6C or 30C** – Joint painful, swollen and distended with fluid; pain worse with the least movement and does not improve with continued motion; worse when jarred or bumped and from cold; better with heat. Dosage: Dissolve 5 pellets under the tongue, two to three times daily or weekly or as required.

♦ **Ruta 6C or 30C** – Pain feels close to the bone where the tendon inserts; aching pain worse with every movement; swelling of affected part; restlessness; worse in cold, damp weather; injuries from chronic overuse. Dosage: Dissolve 5 pellets under the tongue, two to three times daily or weekly or as required.

## Miscellaneous

♦ **Cold Wet Pack** – Place three layers of wet, cold towels on the affected area. Cover with two layers of dry towels. Keep in place for one hour and do not move the joint. Perform this two times daily. Keep another cold wet pack in place overnight. May prove of good service in reducing joint inflammation of acute bursitis.

♦ Consider **acupuncture** from a qualified practitioner for symptomatic relief.

♦ **Hot compresses** – *Apply only after acute phase and pain have subsided* (if applied during acute phase, heat will worsen the inflammation). Apply compress one time daily, as hot as can be tolerated (not scalding) for one hour. Follow with range-of-motion exercises.

♦ **Ice applications** – During initial phase of bursitis, apply ice pack every 30 minutes for several hours or as required.

♦ **Proteolytic Enzyme Formula** (protein digesting enzymes that include pancreatic protease, bromelain, papain) – Dosage: 3 or more capsules three times daily between meals. When taken between meals, may decrease inflammation and speed healing of tissues; if taken with meals, the enzymes are used for the digestive process.
*Note:* Avoid if there are stomach or duodenal ulcers; proteolytic enzymes may aggravate ulcers and induce bleeding.

\* Most herbal extracts contain alcohol. Avoid use if alcohol sensitive or if there is a history of alcohol abuse. *Note:* Alcohol content can be reduced through evaporation by adding extract to very hot water (just below boiling point) and allowing to stand 5 to 7 minutes before drinking.

# Candidiasis

Candida albicans is a yeast species present in the intestines, vagina, and oral cavity. It normally coexists with the friendly bacteria that help keep it under control in a relationship known as symbiosis. A delicate balance of yeast and bacteria live in the body and serve the purpose of detoxification, digestion, and secretion of natural antibiotics. When the friendly bacteria are reduced due to antibiotics or steroids, candida can multiply rapidly, causing a yeast overgrowth. Also, a compromised immune system, diabetes, and malnutrition may contribute to this condition. Candidial overgrowth may cause chronic vaginal yeast infections, oral and esophageal yeast infections, skin and nail infections, and male genital infections. Many individuals will not have frank symptoms of yeast overgrowth and may suffer from other symptoms related to candida such as bloating, nausea, loose stools, fatigue, headaches, "brain fog", irritability, and skin rashes among other problems. In severe cases, it travels through the blood stream, causing severe illness.

Conventional treatments include antifungal creams, suppositories, tablets, or intravenous antifungal drugs for severe cases.

| EZ Care Program | |
| --- | --- |
| Diet | **Eliminate** sugar, alcoholic beverages, and white flour, because they encourage yeast growth. |

| EZ Care Program | |
|---|---|
| | **Limit** intake of **high carbohydrate foods**, including dried fruits, potatoes, and refined grains. |
| Herbs | **Garlic** (Allium sativum) – Dosage: 1 to 2 capsules per meal of standardized allicin garlic or aged garlic extract. Fresh, raw garlic (a whole, living food) is preferable, but capsules should be considered if raw garlic is not taken consistently.<br>*Beneficial properties:* Has powerful antifungal properties.<br>*Note:* Raw parsley taken with raw garlic helps prevent "garlic breath", and enhances garlic's blood-cleansing effects. |
| | **Pau d'arco** bark (Tabebuia heptophylla) – Dosage: 6 oz. of tea prepared by decoction two to three times daily (see appendix B). Add 15 drops of goldenseal root or echinacea fluid extract to each serving for additional benefit.<br>*Beneficial properties:* Has powerful antifungal properties. |
| Miscellaneous | **Lactobacillus probiotic** (friendly intestinal bacteria that aids digestion, nutrient assimilation, and toxin elimination) – L. acidophilus with bifidobacteria and fructo-oligosaccharides is most preferable. Use according to label directions and always keep refrigerated. |
| | **Capryllic acid** (time-release capsule) – Dosage: 500 mg., two times daily with meals.<br>*Beneficial properties:* May help counteract candida overgrowth. |

# Additional Recommendations

The EZ Care Program consists of basic remedies that are commonly used for candidiasis and have been found to work well in most cases. The remedies are most effective when combined, but can be used individually. The options stated below can supplement or replace EZ Care remedies and may be combined when suggested doses are followed.

## Diet

♦ **Drink** 6 to 8 glasses of pure water daily.

♦ **Identify personal food sensitivities**. Avoid all common allergenic foods (e.g., dairy, eggs, wheat, corn, sugar, and preservatives). Rotate moderately allergic foods on a four-day schedule (see Appendix C).

## Vitamins

♦ **A** (natural, from fish liver oil) – Dosage: 10,000 to 25,000 IU one to two times daily with meals. Required for maintaining the structural and immunological integrity of the mucosal lining of the gastrointestinal and genito-urinary tracts.
*Note:* Consult a physician before using higher doses of vitamin A. Avoid use if pregnant. Discontinue use if nausea, dry skin, sore lips, blurred vision, or other signs of vitamin A toxicity are experienced.

♦ **B complex** (yeast-free, low potency, natural source) – Dosage: 1 capsule two to three times daily with meals. B complex vitamins are required for normal assimilation of carbohydrates and may help assuage moodiness and other emotional symptoms commonly associated with candidiasis.

♦ **C** (mineral ascorbates mixed with bioflavonoids) – Dosage: 500 mg., two to three times daily with meals. May help support immune system response to infection.

## Minerals

♦ **Chromium** (polynicotinate is preferred form) – Dosage: 200 mcg. two times daily with meals. Essential for blood sugar regulation and control of cravings. High blood-sugar peaks contribute to yeast overgrowth that is fueled by sugar excess.

♦ **Magnesium** (elemental from amino acid chelate) – Dosage: 250 to 500 mg. taken in divided doses, separately from zinc, at meals and bedtime. Many individuals with chronic candidiasis have been noted to be magnesium deficient.

♦ **Selenium** – Dosage: 200 mcg. daily from l-selenomethionine. An antioxidant and immune stimulant that may help protect cells from toxins produced by pathogenic microbes and may enhance antibody formation.

♦ **Zinc** (take only if over 14 years of age) – Dosage: 50 mg. elemental zinc from amino acid chelate taken with meals. Zinc is necessary for normal immune function and carbohydrate assimilation and helps utilize and maintain body levels of vitamin A.

## Herbs

♦ **Barberry Root** (Berberis vulgaris) – Dosage: 2 capsules or 50 drops of fluid extract* two times daily on arising and mid-afternoon.
*Beneficial Properties:* Potent anti-infectious. Liver, intestine, and kidney cleansing properties. Contains berberine, which is an alkaloid that inhibits growth of candida albicans.

♦ **Echinacea Root** (Echinacea purpurea) – Dosage: 50 drops of fluid extract two times daily between meals. Use in a pattern of two weeks on, then two weeks off, then two weeks on, etc. May enhance immune system response to candida infection.

♦ **Goldenseal Root** (Hydrastis canadensis) – Dosage: 2 capsules or 50 drops of fluid extract* two times daily with meals, alternating with barberry root (e.g., use barberry root two weeks, then goldenseal root two weeks); both contain berberine. May exert a beneficial effect on sluggish liver and intestines. Powerful tonic for people with food assimilation problems.

♦ **Standardized Extract of Oil of Oregano** – Dosage: one to four 50 mg. tablets three times daily with meals for several weeks; then reduce dosage as required. The emulsified form is preferred. May help counteract candida infection.

### Miscellaneous

♦  **Psyllium seed and husk powder** – Dosage: 2 tsp. in 8 oz. warm water. Follow with another 8 oz. warm water one time daily either on arising or before bed. Helps bind toxins in the bowel and alleviate or prevent constipation; a top priority for treating candidiasis. A toxic, waste-choked bowel is an ideal breeding ground for all types of pathogenic microbes, including candida yeast.

♦  **Liquid bentonite clay** or **French green clay** – Dosage: 1 tsp. clay in 4 oz. warm water taken on rising or before bedtime; daily for three weeks, then stop for one week. Thereafter, alternate daily for one week then stop for one week, etc. May help restore deficient function of the gastro intestinal tract and remove pathogenic microorganisms from the intestines.

*   Most herbal extracts contain alcohol. Avoid use if alcohol sensitive or if there is a history of alcohol abuse. *Note:* Alcohol content can be reduced through evaporation by adding extract to very hot water (just below boiling point) and allowing to stand 5 to 7 minutes before drinking.

# Canker Sores

Canker sores are shallow, open sores that develop in and around the mouth. Burning, pain, tingling and a slight swelling often accompany their appearance. Although the condition usually clears up by itself in one to three weeks, recurrent outbreaks can occur. Possible causes include vitamin or mineral deficiency, and should be considered by a healthcare practitioner.

Conventional treatment may include icing the affected area, rinsing the mouth with warm salt water, avoiding irritating foods, and applying a waterproof ointment to protect and cover the ulcers.

| EZ Care Program | |
|---|---|
| Diet | **Avoid sweets, citrus fruits, and spicy or acidic foods**, because they may aggravate this condition. |
| Herbs | **Goldenseal Root** (Hydrastis canadensis) – Gargle three times daily with 20 drops of goldenseal root fluid extract dissolved in 3 oz. hot (not scalding) water. Option: mix in 1 drop essential oil of geranium, lemon, or sage. Apply goldenseal root powder or tea bag directly to accessible canker sores. |
| Miscellaneous | **L-Lysine** (amino acid) – Dosage: 1000 mg. with meals during outbreak, and 500 mg. with each meal thereafter for one week. May help prevent and heal canker sores. Consider regular supplementation to help reduce recurrence. |

| | **EZ Care Program** |
|---|---|
| | **Reduce** lifestyle **stress** and implement a relaxation program. Harmonizing practices (e.g., visualization, meditation, yoga, Tai Chi exercise) may prove beneficial. |

# Additional Recommendations

The EZ Care Program consists of basic remedies that are commonly used for canker sores and have been found to work well in most cases. The remedies are most effective when combined, but can be used individually. The options stated below can supplement or replace EZ Care remedies and may be combined when suggested doses are followed.

## Diet

♦ **Avoid** alcohol, tobacco, and sugar, because these may suppress immunity and slow the repair process.

♦ **Drink** 6 to 8 glasses of pure water daily.

♦ **Identify personal food sensitivities**. Avoid all common allergenic foods (e.g., dairy, eggs, wheat, peanuts). Rotate moderately allergic foods on a four-day schedule (see Appendix C).

## Vitamins

♦ **A** (natural, from fish liver oil) – Dosage: 10,000 to 25,000 IU daily with meals or **Beta-Carotene** 25,000 IU three to four times daily with meals. Vitamin A is required for maintaining the structural integrity of the epithelial lining of the mouth. Beta- carotene, which converts to vitamin A in the body, does not have the same potential for toxicity from high dosage as pre-formed vitamin A.
*Note:* Consult a physician before using higher doses of vitamin A. Avoid use if pregnant. Discontinue use if nausea, dry skin, sore lips, blurred vision, or other signs of vitamin A toxicity are experienced.

♦ **B complex** – Dosage: 50 to 100 mg. balanced B complex capsule once daily with meals.
*Note:* For highest assimilation, use a multi B complex which contains the vitamins in their coenzyme form and avoid mega-potency B complex products. B vitamins are "anti-stress" nutrients. Stress is often a major factor in canker sores. May help prevent recurrence when taken regularly.

♦ **B3** (niacin) – 100 mg., two to three times daily at end of a meal. Required for forming and maintaining a healthy mouth, tongue, and digestive system tissues. Deficiency may cause canker sores.

♦ **C** (mineral ascorbates mixed with bioflavonoids) – Dosage: 1,000 mg., three to four times daily with meals. Essential for skin health. May be beneficial in healing damaged tissue through its crucial role in producing and maintaining healthy collagen, which is the basis of the connective tissue that holds the epithelial cells together.

### Minerals

♦ **Zinc** (take only if over 14 years of age) – Dosage: 25 mg. elemental zinc from amino acid chelate two times daily with meals. Helps utilize and maintain the body's level of vitamin A. May speed the healing of mouth and tongue lesions. Has properties to inhibit viral reproduction.

### Herbs

♦ **Burdock Root tea** (Arctium lappa) – Dosage: 6 oz. of tea prepared by decoction (see Appendix B), two to three times daily between meals.
*Beneficial properties*: Traditionally used for disease of the skin and mucous membranes, including canker sores.

♦ **Calendula Flowers tea** (Calendula officinalis) – Prepare tea by infusion (see Appendix B). Use as a mouthwash several times daily or as required.
*Beneficial properties*: May help relieve pain and promote healing of canker sores.

### Homeopathy

See Appendix E for proper use and handling instruction prior to administering remedies described below.

♦ **Arsenicum Album 6C** – Canker sores with great dryness and burning heat of the mouth and tongue. Dosage: Dissolve 5 pellets under the tongue, one to two times daily or as required.

♦ **Mercurius Cor. or Mercurius Sol. 6C** – Canker sores with soreness and excessive salivation. Dosage: Dissolve 5 pellets under the tongue, one to two times daily or as required.

♦ **Nitric Acid 6C** – Canker sores with sharp, sticking pains brought on by overindulgence in sweets. Dosage: Dissolve 5 pellets under the tongue, two to three times daily or as required.

### Miscellaneous

♦ **Lactobacillus Probiotic Product** (friendly intestinal bacteria that aid digestion, nutrient assimilation, and toxin elimination) – L. acidophilus with bifidobacteria and fructo-oligosaccharides; powder or capsules. Mix with water and swish in mouth before swallowing.

\* Most herbal extracts contain alcohol. Avoid use if alcohol sensitive or if there is a history of alcohol abuse. *Note:* Alcohol content can be reduced through evaporation by adding extract to very hot water (just below boiling point) and allowing to stand 5 to 7 minutes before drinking.

# Carpal Tunnel Syndrome

This condition occurs when a compression of a nerve in the wrist (Median nerve) causes pain, numbness, and tingling of the thumb and first two fingers. Carpal tunnel syndrome is common among people who constantly use their hands and wrists. This condition may be hereditary. In severe cases of carpal tunnel syndrome, a person may show signs of atrophy of the thumb muscle.

Conventional treatments include using over-the-counter pain relievers, wrist splints, diuretics to reduce fluid accumulation, corticosteroid injections for severe cases, and surgery as a last resort.

| EZ Care Program | |
|---|---|
| Vitamins | **B6** (pyridoxal 5-phosphate is preferred) – Dosage: 100 to 200 mg. daily with meals, along with a balanced B complex supplement. Acts as a natural diuretic and helps with nerve nourishment.<br>*Note:* B6 generally takes at least two months to produce desired results. Always use in conjunction with a complete coenzyme B complex formula, because high doses of one B vitamin may lead to imbalance in the body's pool of the other B vitamins. |
| Homeopathy | **Ruta 12C or 30C** – Pain worse in cold damp weather, after exertion, and from strains; bruised or sore pain; sensation as if wrist broken. Keynote symptom: tremendous stiffness of affected part. Dosage: Dissolve 5 pellets under the tongue, one to two times daily, weekly or as required. |
| Miscellaneous | **Avoid** long hours of repetitive use of the affected joint. |
| | **Bromelain** (enzyme derived from pineapple) – Dosage: 500 to 1,000 mg., three times daily between meals. May help reduce inflammation and speed healing. |
| | **Curcumin** (from turmeric) – Dosage: 250 to 500 mg. between meals. May reduce inflammation and speed healing. |
| | **Practice** wrist-stretching exercises regularly. |
| | Utilize **ergonomically-designed devices,** such as supportive mouse pads and keyboards, as well as wrist supports to reduce heavy bending and straining of wrists. |

## Additional Recommendations

The EZ Care Program consists of basic remedies that are commonly used for carpal tunnel syndrome and have been found to work well in most cases. The remedies are most effective when combined, but can be used individually. The options stated below can supplement or replace EZ Care remedies and may be combined when suggested doses are followed.

## Diet

♦ **Avoid caffeine**, alcohol, and processed sugar.

♦ **Avoid** excessive intake of protein, especially animal protein.

♦ **Drink** 6 to 8 glasses of pure water daily.

## Vitamins

♦ **C** (from mixed mineral ascorbates) – Dosage: 500 to 1000 mg., three to four times daily with meals and at bedtime. vitamin C plays a crucial role in producing and maintaining collagen, which is the intercellular ground substance required for forming tendon tissues.

## Minerals

♦ **Calcium** (elemental calcium from amino acid chelate) – Dosage: 150 to 250 mg., three times daily with meals. Required for developing and maintaining muscle and bone tissue.

♦ **Magnesium** (elemental magnesium from amino acid chelate) –Dosage: 150 to 250 mg., three to four times daily with meals and at bedtime. Required for normal relaxation of skeletal muscles. Also helps promote absorption and metabolism of calcium, and helps in utilization of vitamin C and B complex vitamins, including vitamin B6.

♦ **Zinc** (picolinate or lysinate) – Dosage: 25 to 50 mg. elemental zinc taken daily with food, separately from calcium and magnesium. Found in high concentration in muscle tissue, zinc is required for forming collagen, the ground substance required for forming tendon tissues. Zinc is a vitamin B6 synergist.

## Aromatherapy

Rub a small amount of the following essential oil massage blend into both wrists two to three times daily. Mix in a one-ounce, amber glass, dropper bottle: 1 oz. olive oil, 15 drops **Marjoram** (Origanum marjorana) and 15 drops **Lavender** (Lavendula vera). Shake well before each use. Store in a cool, dark place. Apply at least two hours before or after taking any of the homeopathic remedies described below.

## Homeopathy

See Appendix E for proper use and handling instruction prior to administering remedies described below.

♦ **Causticum 6C or 30C** – Symptoms worse when cold and during overuse, strain, bathing, and dry weather; slowly progressive paralysis of the joint; contraction of muscles and tendons. Dosage: Dissolve 5 pellets under the tongue, one to two times daily or weekly or as required.

♦ **Hypericum 12C or 30C** – Shooting, stabbing pain along nerves, extending from the affected joint; pain appears suddenly and subsides gradually; numbness and crawling sensations; worse when cold, with cold air, dry weather, foggy weather, and changes of weather. Dosage: Dissolve 5 pellets under the tongue, one to two times daily or weekly or as required.

<u>Miscellaneous</u>

♦ **Avoid** all forms of tobacco.

♦ Consider **physical therapy** or **manipulation** from a qualified professional.

♦ **Hot Hand Soak** – Soak hand in water that is as hot as can be tolerated safely (*not scalding*) for 3 to 4 minutes, or less, depending on individual tolerance. While the hand is immersed, exercise the fingers to increase circulation. Then cool the hands with a brief cold-water splash for only a few seconds. Dry hands well. Repeat this procedure three to four times daily.

♦ **Proteolytic Enzyme Formula** (protein digesting enzymes that include protease, bromelain, papain) – Dosage: 3 or more tablets three times daily between meals. When taken between meals, may decrease inflammation and speed healing of tissue; if taken with meals, the enzymes are used for the digestive process.
*Note:* Avoid if there are stomach or duodenal ulcers; proteolytic enzymes may aggravate ulcers and induce bleeding.

# Cataracts

A cataract is the partial or complete clouding of the lens of the eye. The lens is the structure in the eye that focuses on objects. Cataracts are the leading cause of blindness and impaired vision in the United States, with 75% of all people over the age of sixty showing some signs of the disease. Early stages may go unnoticed, and can be detected only with an eye examination, which should be done annually. As the condition advances, vision begins to blur, cloud, and slowly deteriorate.

Conventional treatments include reducing eye exposure to the sun, prescription eye drops, and surgical procedures that include extracting the cataract and performing lens transplantation. Wearing sunglasses with UV coatings may prevent cataracts.

| EZ Care Program | |
|---|---|
| Diet | **Eat a high-water-content diet** consisting of large quantities of fresh fruits and vegetables and comparatively smaller quantities of whole grains, legumes, seeds, nuts, fish, skinless chicken and turkey. |

| EZ Care Program | |
|---|---|
| | *Note:* Fresh fruits and vegetables contain high amounts of antioxidants that are extremely important for this condition. |
| | **Avoid rancid** (i.e. oxidized) **fats** (including vegetable oils) because they contain oxygen-free-radicals. |
| Vitamins | **A** (Emulsified) – Dosage: 25,000 IU daily. Essential nutrient for the development and maintenance of eye tissue. In cases of poor fat digestion and hypothyroidism, beta- carotene is not efficiently converted in the body to vitamin A.  Also available in **eyedrops** (available through a compounding pharmacy by prescription).<br>*Note:* Consult a physician before using higher doses of vitamin A. Avoid use if pregnant. Discontinue use if you experience nausea, dry skin, sore lips, blurred vision, or other signs of vitamin A toxicity. |
| | **Beta-Carotene** – Dosage: 100,000 to 150,000 IU daily. The water-soluble form of vitamin A. |
| | **C** (mineral ascorbates mixed with bioflavonoids) – Dosage: 1,000 mg., three times daily with meals. Exerts antioxidant action that protects against photodamage to the lens.  Also available in **eyedrops** (available through a compounding pharmacy). |
| | **E** (natural d-alpha tocopherol in a base of mixed tocopherols) – Dosage: 800 to 1200 IU daily with meals. Poor vitamin E status may increase risk of eye disease.<br>*Note:* Individuals with high blood pressure should begin with no more than 200 IU daily and increase dosage gradually over time. |
| Minerals | **Selenium** (from l-selenomethionine) – Dosage: 200 mcg. daily. May help protect the lens from free radical damage.<br>*Note:* Selenium and vitamin E are synergists; they enhance each other's activity in the body. |
| | **Zinc** – Dosage: 25 to 50 mg. elemental zinc from amino acid chelate taken with a meal. Vital for normal lens function and integrity. Works together in the body with beta-carotene. Helps maintain normal tissue levels of vitamin A. |
| Herbs | **Bilberry** (Vaccinium myrtillus) standardized to contain 25% anthocyanosides – Dosage: 160 mg., two to four times daily.<br>*Beneficial properties*: Antioxidant that may increase circulation of blood to the eyes. |
| | **Cineraria** (Cineraria maritima) **Eyedrops** – Dosage: 1 drop in each eye three times daily for six months.<br>*Beneficial properties:* Traditionally used in treating cataracts. |

## Additional Recommendations

The EZ Care Program consists of basic remedies that are commonly used for cataracts and have been found to work well in most cases. The remedies are most effective when combined, but can be used individually. The options stated below can supplement or replace EZ Care remedies and may be combined when suggested doses are followed.

### Diet

♦ **Avoid** processed sugars, caffeine, and alcohol.

♦ **Drink** 6 to 8 glasses of pure water daily.

### Vitamins

♦ **B complex** – Dosage: 50 mg. daily.
*Note:* For highest assimilation, use a multi B complex which contains the vitamins in their coenzyme form and avoid mega-potency B complex products.

### Minerals

♦ **Calcium** (elemental calcium from amino acid chelate) – Dosage: 150 to 250 mg., three times daily with meals. Required for proper lens functioning and metabolism.

♦ **Chromium** (from polynictinate) – Dosage: 200 mcg. one to two times daily with meals. Required for proper insulin function. Deficiency may be a secondary factor in cataract changes in the lens of diabetics.

### Herbs

♦ **Dandelion Root** (Taraxacum officinalis) – Dosage: 50 drops liquid extract* or 8 oz. of tea prepared by decoction (see Appendix B) two times daily between meals. May help support liver function. In Chinese medicine, the liver and eye functions are thought to be closely related.

♦ **Eyebright Eyewash** (Euphrasia officinalis) – Dosage: Pour 1/2 cup boiling distilled water over 1 tsp. eyebright herb in a glass or stainless steel cooking pot (avoid aluminum pots). Cover pot and steep 30 minutes. Strain and allow for cooling. Pour into an eyecup and use as eyewash. Eyebright herbs may also be taken orally.

♦ **Eyebright** (2 parts) + **Bayberry Root Bark** (Myrica cerifera) (2 parts) + **Goldenseal Root** (Hydrastis canadensis) (1part) + **Cayenne** (Capsicum annuum) (1/2 part) **eyewash** – Prepare an infusion (see Appendix B) using 1 tsp. of the herb mix to 1 cup water. Strain through a fine cloth to remove solid particles. Using an eyecup, rinse each eye two to three times daily.

♦ **Ginkgo Biloba** – Dosage: 80 mg. of 24% standardized extract two times daily.
*Beneficial properties*: May improve general circulation and blood flow to the eyes.

### Homeopathy

See Appendix E for proper use and handling instruction prior to administering remedies described below.

♦ **Calc Fluor 30C and Sulphur 200C** – Especially indicated in later stages of cataract development when there is dimness of vision, feeling of heat rising toward face, a sinking feeling in pit of stomach, and flickering or sparks before eyes. Dosage: Dissolve 5 pellets Calc Fluor 30C under the tongue, one time weekly for four weeks. Then dissolve 5 pellets Sulphur 200C under the tongue, one time weekly for two weeks. Then revert to Calc Fluor 30C for four weeks; followed by Sulphur 200C for two weeks. Continue this cycle as long or as required.

<u>Miscellaneous</u>

♦ **Avoid** direct exposure to bright lights, and wear protective sunglasses when outside.

**Carrot or Potato Poultice** – Grate carrot or raw potato. Blend with a sufficient quantity of water to make a thick paste. Spread paste on cotton or linen cloth. Lie down and place poultice (vegetable side down) over eyes. Keep in place one hour. Repeat three to four times weekly or as required.

♦ Diabetics must be extra careful to **regulate blood sugar**. High blood sugar has been associated with cataracts and other eye disorders.

♦ **GSH** (reduced glutathione) – Dosage: 75 mg., two times daily with meals. May be one of the most important antioxidants for the eye. Normally found in very high concentrations in the lens of the eye.

♦ **NAC** (N-acetyl-l-cysteine) – Dosage: 600 mg., two times daily with meals. Important nutritional component of body's antioxidant defenses and a precursor to glutathione. May be useful in preventing and treating cataracts.

♦ **Lutein** – Dosage: 20 mg., twice daily. A member of the vitamin A family which can protect the retina, macula, and lens from free radical damage.

# Cervical Dysplasia

Cervical Dysplasia is a potentially serious condition and should never be cared for without the assistance of a licensed healthcare professional. The following information is intended to help you be aware of the options available to you.

Cervical Dysplasia is a precancerous condition of the uterine cervix caused by the human papilloma virus. Dysplasia means that abnormal cells were found by a Pap smear, which classifies the abnormality of cells by stages on a scale from one to four. A higher stage indicates a greater degree of abnormality. Cervical cancer can result if this condition is not reversed at an early stage.

The disease stage predicates the treatment plan. Low-grade dysplasia may require more aggressive follow-up while high-grade lesions may require a procedure known as culposcopy. A culposcopy is a direct microscopic exam of the cervix where biopsy samples may be taken. If the samples indicate cervical cancer, further procedures may be needed to cure the condition.

| EZ Care Program | |
|---|---|
| Diet | **Avoid** all sugar, white flour, fried foods, soda, alcohol, coffee, black tea, and caffeine. |
| | **Eat a high-water-content diet** consisting of large quantities of fresh fruits and vegetables and comparatively smaller quantities of whole grains, legumes, seeds, nuts, fish, skinless chicken and turkey. *Note:* Take an extra precaution to avoid animal fats. |
| Vitamins | **Beta-Carotene** – Dosage: 150,000 to 200,000 IU daily with meals. Boosts the immune system. Deficiency of beta-carotene and vitamin A may increase the risk and severity of cervical dysplasia. |
| | **B6** (pyridoxal 5-phosphate) – Dosage: 25 to 50 mg., two to three times daily. Take with B complex. B6 status may be decreased in a significant number of women with cervical dysplasia, thus impacting both their estrogen metabolism and immune response. *Note:* Always use a complete B complex formula in conjunction with vitamin B12 and B6 supplementation, because high doses of one of the B vitamins may lead to imbalance in the body's pool of the other B vitamins. *Note:* For highest assimilation, use a multi B complex which contains the vitamins in their coenzyme form and avoid mega-potency B complex products. |
| | **B12** – Dosage: 2,000 mcg. Sublingually four times daily. Reduce to one time daily when folic acid dosage is reduced to 800 mcg. B12 is a folic acid synergist, which also is essential for normal production of DNA and RNA, essential components of normal cellular reproduction. |
| | **C** (mineral ascorbates mixed with bioflavonoids) – Dosage: 1,000 mg., three to four times daily with meals. Inadequate levels of vitamin C may be a risk factor in cervical dysplasia. |
| | **Folic acid** – Dosage: 1 mg., three times daily for 90 days with meals. Then decrease to 800 mcg. daily. Green, leafy vegetables are an excellent source also. Folic acid is commonly taken with vitamin B12, because as they are intimately related regarding red blood cell production. *Note:* Folic acid is often deficient in women with cervical dysplasia. Supplementation in these women may help regress cervical dysplasia |
| Herbs | **Garlic suppository** – Peel, but don't nick, a garlic clove. Wrap in gauze that has a clean string attached to it, forming a tampon like suppository. Insert once daily at bedtime. |

## Additional Recommendations

The EZ Care Program consists of basic remedies that are commonly used for cervical dysplasia and have been found to work well in most cases. The remedies are most effective when combined, but can be used individually. The options stated below can supplement or replace EZ Care remedies and may be combined when suggested doses are followed.

## Diet

♦ **Eat generous amounts of raw garlic and onions**, which are considered to be blood cleansers.

♦ **Protein** intake should come from soy products and **fish** such as mackerel, herring, salmon, and sardines.

♦ **Use cold-pressed oils** such as extra-virgin olive oil or flaxseed oil.

♦ **Drink** 6-8 glasses of pure water daily.

## Herbs

♦ Herbal tea: 4 parts **Red Clover** (Trifolium pratense) + 2 parts **Burdock Root** (Arctium lappa) + 2 parts **Astragalus Root** (Astragalus membranaceus) + 1 part Chinese **Licorice Root** (Glycyrrhiza uralensis) + 1 part **Jamaican Sarsaparilla Root** (Smilax officinalis) + 1/2 part **Goldenseal Root** (Hydrastis canadensis). Place 2 tbsp. of the herb blend in a glass or stainless steel cooking pot (avoid aluminum pots). Pour 3 cups boiling distilled water over the herb blend. Cover and let steep for one hour. Strain. Drink 6 oz., three to four times daily between meals.
*Beneficial properties*: May help purify the blood, detoxify the liver, and stimulate the immune system.

## Minerals

♦ **Selenium** – Dosage: 200 mcg. daily from l-selenomethionine. Low serum selenium levels have been observed in women with cervical dysplasia.

♦ **Zinc** (take only if over 14 years of age) – Dosage: 25 to 50 mg. elemental zinc from amino acid chelate taken with meals. Important to the immune system and for maintaining normal vitamin A levels and usage.

## Homeopathy

See Appendix E for proper use and handling instruction prior to administering remedies described below.

♦ **Conium 12C** – Bearing down pain during and after menses; whitish, acrid, or bloody vaginal discharge; cancer of the ovaries and uterus. Dosage: Dissolve 5 pellets under the tongue, one to two times daily or as required.

♦ **Kreosotum 12C** – Putrid, green, corn-like, irritating vaginal discharge, accompanied by a great deal of itching; heavy menstrual flow, with clotting and offensive odor; malignancy of the cervix, uterus, or vagina. Dosage: Dissolve 5 pellets under the tongue, one to two times daily or as required.

♦ **Thuja 12C** – Genital herpes; ovarian cysts, especially left-sided; profuse, greenish vaginal discharge; uterine tumors or polyps. Dosage: Dissolve 5 pellets under the tongue, one to two times daily or as required.

**Miscellaneous**

♦ **Discontinue smoking** and avoid second-hand smoke.

♦ **Use condoms** when having sexual intercourse.

♦ **Warm Sitz Bath with Kombu Seaweed** (Laminaria spp.) **tea** followed by **Lemon Juice Douche** – three to four times weekly on rising. To prepare kombu tea: Simmer 4 tbsp. kombu broken in pieces in 4 cups pure water for 20 minutes. Add tea to warm water in tub. Water level should reach to just below navel. Remain in the sitz bath for 20 minutes. Follow with a dilution of **lemon juice douche** (1 to 2 tbsp. lemon juice : 1 qt. warm water).

# Colds & Flu

Colds and flu are caused by a wide variety of viruses. Occasional colds are common, but frequent colds may be a sign of a weakened immune system. The symptoms may include general malaise, headaches, sneezing, fever, runny nose, cough, sinus congestion, stomach and intestinal cramping, diarrhea, and more. Many holistic practitioners believe that fever is the body's way of stimulating the immune system, and should not be suppressed. It is also believed that bacteria and viruses have difficulty replicating at higher temperatures. Contact a physician if the fever is 102°F or higher, if you become dehydrated, or experience shortness of breath. A frequent complication of influenza is pneumonia, especially in the elderly or immunocompromised individuals.

Conventional treatments to reduce fever and discomfort may include using anti-pyretics such as acetaminophen, or anti-inflammatory drugs such as ibuprofen, naproxen sodium. Decongestant, expectorant, and anti-histamine medicines are also used as well as increasing fluids and rest. Antibiotics should not be used to treat a cold or flu.

*Note:* Avoid aspirin, because this may cause Reye's Syndrome in children with influenza.

| EZ Care Program | |
|---|---|
| Diet | **Drink a minimum of 8-10 glasses of pure, room-temperature water** daily upon arising and between meals. Herbal teas or raw vegetable |

## EZ Care Program

| | |
|---|---|
| | juices are also acceptable. Fresh juices, such orange or carrot juice, should be diluted before consuming. |
| | **Avoid sugar** in any form (including undiluted fruit juices if possible), because this may suppress immunity and increase fever. |
| Vitamins | **C** (mineral ascorbates mixed with bioflavonoids) – Dosage: 1,000 to 2,000 mg., every two hours or to bowel tolerance. The body's requirements for C increase to 7000 mg. during viral illness. vitamin C has antiviral and antibacterial properties. It strengthens the body's resistance. |
| Herbs | **Echinacea** (Echinacea purpurea) – Dosage: 2 to 4 capsules or 50 drops liquid extract* three to four times daily for two weeks. *Beneficial Properties:* Antiviral and immune stimulant. Boosts virus-killing T cells. *Note:* It is important to begin at the first sign of a cold or flu. |
| | **Garlic** (Allium sativum) – Dosage: 1 to 2 capsules every two hours of standardized allicin garlic or aged garlic extract until the cold or flu dissipates. Fresh, raw garlic (a whole, living food) is preferable. Eat two chopped cloves of garlic at the first sign of a cold or flu. The cloves can be swallowed like a pill without chewing, or chopped and sprinkled over food, such as applesauce. *Beneficial properties:* Powerful antibiotic and antiviral. *Note:* Raw parsley taken with raw garlic helps prevent "garlic breath" and enhances garlic's blood-cleansing effects. |
| | **Goldenseal** (Hydrastis canadensis ) – Dosage: 2 to 4 capsules or 40-50 drops liquid extract* three times daily for up to 14 days. Take in combination with echinacea. *Beneficial properties:* Antiviral and immune stimulant. *Note:* Decrease dosage if nausea, loose stools, or other gastrointestinal symptoms are experienced. |
| Miscellaneous | **N-Acetyl Cysteine** (NAC) – Dosage: 600 mg. three times daily. NAC, a precursor to the antioxidant glutathione, is a natural mucolytic, aiding in the thinning and expelling of mucus secretions. |
| | **Rest, sleep, and quiet.** Enables the body to meet the energy requirements of acute cleansing and restoration. Adequate rest and sleep are essential for rapid and complete resolution of a viral illness. |

## Additional Recommendations

The EZ Care Program consists of basic remedies that are commonly used for colds and flu and have been found to work well in most cases. The remedies are most effective when combined, but can be used individually. The options stated below can supplement or replace EZ Care remedies and may be combined when suggested doses are followed.

### Vitamins

♦ **A** (natural, from fish liver oil) – Dosage: 50,000 IU daily for five days with meals. Essential for maintaining the functional integrity and immunological activity of the mucosal lining of the respiratory tract.

*Note:* Consult a physician before using higher doses of vitamin A. Avoid use if pregnant. Discontinue use if nausea, dry skin, sore lips, blurred vision, or other signs of vitamin A toxicity are experienced.

## Minerals

♦ **Zinc** (take only if over 14 years of age) – Dosage: 50 mg. elemental zinc from amino acid chelate with meals, or suck on zinc lozenges containing 23 mg. elemental zinc every two hours while awake. Do not use lozenges this frequently for more than one week or if nausea occurs from use.
*Note:* Zinc helps the body utilize and maintain the body's level of vitamin A and is crucial for normal immune function.

## Herbs

♦ **Astragalus** (Astragalus membranaceus) – Dosage: 2 capsules 4 times daily.
*Beneficial properties:* Antiviral and immune stimulant.

♦ **Cayenne Pepper** (Capsicum annuum) – Sprinkle on foods and/or in broths.
*Beneficial properties:* May help to temporarily alleviate nasal congestion.

♦ **Cinnamon** (Cinnamomum zeylanicum) + **Sage** (Salvia officinalis) + **Bay leaves** (Laurus nobilis) **Combination tea** – Prepare tea by infusion using equal parts of the three herbs. Dosage: 1 heaping tsp. of the herb blend to 8 oz. pure water. Steep 30 minutes, then strain. Drink freely throughout the day.
*Beneficial properties:* Traditional formula for colds.

♦ **Elder Flower** (Sambucus spp.) + **Peppermint** (Mentha piperita) + **Yarrow** (Achillea millefolium) **Combination tea** – Prepare tea by infusion using equal parts of the three herbs. Dosage: 1 heaping tsp. of the herb blend to 8 oz. pure water. Steep for 30 minutes and strain. Drink freely throughout the day. Traditional formula for colds and flu. Because this tea-blend promotes perspiration, it is an excellent treatment option for colds, flu, and/or fever; take it before, during, and immediately after a hot epsom salt bath.

♦ **Ginger Root** (Zingiber officinalis) – Dosage: 2 capsules three times daily or 6-8 oz. dried ginger root tea three times daily (see Appendix B; Jamaican ginger root is preferred). For enhanced effect, add a pinch of cayenne to each serving.
*Beneficial properties:* May benefit colds accompanied by fever and flu.

♦ **Pleurisy Root** (Asclepias tuberosa) – Prepare tea by decoction (see Appendix B). Drink 6 oz. warm tea three to four times daily or as required. Add a pinch of cayenne to each serving. Consider using in conjunction with the Hot Foot Bath and/or Epsom Salts Bath described below
*Beneficial properties:* Promotes perspiration, equalizes circulation, and relaxes spasm; specific for pains in the chest from coughing.

♦ **Yarrow tea** (Achillea millefolium) – Prepare by infusion (see Appendix B). Add a pinch of cayenne to each serving. Drink 6 oz. warm tea three to six times daily or as required.

*Beneficial properties*: May benefit colds accompanied by fever and flu. May encourage fever to break. Since yarrow tea promotes perspiration, it is an excellent treatment option for colds, flu, and fever; take before, during, and immediately after a hot epsom salt bath.

## Aromatherapy

Use the following undiluted essential oil combination. Blend and store in an amber glass bottle. Use the blend as an adjunct to suggested hydrotherapies, as well as local massage oil. Also, several times daily, tap 3 to 4 drops of the blend onto a palm. Rub the palms together. Take 10-15 deep breaths from the cupped palms, turning the head to the side when exhaling.

1 part **Lemon** (Citrus limonum) + 2 parts **Eucalyptus** (Eucalyptus globulus) + 1 part **Peppermint** (Mentha piperita)

Prepare massage oil using the following proportion: 25 drops of a given blend to 1 oz. jojoba or sweet almond oil. Shake well before each use. Rub the massage blend into the upper chest, upper back, neck, and throat two to three times daily.

## Homeopathy

See Appendix E for proper use and handling instruction prior to administering remedies described below.

♦ **Aconitum 6C** – Cold or flu brought on by exposure to dry, cold weather; dry, croupy cough that is worse at night, especially after midnight; dry mouth, shortness of breath; sudden onset of fever with chills; rapid, hard pulse with face either flushed or alternates between flushed and pale; tingling in the nostrils; restless. Dosage: Dissolve 5 pellets under the tongue, every two to four hours or as required.
*Note:* Use primarily during the first 24-hour onset period of a cold or flu.

♦ **Allium Cepa 6C** – Colds with profuse, watery, burning nasal discharge; worse in a warm room; better outdoors; nasal discharge irritates the nostrils; profuse flow of tears from eyes; reddened eyes, raw feeling and tingling sensation in the nose, with tendency to violent sneezing; sensitive to scent of flowers. Dosage: Dissolve 5 pellets under the tongue, every two to four hours or as required.

♦ **Belladonna 6C** – When nasal discharge stops suddenly and is replaced by a congestive, throbbing headache and high fever; flushed face and reddened lips and gums; sudden onset of high fever with hot head and cold extremities; strong pounding pulse; hallucinations when eyes are closed; toss and turn in sleep and have frightening dreams. Dosage: Dissolve 5 pellets under the tongue, every two to four hours or as required.

♦ **Gelsemium 6C** – Flu with great weakness and heavy sensation of the body; can open the eyes only halfway because the eyelids feel heavy; bland, thick nasal discharge; general aching with headache at back of head; chilly and thirstless; great fatigue that lingers even after flu otherwise resolved; feel better after urinating; frequent sneezing and great chilliness in back. Dosage: Dissolve 5 pellets under the tongue, every two to four hours or as required.

♦ **Pulsatilla 6C** – Thick, yellowish or greenish mucus discharge; nasal congestion; worse at night, especially when lying down; nasal congestion alternates between nostrils; dry mouth, but thirstless; loss of smell and taste; cold or flu brought on by overindulgence in fatty or rich foods. Dosage: Dissolve 5 pellets under the tongue, every two to four hours or as required.

<u>Miscellaneous</u>

♦ **Antibiotics** do not have a significant effect on colds and flu and should not be used.

♦ **Be sure there is a good supply of fresh air in the room at all times**. However, be properly situated and well-covered, so as to avoid drafts.

♦ **Check the household's humidity.** Dry air, especially in winter, dries mucus membranes and allows foreign particles to enter the body, which may cause colds and flu. Keep household humidity at a minimum of 40%. A whole-house humidifier may be needed.

♦ **Epsom Salt Bath** (see Appendix D) – To encourage free perspiration, drink several cups of either peppermint, yarrow or pleurisy root tea or the elder flower/ peppermint/ yarrow combination before entering the tub and while in the tub.
After soaking, do not dry. Wrap in a cotton sheet, go to bed, and cover well for at least one hour. After another round of sweating, take a tepid shower and follow with a brisk towel rub. Rest at least one hour after.
*Note:* Sweating assists the body in reducing elevated toxic loads.

♦ **Hot Foot Bath** (see Appendix D) – Continue the foot bath for 15 to 20 minutes. May help relieve head and nasal congestion.

# Cold Sores

Cold sores, also known as fever blisters, are usually found on the mouth or lips. They may be caused by the Herpes Simplex 1 virus and usually are a sign of a weakened immune system. The virus lies dormant in approximately 98% of people. However, stress, anxiety, temperature changes, other illnesses, and nutrient deficiencies activate this virus and allow it to replicate.

Flu-like symptoms may accompany the attack. Tingling, tenderness, and itchiness in the area where the eruption will be often precipitate cold sores. The tingling or tender area may become a small pus-filled blister, then ulcerate and scab over. These lesions are contagious until crusted over, and may spread from mouth to mouth or mouth to genitalia contact.

Conventional treatments include topical and oral prescriptions of anti-viral drugs such as acyclovir. Some alternative medicine physicians can produce anti-viral vaccines to help prevent future outbreaks.

| EZ Care Program | |
|---|---|
| Diet | **Avoid arginine-rich foods**. These include chocolate, peanuts, other nuts and seeds, cereal grains, and carob. Arginine is an amino acid that may promote herpes outbreaks. |
| Minerals | **Zinc** (take only if over 14 years of age) – Dosage: 50 mg. elemental zinc from amino acid chelate with meals. May reduce symptoms and help prevent recurrence by enhancing cell-mediated immunity. |
| Herbs | **Licorice Root** (Glycyrrhiza uralensis or glabra) – Dosage: 2 capsules or 40-50 drops liquid extract * two times daily.<br>*Beneficial properties*: Contains glycyrrhizic acid that inhibits the growth and pathological actions of the Herpes Simplex virus. May also be used topically as a gel.<br>*Note:* Avoid use if you have kidney or heart disease. If you have high blood pressure, consult a physician before using this herb because it may increase blood pressure via increased water retention. Chinese licorice root (uralensis) is less problematic in this regard than the western variety (glabra). |
| Aromatherapy | **Melissa** (Melissa officinalis) – Apply topically 3 drops essential oil diluted in ¼ tsp. aloe vera gel two to three times daily. Exerts an antiviral action. |
| Miscellaneous | **L-lysine** – Dosage: 1,000 to 2,000 mg. between meals three times daily while acute.<br>*Lysine ointment* – Apply topically three times daily or as required.<br>*Note:* When taken regularly (500 mg. daily), may prevent future outbreaks. In addition, a diet rich in foods containing lysine may be beneficial including beans, eggs, brewer's yeast, potatoes, and fish. |
| | **Reduce** lifestyle **stress** and implement a relaxation program. Harmonizing practices (e.g., visualization, biofeedback, meditation, Tai Chi exercise) may prove beneficial. |

## Additional Recommendations

The EZ Care Program consists of basic remedies that are commonly used for cold sores and have been found to work well in most cases. The remedies are most effective when combined, but can be used individually. The options stated below can supplement or replace EZ Care remedies and may be combined when suggested doses are followed.

### Diet

♦ **Identify personal food sensitivities**. Avoid all common allergenic foods (e.g., dairy, eggs, wheat, corn, preservatives, sugar). Rotate moderately allergic foods on a four-day schedule (see Appendix C).

## Vitamins

- **B12** – Dosage: 2,000mcg. sublingually two times daily. Necessary for the metabolism and integrity of nerve tissue. Herpes viruses have an affinity for nerve tissue.

- **Bioflavonoids** (full potency) – Dosage: 500 mg., two times daily with vitamin C doses. In combination with vitamin C, may help resolve herpes infection.

- **C** (mineral ascorbates mixed with bioflavonoids) – Dosage: 1,000 mg., three to four times daily with meals. Exerts an antiviral action and strengthens the body's resistance.

- **E** (natural d-alpha tocopherol in a base of mixed tocopherols) – Dosage: 800 IU daily with meals. May decrease pain and decrease healing time of cold sores.

## Minerals

- **Selenium** – Dosage: 200 mcg. daily from l-selenomethionine. May exert a useful immuno-stimulating effect.
  *Note:* Selenium and vitamin E are synergists; thus, they enhance each other's activity in the body.

## Herbs

- **Goldenseal Root** (Hydrastis canadensis) – Dosage: 2 capsules or 50 drops liquid extract* two times daily. Also dab liquid extract directly on the cold sore several times daily. May help control infection and reduce inflammation.

- **Lomatium Root** (Lomatium dissectum) – Dosage: 2 capsules or 50 drops of a liquid extract* two times daily. Potent antiviral properties.

- **Myrrh** (Commiphora myrrha) – Dosage: 2 capsules or 50 drops liquid extract* two times daily. Also dab liquid extract directly on the cold sore several times daily. May exert useful astringent and antiseptic effects.

### Aromatherapy

**Essential Oils mixed in Aloe Vera Gel** – Mix a total of 6 drops of one or more of the following essential oils in 1/2 tsp. aloe vera gel. Apply several times daily to cold sores. Using two of these oils or in combination may prove more effective than a single oil: **Lavender** (Lavendula vera), **Tea Tree** (Melaleuca alternifolia). Alternate applications of the diluted mix with dabbing undiluted lavender oil on the cold sore.

### Homeopathy

See Appendix E for proper use and handling instruction prior to administering remedies described below.

♦   **Arsenicum 6C** – Cold sores with burning and shooting pain that are worse at night; crusts are large and deep and bleed when removed. Dosage: Dissolve 5 pellets under the tongue, two to three times daily. If results are noticeable after three days, continue until lip is clear; otherwise discontinue.

♦   **Hepar Sulph 6C** – Cold sores in center of lower lip; upper lip swollen and tender. Dosage: Dissolve 5 pellets under the tongue, two to three times daily. If results are noticeable after three days, continue until lip is clear; otherwise discontinue.

♦   **Mercurius 15C** – Herpes outbreak is accompanied by drooling and fevers. Dosage: Dissolve 5 pellets under the tongue, two to three times daily. If results are noticeable after three days, continue until lip is clear; otherwise discontinue.

### Miscellaneous

♦   **Ice** (during early stages of outbreak) – Apply to affected area for 10 minutes *on* and 5 minutes *off*. May help soothe and reduce itching.
    *Note: Rubbing an emerging cold sore with an ice cube may halt its eruption.*

*   Most herbal extracts contain alcohol. Avoid use if alcohol sensitive or if there is a history of alcohol abuse. *Note:* Alcohol content can be reduced through evaporation by adding extract to very hot water (just below boiling point) and allowing to stand 5 to 7 minutes before drinking.

# Colic

Never attempt any home remedies with infants without consulting your pediatrician first. The information contained here should be used only in consultation with your pediatrician.

Colic is defined as persistent crying of two hours or more at least two times daily for two weeks. Symptoms include excessive crying, tightness of the abdominal muscles, and irritability. This condition occurs in infants between the age of two weeks and one year.

Conventional treatments include determining the underlying problem, which may include constipation, volvulus (twisting of the bowel), intusseption (telescoping of the bowel), infection, or indigestion. Then treat the underlying cause accordingly. However, formula changes are usually recommended as first line therapy.

| EZ Care Program | | |
|---|---|---|
| Diet | **Replace cow's milk formula with soy formula**. If the baby is allergic to both, look for alternatives and predigested formulas. | |
| | **If breast-feeding**, eliminate milk, soy, corn, wheat, sugar, caffeine, and eggs from the mother's diet; also consider eliminating garlic, onions, cabbage, and beans because these may cause gas. Breast-fed babies may receive antigens through the mother's milk. | |
| Herbs | *Consult your pediatrician before administering to an infant or child:* **Herbal teas** can help reduce colic symptoms. **Catnip** (Nepeta cataria) and **Fennel Seed** (Foeniculum vulgare) are commonly used to help expel gas, relieve gas pain, and calm an infant. Prepare an infusion (see Appendix B) using 1/2 tsp. of each herb : 8 oz. pure water. Administer 1/2 to 1 tsp. of the infusion every 15 minutes until the symptoms abate. **Chamomile** (Matricaria chamomilla) also may help quiet the baby's nerves and relieve spasm. To prepare, pour 4 oz. boiling pure water over 1 tsp. of the fresh herb in a glass or stainless steel cooking pot (avoid aluminum pots). Cover and let steep 30 minutes. Strain. Administer 1/2 to 1 tsp. warm (not hot) tea every 15 minutes when symptoms occur and until relief is obtained. *Note:* As a maintenance dose during quiet periods, 1/2 to 1 tsp. of either herbal tea administered 30 minutes before feedings may help avert acute colic episodes. | |
| Miscellaneous | **Abdominal massage with Essential Oil of Peppermint** (Mentha piperita)   May help decrease spasm of the intestines via dispersal breakup of gas pockets and stimulation of bowel movements. Lubricate your hands with equal parts warm olive oil mixed with peppermint oil. *To prepare dilution:* Add 1 oz. olive oil to a small bottle. Add 25 drops peppermint oil. Before each use, gently warm bottle on stove in a small amount of warm water. Shake bottle well before each use. Warm hands before beginning massage. Gently massage abdomen in a clockwise direction. Massage upward on right side of navel, from right to left above navel, and downward on left side of navel. Although this can be performed during acute episodes (except if child's abdomen is very sensitive), it is best done two times daily during quiet periods | |

# Additional Recommendations

The EZ Care Program consists of basic remedies that are commonly used for colic and have been found to work well in most cases. The remedies are most effective when combined, but can be used individually. The options stated below can supplement or replace EZ Care remedies and may be combined when suggested doses are followed.

### Diet

♦  All infants should be **breastfed for at least 6 months to 1 year**. This practice may help prevent many problems, because commercial baby formulas and introduction of inappropriate foods into the baby's diet may cause colic.

♦  Avoid **over-feeding** infant.

◆ Breast-feeding mother should **adhere to a simple diet**. Complex, chaotic diets may encourage colic in the infant.

◆ Do not introduce **solid food** into the baby's diet before 6 months of age.

◆ To **feed**, position the baby **in a sitting position**. Burp after each ounce of fluid.

## Vitamins

◆ **Vitamins** and other nutritional supplements, herbal products, etc. may act as allergens. If breast-feeding, mother should eliminate her supplements for 7 days and observe the baby's condition. If the colic subsides, one or more of the supplements may have been causing the colic response. Next, reintroduce 1 type of supplement every two days to see which one aggravates the baby's symptoms. Permanently eliminate the offending supplements, and seek well-tolerated alternatives.

## Homeopathy

See Appendix E for proper use and handling instruction prior to administering remedies described below.

◆ **Belladonna 6C** – Abdomen greatly distended; regurgitation of even small drinks of liquid; spasms that come and go quickly; slightest touch causes great pain; baby shrieks and bends forward or arches back; abdomen hot to the touch; constipation and great agitation. Dosage: 3 pellets dissolved in 1/2 tsp. warm water two times daily. During acute episodes, administer 1/4 tsp. of this solution every 15 minutes until relief is obtained.

◆ **Chamomila 6C** – Especially indicated if the baby is irritable, desires to be carried, and is teething at the same time; abdomen sensitive to touch, distended, and passing of flatus does not relieve symptoms; the stool may also be loose, green, foul-smelling, and contain undigested food; colic from anger; pain relieved by belching. Dosage: 3 pellets in 1/2 tsp. warm water two times daily. During acute episodes, administer 1/4 tsp. every 15 minutes until relief is obtained.

◆ **Colocynthis 6C** – Infant doubles up and cries or screams if an effort is made to change position; restless, irritable, writhing in pain; colic often accompanied by diarrhea; both may be brought on by undigested food, eating fruit, exposure to cold or cold foods and drinks, or a fit of anger; pressure applied to the abdomen relieves colic pain. Dosage: 3 pellets in 1/2 tsp. warm water two times daily. During acute episodes, administer 1/4 tsp. every 15 minutes until relief is obtained.

◆ **Pulsatilla 6C** – Colic with chilliness and abdominal distention in the evening after feeding, especially if infant or breast-feeding mother eats fruit, pastries, ice cream, or fatty foods; loud rumbling and gurgling in the abdomen; constipation alternating with diarrhea; no two stools alike; diarrhea may be watery and greenish and worse at night; baby feels better when picked up and rocked. Dosage: 3 pellets in 1/2 tsp. warm water two times daily. During acute episodes, administer 1/4 tsp. every 15 minutes until relief is obtained.

## Miscellaneous

♦ **Charcoal Powder** – Stir 1 tbsp. activated charcoal powder into 4 oz. pure warm water. Administer 1 to 2 tbsp. of the mixture two to four times daily or as required. May help relieve gas pressure and resultant pain. Avoid using for extended periods of time.

♦ **Hot Water Bottle** – Fill hot water bottle *partially* with warm water. Apply to the abdomen. May relieve colic spasms.
*Note:* Only partially fill the hot water bottle so it is not too heavy when laid on the baby's abdomen. Check temperature of water bottle for safety.

♦ **Probiotic Supplement** (friendly intestinal bacteria that aid digestion, nutrient assimilation, and toxin elimination) (Lactobacillus bifudus, powder or capsules)  Add 1/4 tsp. to baby's formula every day. Nursing mothers may take 5 capsules of L. bifudus per meal for 1 week. L. bifudus is the species of lactobacillus initially implanted in the child's gut via the colostrum. Babies that are not breast-fed are susceptible to intestinal flora imbalances and a predomination of undesirable gas-forming species.

♦ **Warm, Shallow Sitz Bath** (see Appendix D) – Water should be quite warm, yet comfortable. Gently massage the baby's abdomen in a clockwise direction with the warm water. Continue the bath for 5 to 15 minutes or as required. The Warm Sitz Bath helps relieve colic spasms via reflex action. Option: follow the sitz bath with Abdominal Massage with essential oil of peppermint described above.

# Constipation

Constipation refers to infrequent and painful bowel movements. Stools generally become hard and are difficult to pass. Bloating, gas, and discomfort often accompany this condition. Unexplained changes in bowel frequency or severe abdominal pain should be discussed with a physician, because it could be a sign of an underlying disorder.

Conventional treatments include the use of laxatives, increasing fiber and water intake, and eliminating constipating medications such as calcium channel blockers.
*Note:* **(1)** Avoid prolonged use of laxatives, natural or chemical, because they tend to cause improper gut motility and a condition known as *melanosis coli*, leading to further problems with constipation. **(2)** Certain medications and supplements may have side-effects (including constipation), such as iron pills, antihypertension drugs, tricyclic antidepressants, narcotics, and atropine. Check with a healthcare practitioner if taking any medication.

| EZ Care Program | |
|---|---|
| Diet | **Chew foods well**. Chewing breaks down foods and encourages salivation. Saliva contains digestive enzymes and lubricates the gastrointestinal (g.i.) tract. |
| | **Drink** 6 to 8 glasses of pure water daily. |
| | **Eat high fiber foods**, such as whole grains, legumes, broccoli, raw cabbage, and dark green, leafy vegetables. **Include fruits,** such as apples, apricots, blueberries, figs, papaya, and pears. |
| | Eat a **high-water-content** diet consisting of large quantities of fresh fruits and vegetables and comparatively smaller quantities of whole grains, legumes, seeds, nuts, fish, skinless chicken and turkey. |
| Vitamins | **C** (mineral ascorbates mixed with bioflavonoids) – Dosage: 1,000 mg., three to four times daily with meals. High doses may pull water into the intestines and act as a laxative and stools softener. |
| Minerals | **Magnesium** – Dosage: 150mg. elemental magnesium from amino acid chelate or magnesium citrate four times daily with meals and at bedtime. High doses may draw water into the intestines and exert a laxative action. Required for relaxation of the smooth muscles in the g.i. tract. |
| Herbs | **Triphala** – Dosage: 2 to 6 grams daily 1/2 hour before bedtime one to seven times weekly. *Beneficial properties:* Popular Ayurvedic remedy consisting of 3 tropical fruits. Nourishes and cleanses the digestive tract and is non-habit forming. Considered safe for long-term use. May stimulate digestion and elimination. |
| Miscellaneous | **Fiber Supplement** – Dosage: 1 to 3 tsp. Psyllium Husk fiber: 8 oz. pure water one to two times daily between meals. *Note:* Carefully read label. Some brands require additional water. |
| | **Morning Cold Water Draught** – Drink 16 oz. to 32 oz. cool water (*not iced or refrigerated*) on rising each morning. Wait at least one hour before breakfast. This procedure stimulates blood circulation in the g.i. tract and is one of the simplest and easiest methods to help overcome chronic constipation. |
| | **Omega-3 Fatty Acids** – Dosage: 300 mg. of EPA and DHA from marine lipid concentrate one to four times daily with meals. Aids bowel function and decreases bowel inflammation. |
| | **Regular exercise** – at least 30 minutes daily. Supports blood circulation and stimulates the digestive system. Be sure to take brisk walks morning and evening. |

## Additional Recommendations

The EZ Care Program consists of basic remedies that are commonly used for constipation and have been found to work well in most cases. The remedies are most effective when combined, but can be used individually. The options stated below can supplement or replace EZ Care remedies and may be combined when suggested doses are followed.

## Diet

♦ **Add ground flaxseed** to the diet, which is high in fiber and omega-3 fatty acids. 1 tbsp. per meal.

♦ **Avoid dairy products,** such as milk and cheese, because they may cause constipation. Avoid flour products, such as bread, pastry, and pasta. Even whole-grain flour products may be congestive for people prone to constipation.

♦ **Avoid** refined foods and sugar, excessive salt, and fried foods.

♦ **Eat** 1 serving black mission figs daily. Place 10 figs in a bowl. Cover with pure water and let soak overnight (cover soaking bowl). Serve the next day with chopped apples and 1 tbsp. ground flaxseed. *Note:* Figs mixed with 1 tbsp. olive oil and 1 tbsp. ground flaxseed may prove of good service.

♦ **Identify personal food sensitivities**. Avoid all common allergenic foods (e.g., dairy, eggs, wheat, corn, sugar, preservatives). Rotate moderately allergic foods on a four-day schedule (see Appendix C). This is usually necessary for patients with chronic constipation.

## Herbs

♦ **Aloe Vera Juice** – Dosage: 2 to 3 tbsp. juice from organically-grown, whole-leaf, cold-pressed aloe vera in 8 oz. pure water two times daily between meals.
*Beneficial properties*: May soothe and heal dysfunctional bowels and encourage return of natural bowel movements.

♦ **Butternut Bark** (Juglans cinerea) – Dosage: 50 drops of extract* in 4 oz. water two times daily on rising and at bedtime.
*Beneficial properties*: May act as a gentle laxative, especially for elderly and middle-aged adults and weakly children. Adjust dosage in accordance with tolerance and vitality of the individual.

♦ **Dandelion Root** (Taraxacum officinalis) – Dosage: 1 to 2 capsules with each meal.
*Beneficial properties*: Liver tonic that may help stimulate digestion.

♦ **Gentian Root** (Gentiana lutea) – Dosage: 1 to 2 capsules or 40 drops of extract* in 4 oz. water two times daily 1/2 hour before a meal.
*Beneficial properties*: Tonic bitter; traditionally used to aid digestion and elimination and as a liver cleanser.
*Note:* Extract may be preferable in this case, because actual perception of the bitter taste will enhance the body's response.

♦ **Ginger Root** (Zingiber officinalis) – Dosage: 2 capsules three times daily with dandelion root capsules.
*Beneficial properties*: May aid circulation, digestion, and expulsion of gas.

## Homeopathy

See Appendix E for proper use and handling instruction prior to administering remedies described below.

- **Calc Carb 6C** – Feel better when constipated; sour-smelling stools; physically lethargic, lack stamina; allergic to milk; crave iced drinks, eggs, ice cream, sweets, and salt; averse to warm foods. Dosage: Dissolve 5 pellets under the tongue, one to two times daily or as required.

- **Lycopodium 6C** – Severe constipation with ineffective urging, accompanied by acidity and burning in stomach; relieved by belching. Dosage: Dissolve 5 pellets under the tongue, one to two times daily or as required.

- **Nux Vomica 6C** – Constipation with constant ineffective urge to pass stools, but feeling of never being finished; pain in bowels with great straining; may be accompanied by irritability, nausea, vomiting, bloating, heartburn, and/or headache; constipation related to overindulgence in rich foods, coffee, alcohol, drugs, or to protracted emotional stress. Dosage: Dissolve 5 pellets under the tongue, one to two times daily or as required.

- **Sepia 30C** – Constipation in women, with ineffective urging; difficulty passing even soft stools; bearing down pains in rectum, sensation as if a ball lodged in rectum or as if rectum dilated and will not contract; allergic to milk and milk products. Dosage: Dissolve 5 pellets under the tongue, one to two times daily or as required.

- **Sulphur 6C** – Constipation with hard, knotty, painful stools; child afraid to have a bowel movement on account of pain. Dosage: Dissolve 5 pellets under the tongue, one to two times daily or as required.

## Miscellaneous

- **Alternating Hot and Cold Shower Directed at the Abdomen** – Begin with 2 minutes of hot water spray. Follow with 30 seconds cold. Repeat cycle one to two more times, finishing with cold. Then perform deep clockwise massage of the abdomen with the aromatherapy massage blend described above. Perform this procedure three to four times weekly. May help tone the organs of digestion and elimination.

- **Always respond promptly to the natural urge to move bowels**. "Holding it in" disrupts natural bowel rhythms and overrides autonomic nerve stimulation of the bowels.

- **Avoid caffeine and tobacco.**

- **Avoid commercial laxatives.** They artificially stimulate and irritate the bowels and ultimately may lead to dependency and worsen constipation.

- **Avoid coffee and regular tea**, which may worsen constipation.

- **Betaine HCL and Pepsin** – Dosage: one to two 700 mg. capsules at beginning of all meals with protein. Provides hydrochloric acid and pepsin to aid stomach phase of digestion. Many older individuals no longer produce adequate amounts of these two digestive substances; hence, their digestion is sluggish and they are subject to constipation.

*Note:* Avoid if suffering from stomach or duodenal ulcers. Discontinue use if experience a burning sensation in stomach.

♦ **Brewer's Yeast** – Dosage: 1 tsp. two to three times daily with meals. A rich source of natural B-vitamins which are important for relieving nervousness and tension due to stress that is often a major factor in constipation.

♦ **Deep Breathing Exercises** – These exercises involve strong movement by the diaphragm and abdominal muscles, thus exerting a massaging action on the intestines. Following is a yoga breathing exercise: Inhale through the nose for a count of 4, hold for a count of 7, exhale through the mouth for a count of 8. Practice twice daily, four to eight repetitions each session.

♦ **Maintain a normal, regular pattern of rest and sleep.** Disruption of healthy, wake/sleep cycles disrupts all body rhythmic processes, including the peristaltic movement of food along the gastro intestinal tract.

♦ **Ox Bile Extract/ Whole Beet Concentrate Capsules** – Dosage: one 250 mg. capsule with meals or as required. May be useful for constipated individuals who have had gall bladder removed or for anyone with fat digestion problems.

♦ **Probiotic Supplement** – Non-dairy, L. acidophilus capsules or powder with bifidobacteria and fructo-oligosaccharides – Dosage: 1 to 2 times daily in accordance with label instructions. Avoid commercial laxatives.

♦ **Proteolytic Enzyme Formula** (protein digesting enzymes that include pancreatic protease, bromelain, and papain) – Dosage: 2 capsules three times daily with meals. *Beneficial properties:* When taken with meals, these enzymes aid the digestive process. Underactive digestion is a primary factor in constipation.

♦ **Raw Sauerkraut** – This item is stocked in the cooler in many health food stores. It is made with raw, rather than cooked, sauerkraut and does not contain vinegar. It is a rich source of probiotic bacteria. Dosage: 2 tbsp. one to two times daily with meals. Keep refrigerated, even when unopened, because it is perishable.

♦ **Reduce** lifestyle **stress** and implement a relaxation program. Harmonizing practices (e.g., biofeedback, meditation, yoga, Tai Chi exercise) may prove beneficial.

♦ **Retrain bowels** – Drink 1 glass of pure water upon arising and immediately sit on toilet, in a relaxed manner. The water helps stimulate the bowels. This may retrain the bowels to move regularly at the start of each day.

\*   Most herbal extracts contain alcohol. Avoid use if alcohol sensitive or if there is a history of alcohol abuse. *Note:* Alcohol content can be reduced through evaporation by adding extract to very hot water (just below boiling point) and allowing to stand 5 to 7 minutes before drinking.

# Cough

Coughs occur for many reasons. Viral infection and the inhalation of allergenic particles are two common causes of coughing. Coughs can be characterized in two general ways, either productive or nonproductive. Productive coughs that are not severe can be helpful because they help expel phlegm or mucus from the lungs and may not need to be suppressed. Nonproductive coughs do not expel mucus; these uncomfortable coughs can be irritating to the throat and are generally safe to suppress. A chronic cough may be a sign of a more serious underlying illness such as asthma, emphysema, pneumonia, or allergies.

*Warning signs of a more serious illness include shortness of breath, night sweats, weight loss, fever, and coughing of blood. If you have these symptoms or a cough that has not resolved within one week, contact a physician immediately.*

Conventional therapies involve determining the underlying causes, as well as use of expectorants, nasal decongestants, oral bronchodilators, vaporizers/humidifiers, and antibiotics.

| EZ Care Program | |
|---|---|
| Diet | **Avoid milk** and all milk products, because they increase mucus formation. Consider dairy alternatives, such as soy or nut milks and cheeses. |
| Vitamins | **C** (mineral ascorbates mixed with bioflavonoids) – 1,000 - 2000 mg., three to four times daily with meals. May help control infection and lessen the severity of coughs. |
| Herbs | **Mullein** (Verbascum thapsus) – Dosage: 2 to 4 capsules or 6 oz. warm tea prepared by infusion (see Appendix B) four times daily. *Beneficial properties*: May soothe respiratory tract and help bring up mucus. |
| | **Wild Cherry Bark** (Prunus virginiana) – Dosage: 2 to 4 capsules or 6 oz. of tea prepared by decoction (See appendix B) four times daily until the cough is resolved. Take each serving with 1 tsp. raw honey and a pinch of cayenne. *Beneficial properties:* May be beneficial to soothing coughs, and reducing bronchial spasms and throat irritation. |

| EZ Care Program | |
|---|---|
| Miscellaneous | **N-Acetyl Cysteine** (NAC) – Dosage: 600 mg. three times daily. NAC, a precursor to the antioxidant glutathione, is a natural mucolytic, aiding in the thinning and expelling of mucus secretions. |
| | **Head Vapor** (i.e., steam inhalation) (see appendix D for complete instructions) – Dosage: Add 8 drops each of one of the essential oil blends listed below to water, just before beginning inhalation of steam, two to three times daily or as required. May increase oxygenation, loosen phlegm, and reduce infection. |

# Additional Recommendations

The EZ Care Program consists of basic remedies that are commonly used for coughs and have been found to work well in most cases. The remedies are most effective when combined, but can be used individually. The options stated below can supplement or replace EZ Care remedies and may be combined when suggested doses are followed.

## Diet

♦   **Avoid all sugar**, as it may weaken the immune system.

♦   **Identify personal food sensitivities**. Avoid all common allergenic foods (e.g., dairy, eggs, wheat, corn, preservatives, sugar). Rotate moderately allergic foods on a four-day schedule (see Appendix C).

♦   If cough is part of a cold, flu, or other acute disorder, **eat lightly** until the acute disorder passes. Drink large amounts of warm fluids, which help with mucus expectoration.

♦   **Avoid starchy foods** (e.g., grains, potatoes, yams, sweet potatoes, bread, pasta, and other flour products), because these may worsen irritation of the mucous membranes of the respiratory tract. Ideal intake during this period consists of fresh fruit meals with a few tbsp. of nuts or seeds, raw vegetable salads with lemon juice, and a few tbsp. of sunflower or sesame seeds or sliced avocado.

## Vitamins

♦   **A** (natural, from fish liver oil) – Dosage: 25,000 to 50,000 IU daily with meals for up to two weeks. Vitamin A is required for maintaining the structural integrity and lubrication of the epithelial tissues that line the lungs, nose, and throat.
*Note:* Consult a physician before using high doses of vitamin A for longer than two weeks. Avoid use if pregnant. Discontinue use if nausea, dry skin, sore lips, blurred vision, or other signs of vitamin A toxicity are experienced.

♦   **Beta-Carotene** – Dosage: 20.000 to 50,000 IU three times daily with meals. A potent antioxidant that protects lung tissue and converts to vitamin A in the body. Unlike vitamin A, however, it generally does not have the risk of side effects from high doses or extended use.

## Minerals

♦ **Zinc** (take only if over 14 years of age) – Dosage: 25 to 50 mg. elemental zinc from amino acid chelate one to two times daily with meals for one week, or one 25 mg. zinc lozenge two to three times daily for one week. Zinc supports the immune function. Requirement increases during acute or chronic infection.
*Note:* Zinc helps utilize and maintain the body's level of vitamin A; they work well together in this context.

## Herbs

♦ **Astragalus Root** (Astragalus membranaceus) – Dosage: 2 capsules three times daily with meals until the cough subsides.
*Beneficial properties:* Antiviral and an immune stimulant.

♦ **Echinacea** (Echinacea purpurea) – Dosage: 2 to 4 capsules or 50 drops liquid extract* three times daily for two weeks.
*Beneficial Properties:* Used to fight infections and stimulate the immune system.

♦ **Garlic** (Allium sativum) – Dosage: 1 to 2 capsules per meal of standardized allicin garlic or aged garlic extract. Fresh, raw garlic (a whole, living food) is preferable, but capsules should be considered if raw garlic is not taken consistently.

♦ **Garlic or Onion** (Allium cepa) **Syrup** – Garlic juice mixed at a ratio of 1 to 2 with raw honey or several garlic cloves (or a similar quantity of raw onion) pureed. (Mixing with a sufficient quantity of raw honey to make a thick syrup may also prove of good service.) Take 1 tbsp. of syrup every one to two hours or as required.
*Beneficial properties:* Garlic exerts a powerful antibiotic action and has a special affinity for the respiratory tract where it helps to limit infection, act as an expectorant, and positively influence bronchial secretions.
*Note:* Raw parsley taken with raw garlic helps prevent "garlic breath" and enhances blood-cleansing effects.

♦ **Marshmallow Root** (Althea officianlis) – Dosage: 6 oz. of tea three to four times daily (see Appendix B). Take each serving with 1 tsp. raw honey. May be prepared in combination with wild cherry bark (1 part marshmallow root to 1 part wild cherry bark).
*Beneficial properties:* May soothe coughs and reduce throat and bronchial irritation.

♦ **Pleurisy Root** (Asclepia tuberosa) – Prepare tea by decoction (see Appendix B). Drink 6 oz. warm tea three to four times daily or as required. Add a pinch of cayenne to each serving. Consider using in combination with yerba santa described below.
*Beneficial properties:* Relaxes spasms; specific for pains in the chest from coughing.

♦ **Slippery Elm Bark tea** (Ulmus fulva) – Dosage: 6 oz. tea prepared by decoction (see Appendix B) three to four times daily between meals. Serve warm with a pinch of ginger root powder.
*Beneficial properties:* Contains abundant mucilage that may soothe and quiet inflamed mucosal lining of the respiratory tract.

- **Thyme tea** (Thymus vulgaris) **with Lobelia** (Lobelia inflata) – Dosage: 6 oz. of tea prepared by infusion (see Appendix B) three to four times daily between meals. Add 10 drops liquid extract of lobelia to each serving.
  *Beneficial properties:* May exert a healing, antispasmodic, antiseptic action in the respiratory tract. Thyme forms the basis of the Listerine antiseptic compound. Lobelia exerts a potent antispasmodic action that may help relax bronchial spasms and ameliorate spasmodic coughing.

- **Yerba Santa (Eriodictyon glutinosum)** – Dosage: 6 oz. of tea prepared by infusion (see Appendix B) three to four times daily between meals. May be of value in treating all coughs when there is dryness of the mucous membranes of the respiratory tract. Consider using in combination with pleurisy root.

## Aromatherapy

Use the following undiluted essential oil combination. Blend and store in an amber glass bottle. May be used as an adjunct of suggested hydrotherapies, as well as local massage oil.

2 parts **Eucalyptus** (Eucalyptus globulus) + 1 part **Marjoram** (Origanum marjorana) + 2 parts **Lavender** (Lavendula vera) + 1/2 part **Thyme** (Thymus vulgaris)

Also, several times daily tap 3 to 4 drops of the blend onto a palm. Rub the palms together, then take 10-15 deep breaths from the cupped palms, turning the head to the side when exhaling.

*Prepare massage oils using the following proportion:* 25 drops of the blend for each 1 oz. jojoba or sweet almond oil. Shake well before each use. Rub the massage blend into the upper chest, upper back, neck, and throat two to three times daily.

## Homeopathy

See Appendix E for proper use and handling instruction prior to administering remedies described below.

- **Aconitum 6C** – Dry, croupy, loud, suffocating cough; worse at night and after midnight; cough brought on by dry wind or dry, cold weather; worse with cold temperature, cold applications, cold drinks, and lying on side, thirsty, anxious, and restless. Dosage: Dissolve 5 pellets under the tongue, every two to four hours or as required.

- **Antimonium Tart. 6C** – Chest feels very heavy, as if a weight placed on it, mental depression and hoarseness; wheezing and rattling loose cough, but unable to raise mucus; labored breathing; white, creamy coating on tongue; aversion to food; worse in early morning about four a.m. Dosage: Dissolve 5 pellets under the tongue, every two to four hours or as required.

- **Belladonna 6C** – Short, rapid, difficult breathing; dry, spasmodic cough with hoarseness or complete loss of voice; restlessness, drowsiness, and wild dreams; face turns red when coughing; symptoms worse at night. Dosage: Dissolve 5 pellets under the tongue, every two to four hours or as required.

♦ **Drosera 6C** – Spasmodic, tickling, choking cough that is worse after midnight, especially about two a.m.; cough dry, loud, barking, deep sounding, and painful; hold chest while coughing to control pain; chilly yet perspire profusely. Dosage: Dissolve 5 pellets under the tongue, every two hours *or* two to four times daily or as required.

♦ **Pulsatilla 6C** – Dry cough during the day and loose cough at night, yellow or greenish expectoration at night and on waking; worse in a warm room, warm weather, at night, lying down; better in the open air. Dosage: Dissolve 5 pellets under the tongue, every two to four hours or as required.

♦ **Rumex 6C** – Spasmodic cough, tickling in the throat, and difficulty raising phlegm; feeling of soreness all the way down the trachea and underneath the breastbone; extremely sensitive to cold air; may place blanket over head to avoid breathing cold air; symptoms worse at night and with motion. Dosage: Dissolve 5 pellets under the tongue, every two to four hours or as required.

♦ **Spongia 6C** – Dry, barking, croupy cough; dry air passages and no phlegm; worse with cold air, cold fluids, sweets, tobacco smoke, warm room, lying with head low, and talking; better with warm food and drinks, sitting up, and leaning forward. Dosage: Dissolve 5 pellets under the tongue, every two to four hours or as required.

## Miscellaneous

♦ **Check air quality** for chronic coughs. Use high quality HEPA air purifier in home. Change household air filters regularly in accordance with manufacturer's specifications.

♦ **Lemon Juice and Raw Honey Gargle** – Mix the juice of 2 lemons + 2 tbsp. raw honey + 6 oz. warm water. Gargle with, then swallow 1/3 of this mixture three times daily. May ease dry coughs.

♦ **Steam Pack** (see Appendix D for complete instructions) – over chest and throat 1 to 2 times daily or as required. After removing pack, massage the aromatherapy oil blends described above into chest, upper back, and under nose diluted as follows: Add 1 oz. olive oil to a small bottle (preferably amber glass). Add 40 drops of the essential oil blend as noted in Aromatherapy section above. Shake well before each use. Store in a dark place if an amber glass bottle is not used.

\* Most herbal extracts contain alcohol. Avoid use if alcohol sensitive or if there is a history of alcohol abuse. *Note:* Alcohol content can be reduced through evaporation by adding extract to very hot water (just below boiling point) and allowing to stand 5 to 7 minutes before drinking.

# Cuts

Minor cuts and scrapes are a common occurrence. Often they can be treated safely in the home setting. However, evaluation of the cut is necessary to insure immediate medical attention is not needed. Guidelines of a more serious condition include a deep wound with any exposure of ligaments, tendons, or underlying tissue which requires suturing to close, location in joint spaces which can become infected, or profuse bleeding which does not stop with simple application of pressure. Any cut or laceration that produces numbness, loss of strength or range of motion should be seen immediately by a physician.

Conventional treatment is to irrigate the wound and clean with antibacterial soap and water. An application of antibiotic ointment is commonly used to prevent infection. Cuts, wounds, and scrapes that are kept covered in a moist environment heal more quickly than when left uncovered. More serious cuts may require stitches or surgical intervention.

| EZ Care Program | |
|---|---|
| Vitamins | **E** (natural d-alpha tocopherol) – After the wound seals, puncture a natural vitamin E capsule and apply topically. May speed healing and prevent scar tissue. Apply two times daily or as required. Do not use on open wounds as it may sensitize the surrounding skin. |
| Herbs | **Calendula** oil or cream – Apply externally four to six times daily. *Beneficial Properties:* May promote healing of tissue and prevent infection. |
| | **Cayenne Pepper** (Capsicum annuum) – For minor bleeding, wash wound well; sprinkle cayenne directly on the cut. *Beneficial properties*: May stop bleeding. |
| | **St. John's Wort Oil** – Apply two to three times daily in alternation with calendula, especially if there is an unusual amount of pain. |
| | **Tea Tree Oil** (Melaleuca alternifolia) – Apply undiluted 1 to 2 drops or more according to size of cut each time wound is washed. Tea tree oil may be mixed into St. John's wort oil as well. |
| Homeopathy | **Arnica 6C or 30C** – Dosage: Dissolve 5 pellets under the tongue, immediately after injury. Repeat one to three times daily for two days in accordance with severity of injury. |
| Miscellaneous | **Hydrogen Peroxide** (3%) – may be used to disinfect. Pour into wound, let foam, then repeat and pat dry with clean gauze or cotton. May be used to cleanse wound before each application of oils or cream listed above. |

# Additional Recommendations

The EZ Care Program consists of basic remedies that are commonly used for cuts and have been found to work well in most cases. The remedies are most effective when combined, but can be used individually. The options stated below can supplement or replace EZ Care remedies and may be combined when suggested doses are followed.

## Vitamins

♦ **C** (mixed mineral ascorbates) – Dosage: 1,000 mg., three to four times daily or as required. May help prevent infection and speed wound healing.

## Minerals

♦ **Zinc** (take only if over 14 years of age) – Dosage: 50 mg. elemental zinc from amino acid chelate with meals for one week or until wound completely heals. Essential nutrient for healthy skin. May speed wound healing.

## Aromatherapy

Choose one of the following essential oils: **Chamomile** (Matricaria chamomilla) or **Lavender** (Lavendula vera). Place a few drops of the oil on an adhesive bandage or strip of gauze and place over the wound. Repeat or as required.

## Homeopathy

See Appendix E for proper use and handling instruction prior to administering remedies described below.

♦ **Hypericum 6C or 30C** – Cuts in areas rich in nerves, such as fingertips, and particularly if pain shoots centrally; consider if cut is infected, or deep, and there is much cutting or shooting pain. Dosage: Dissolve 5 pellets under the tongue, one to three times daily or as required.

♦ **Ledum 30C** – For puncture wounds inflicted by a sharp instrument or after injection and area is sore; particularly useful when extremities are cold. Dosage: Dissolve 5 pellets under the tongue, one to three times daily or as required.

## Miscellaneous

♦ **Green or Semi-ripe Papaya** – Slice papaya and place directly over cut. May speed healing and help prevent infection.

*Note:* The enzymes in papaya that effect healing are used up by the fruit in the ripening process; thus, use only green or semi-ripe papaya.

# Dandruff

Dandruff is a common condition where the scalp is covered with small flakes of dead skin. It occurs in over 15% of the population, and those afflicted may have scalp itching and irritation. These flakes represent an increase in the normal loss of the outermost layer of skin. The condition is known as seborrheic dermatitis.

Conventional treatments generally include dandruff shampoos, cleansing lotions that contain a drying agent, or soothing creams. It is best also to take short, cool showers to prevent an overdrying of the scalp.

| EZ Care Program | |
|---|---|
| Diet | **Eat fish**, such as mackerel, herring, trout and salmon, because they are high in omega-3 fatty acids. Dandruff may be related in part to a deficiency of essential fatty acids. |
| | **Include flaxseed oil**: 1 tbsp. or 1250 mg. capsule, one – two times daily. Flaxseed oil contains omega-3 fatty acids that are beneficial for skin health. Add contents of one capsule of vitamin E to flaxseed oil and keep in refrigerator for storage. This helps prevent against rancidity. |
| Vitamins | **Vitamin A** (Emulsified) – 10,000 to 25,000 IU daily as tolerated. Discontinue use if nausea, dry skin, sore lips, blurred vision, or other signs of vitamin A toxicity are experienced. Emulsified form is preferred because dandruff is often a sign of faulty fat assimilation. Vitamin A is required for maintaining normal function of skin cells. *Note:* Consult a physician before using higher doses of vitamin A. Avoid use if pregnant. |
| Herbs | **Black Currant Oil** (Ribies nigrum) – Dosage: 500 mg., two times daily. *Beneficial properties*: Excellent source of omega 6 fatty acids that may be beneficial for good skin health. |

## Additional Recommendations

The EZ Care Program consists of basic remedies that are commonly used for dandruff and have been found to work well in most cases. The remedies are most effective when combined, but can be used individually. The options stated below can supplement or replace EZ Care remedies and may be combined when suggested doses are followed.

### Vitamins

♦ **B complex** – Dosage: 25 to 50 mg. daily of a natural, balanced B complex formula. *Notes:* (1) For highest assimilation, use a multi B complex which contains the vitamins in their coenzyme form and avoid mega-potency B complex products. (2) B vitamins are "anti-stress" nutrients. Stress is often a major factor in skin disease.

♦ **Biotin** – Dosage: 500 – 1000 mg. twice daily. Biotin is a member of the B vitamin family, essential for hair and skin health.

♦ **C** (mineral ascorbates mixed with bioflavonoids) – 1,000 mg., three to four times daily with meals. Vitamin C is essential for skin health.

## Minerals

♦ **Zinc** (take only if over 14 years of age) – 50 mg. elemental zinc from amino acid chelate with meals. Helps utilize and maintain the body's level of vitamin A; they work well together in this context.

## Herbs

♦ **Burdock Root** (Arctium lappa) – Dosage: 1 to 2 capsules or 30-60 drops liquid extract* in 4 oz. water three times daily.
   *Beneficial properties*: May exert a direct cleansing influence on the blood and skin.

♦ **Kelp** (Laminaria spp.) – Dosage: 1 to 2 tablets two to three times daily.
   *Beneficial properties:* Rich source of nutrition that may exert a positive balancing influence on the glandular system and skin health.

♦ **Nettle** (Urtica urens) – Dosage: 1 to 2 capsules or 30-60 drops liquid extract* in 4 oz. water three times daily. Also, prepare a tea by infusion (see Appendix B) and use as a rinse after shampooing.
   *Beneficial properties:* Traditionally used in treating dandruff and other skin disorders.

## Aromatherapy

Mix a total of 4 to 5 drops of **Rosemary** (Rosmarinus officinalis) with 1 tsp 1/4 tsp. aloe vera gel. Massage into scalp once daily.

## Homeopathy

See Appendix E for proper use and handling instruction prior to administering remedies described below.

♦ **Graphites 6C** – Dandruff accompanied by eczema and other eruptions; scalp very scaly and itchy, with burning sensation at top of head. Dosage: Dissolve 5 pellets under the tongue, one to two times daily or as required.

♦ **Sulphur 6C** – General homeopathic remedy for thick dandruff, especially if worse in warm weather and if itching relieved by scratching. Dosage: Dissolve 5 pellets under the tongue, one to two times daily or as required.

## Miscellaneous

♦ **Avoid** hot hair drying, hair sprays, hair dyes, and perms.

♦ **Brush hair daily** to clean hair and stimulate scalp.

♦ **Clean** brush and comb daily.

♦ **Massage scalp** 5 to 10 minutes daily with fingertips. Avoid scratching scalp with fingernails. Be sure fingernails are clean.

\* Most herbal extracts contain alcohol. Avoid use if alcohol sensitive or if there is a history of alcohol abuse. *Note:* Alcohol content can be reduced through evaporation by adding extract to very hot water (just below boiling point) and allowing to stand 5 to 7 minutes before drinking.

# Depression

Depression is a common disorder affecting more than twenty million people annually in the United States. It can present in a variety of ways, including fatigue, loss of interest, insomnia or oversleeping, decreased libido, negative feelings about self, mood swings, changes in appetite, and a poor ability to concentrate and make decisions. Depression can affect relationships with friends, family, and coworkers. It can reduce job productivity and, in some cases when severe, can cause suicidal thoughts. Because of the complex and serious nature of depression, early recognition and treatment are necessary

Conventional evaluation entails a thorough history, physical, and mental status evaluation. Treatments may include pharmacological agents, behavior modification, and psychiatric counseling. A trial of ECT (electric convulsant therapy) is reserved for more serious cases of depression.

| EZ Care Program | |
|---|---|
| Diet | **Avoid** all processed sugar, artificial sweeteners, caffeine, and alcohol, because they all can act as depressants. |
| Vitamins | **B complex** – Dosage: 50 - 100 mg. daily of a natural, balanced B complex formula. *Note:* For highest assimilation, use a multi B complex which contains the vitamins in their coenzyme form and avoid mega-potency B complex products. Other B vitamins (including B1, B2, B3) also have proven of value in treating depression. Also, a complete B complex compensates for the fact that intake of high doses of one of the B vitamins may lead to imbalance in the other B vitamins. |
| Minerals | **Magnesium** (elemental magnesium from amino acid chelate) – Dosage: 250 mg. with breakfast and dinner, and 500 mg. at bedtime. Deficiency of magnesium, considered an "antistress" tranquilizing mineral, is an important factor in depression. |

| EZ Care Program | |
|---|---|
| | **Zinc** – Dosage: 50 mg. elemental zinc from amino acid chelate taken separately from calcium with meals. <br> *Note:* Zinc and calcium should not be taken at the same meal, because they compete in the gut for absorption. |
| Herbs | **St. John's Wort** (Hypericum perforatum) – Dosage: 1 to 3 capsules of standardized extract (0.3% hypercin) or 8 oz. tea three times daily. <br> *Beneficial properties:* Clinically proven antidepressant. <br> *Note:* Allow 4-6 weeks to take affect. Avoid use if taking antidepressants or any other medication. Consult with a physician before using. |
| Amino Acids | **L-5 HTP** (hydroxytryptophan) 100 mg twice daily. L-5 HTP, a derivative of the amino acid tryptophan, naturally increases the production of serotonin, a powerful brain chemical. It has relaxing and antidepressant properties. |
| | **S-adenosylmethionine** (SAMe) Dosage: 1600 mg per day of enteric coated tablets in the butanedisulfonate form, on at empty stomach. May positively influence mood regulating hormones and neurotransmitters such as serotonin, melatonin, adrenaline and dopamine. May be used in conjunction with St. John's wort. |
| Miscellaneous | **Regular exercise** – 30 minutes daily of aerobic exercise may help reduce depression by increasing levels of mood-elevating chemicals in the blood, building self-esteem, and reducing stress. <br> *Note:* Results generally take 4-6 weeks. |
| | **Reduce** lifestyle **stress** and implement a relaxation program. Harmonizing practices (e.g., biofeedback, meditation, Tai Chi exercise) may prove beneficial. |

# Additional Recommendations

The EZ Care Program consists of basic remedies that are commonly used for depression and have been found to work well in most cases. The remedies are most effective when combined, but can be used individually. The options stated below can supplement or replace EZ Care remedies and may be combined when suggested doses are followed.

## Diet

♦ **Avoid** refined sugars, caffeine, chocolate, and alcohol.

♦ **Identify personal food sensitivities**. Avoid all common allergenic foods (e.g., wheat, milk, cheese). Rotate moderately allergic foods on a four-day schedule (see Appendix C). *Note:* Wheat is the most common food depressant. Food allergies can affect brain chemistry and give rise to depression and other emotional symptoms.

## Vitamins

♦ **B6** (pyridoxal 5-phosphate is preferred) – Dosage: 25 to 50 mg., two times daily with meals until symptoms subside. B6 is required for converting tryptophan to serotonin that, when deficient, may cause depression.

♦ **B12** – Dosage: 1,000 to 2,000 mcg. sublingual daily. Deficiency of this vitamin may be present, even in the absence of anemia.

♦ **C** (mixed mineral ascorbates) – Dosage: 1,000 mg., three times daily with meals. Depression and fatigue may be related to vitamin C deficiency. The body requires greater amounts of vitamin C during times of stress.

♦ **Folic Acid** – Dosage: 800 mcg., two times daily with meals. Depression is a prominent symptom of folate deficiency and among the most common nutrient deficiencies.

## Minerals

♦ **Calcium** (elemental calcium from amino acid chelate) – Dosage: 250 mg. with breakfast and dinner, and 500 mg. at bedtime. May be particularly important in post-partum or post-menopausal depression and depression in the elderly.
*Note:* Calcium and magnesium can be taken together, because they exert a synergistic relaxation effect.

♦ **Chromium** (elemental chromium from polynicotinate) – Dosage: 200 mcg. one to two times daily with meals. Because brain cells require a great deal of glucose, chronic hypoglycemia can be an important factor in depression. Chromium is essential for blood-sugar regulation.

♦ **Potassium** (elemental potassium from citrate or aspartate) – Dosage: 99 mg., two to three times daily with meals. Crucial for nerve function. Depressed patients may have low intracellular levels of potassium despite normal blood levels.

## Herbs

♦ **Black Cohosh** (Cimicifuga racemosa) – Dosage: 1 to 2 capsules three times daily with meals.
*Beneficial properties:* May help depression related to menopause.

♦ **Gotu Kola** (Centella asiatica) – Dosage: 1 to 2 capsules or 30 - 50 drops of extract* in 4 oz. water three times daily.
*Beneficial properties*: May improve mental function and mood by increasing circulation to the brain.

♦ **Kava Kava** (piper methysticum) – Dosage: 250 mg. of a standardized extract or 30 drops liquid extract* in 4 oz. water two to three times daily.
*Beneficial properties:* Significant relaxant and mood-enhancing properties.
*Note:* Do not mix with any other herb that affects mental functioning without consulting a healthcare professional.

## Aromatherapy

There are many different essential oils that may prove of value in depression. The following list is a very general categorization of some of the more common oils used.

**Blue Chamomile** (Matricaria chamomilla) + **Clary Sage** (Salvia Sclarea) + **Lavender** (Lavendula vera) + **Sandalwood** (Santalum album) + **Ylang-Ylang** (Cananga odorata)

Add to warm bath 6 to 8 drops of one or a combination of 2 to 3 of these oils. Add a blend of 2 or more of these oils to an essential oil diffuser and disperse into the air 2 hours twice daily and throughout the night. Also, several times daily tap 3 to 4 drops of one of these oils, or a blend of 2 or more, onto a palm. Rub the palms together, then take 10 to 15 deep breaths from the cupped palms, turning the head to the side when exhaling.

## Homeopathy

See Appendix E for proper use and handling instruction prior to administering remedies described below.

*Please note:* The treatment of depression with homeopathy is very complex. There are literally hundreds of remedies that may be relevant. The following are some of the more common ones used. In cases of chronic depression, professional guidance is advised.

- **Aurum Metallicum 30C** – Severe depression with a feeling of hopelessness so great as to drive toward thoughts of suicide; deep love of music; fear of failure; spiritual inclination and desire for prayer and meditation. Dosage: Dissolve 5 pellets under the tongue, one to two times weekly or as required.

- **Ignatia 30C** – Depression from grief, worry, or romantic disappointments; menopausal depression; easily hurt feelings; aversion to consolation; alternating moods; desire to avoid crying gives way to sobbing. Dosage: Dissolve 5 pellets under the tongue, one to two times weekly or as required.

- **Nat Mur 30C** – Depression during menstrual period; apprehension about future; depression accompanied by ravenous hunger and heart palpitations; depression and suicidal ideas from grief or disappointed love; dwell on past grief and humiliation; serious and overly proper; aversion to consolation; sad yet unable to weep, or involuntary and hysterical weeping; depression is worse when lying down at night or after eating. Dosage: Dissolve 5 pellets under the tongue, one to two times weekly or monthly, or as required.

- **Sepia 30C** – Predominantly a female remedy; tearful and careworn; irritability, angered by the least disturbance; weeping, but does not know why; disconnected and indifferent to family; premenstrual depression; sadness during menopause; aversion to husband and company, yet dreads being alone; fear of poverty; despair of recovery. Dosage: Dissolve 5 pellets under the tongue, one to two times monthly or as required.

## Miscellaneous

- Be sure to get plenty of **rest** and **sleep**.

- **Breathing exercise** – Following is a yoga breathing exercise for calming the mind: Inhale through the nose for a count of 4, hold for a count of 7, exhale through the mouth for a count of 8. Practice two times daily, four to eight repetitions each session. Concentrate on something positive or enjoyable while doing this exercise.

*Note:* To enhance concentration and be certain the exercise is performed properly, you might lie down, place a lightweight book on your abdomen, then peacefully observe the book's rise-and-fall-motion as you breathe deeply.

♦ **Consider possible drug side-effects.** Consult your licensed healthcare professional concerning possible interactions or side effects of prescriptions or over-the-counter medications, including antihistamines, beta blockers, sleeping pills, narcotics, tranquilizers, and recreational drugs.

♦ **Cultivate a positive mental outlook.** Concentrate on something positive on waking each morning.

♦ **Express emotions freely** – Suppressed emotions may cause stress or depression and may lead to other physical illnesses.

♦ **Full-spectrum fluorescent lights** – Use 1 hour daily as supplement for decreased levels of sunlight in winter. Full-spectrum fluorescent lights contain the ultra-violet wavelength found in natural sunlight, but is missing in standard fluorescent tubes. Deficiency of natural light is a factor in both physical and emotional disorders such as depression and hyperactivity. Replace standard fluorescent tubes in your home and workplace with full-spectrum tubes (the latter can be used in the same standard fixtures).

♦ **Low thyroid** and/or **adrenal function** may be a pivotal factor in depression. If necessary, consult a physician in this regard.

♦ **Melatonin** – Dosage: 0.5 mg., thirty minutes before bed. A powerful antioxidant that may relieve symptoms of Seasonal Affective Disorder (SAD), a depressive condition resulting from lack of sufficient sunlight.

\* Most herbal extracts contain alcohol. Avoid use if alcohol sensitive or if there is a history of alcohol abuse. *Note:* Alcohol content can be reduced through evaporation by adding extract to very hot water (just below boiling point) and allowing to stand 5 to 7 minutes before drinking.

# Diabetes

Diabetes is a potentially serious condition and should never be cared for without the assistance of a licensed healthcare professional. The following information is intended to help you become aware of available treatment options.

Diabetes Mellitus is a condition characterized by a high blood sugar level, with fasting values measuring over 110 mg/dl. Symptoms include frequent thirst, frequent urination, and extreme hunger. Patients with blood sugar over 300 mg/dl. may have nausea, fatigue, confusion, and even coma.

There are two types of diabetes: Type 1, or insulin dependent diabetes (IDDM), also know as juvenile diabetes; and Type 2, non-insulin dependent diabetes (NIDDM). Type 1 diabetes usually afflicts those in childhood or adolescence. It is an autoimmune disease resulting in failure of the beta cells in the pancreas to secrete insulin. Therefore, regular insulin injections are required for blood sugar control. Type 2 diabetes is most prevalent in middle aged and older people, although, it is becoming more common among younger people due to the rising incidence of childhood obesity. Type 2 diabetes results from a resistance of cells to use insulin. Because of the potentially dangerous nature of this disease, it is recommended that all diabetics be under the care of a physician.

Conventional treatments for Type 1 patients include strict management of insulin injections, caloric consumption and regular monitoring of blood sugar levels. Weight control—along with a low fat, high-fiber diet—is recommended for all patients, but serves as initial management of patients with Type 2 diabetes. If diet and exercise fail to control blood sugar levels, oral hypoglycemic drugs and/or insulin injections may be prescribed. Through proper management, regular monitoring of blood sugar levels and weight reduction, it is possible for people with Type 2 diabetes to reduce or eliminate medication and obtain good blood sugar control. Diabetics have a high risk of blindness, foot ulceration, nerve and kidney damage; therefore yearly eye exams with an ophthalmologist, 6 month visits with a podiatrist, and careful medical follow-up is highly recommended.

| EZ Care Program | |
|---|---|
| Diet | **Avoid** all processed sugar and high-glycemic foods (e.g., grapes, dates, prunes, raisins, dried fruits, white flour products; and starchy vegetables like corn, peas, and white rice). Avoid a high-fat diet (e.g., red meat and high fat cheese) because diabetics are at high risk of heart attack. |
| | **Eat high fiber foods**, such as whole grains, legumes, broccoli, raw cabbage, and dark green, leafy vegetables. Fiber helps slow down glucose absorption, which may result in increased utilization and the possible normalization of blood sugar. |
| | **Eat fish**, such as mackerel, herring, trout, and salmon, because they are high in omega-3 fatty acids. |
| Minerals | **Chromium** (polynicotinate is preferred form) – Dosage: 200 to 500 mcg. two times daily with meals. <br> *Note:* Chromium is essential for blood-sugar regulation. |
| | **Vanadium** – Dosage: 1.4 mg. elemental vanadium derived from vanadyl sulfate with meals. This trace element plays a role in blood sugar and lipid metabolism. Aids in cellular insulin uptake. |

| EZ Care Program | |
|---|---|
| Vitamins | **Alpha-Lipoic Acid** – Dosage: 100 mg., 1 to 2 times daily with meals. This antioxidant helps transport glucose into cells, thereby helping maintain proper blood sugar metabolism. Can be used to prevent and treat diabetic neuropathy. |
| Herbs | **Blueberry Leaf tea** – Dosage: 6 oz. in the morning and 1 cup in the evening for several months. To prepare: Place 4 tsp. blueberry leaves in a glass or stainless steel cooking pot (avoid aluminum). Pour 2 cups boiling water over the herbs, cover, and let steep for 1/2 hour. Strain. *Beneficial properties*: A mild regulator of blood sugar; considered to be extremely safe. *Note:* Best results are achieved with steady, long-term use. |
| Miscellaneous | **Fiber Supplement** – Dosage: 1 to 3 tsp. Psyllium seed and husk fiber in 8 oz. pure water one or two times daily between meals. *Note:* Carefully read label; some brands require additional water. |
| | **Omega-3 Fatty Acids** (Max EPA) – Dosage: 1000 to 4000 mg. twice daily with meals. *Beneficial properties:* Contains eicosapentacnoic acid (EPA) and docosahexanoic acid (DHA) which inhibit inflammatory processes. Aids blood sugar control and may help prevent diabetic complications. |
| | **Regular exercise** – 20 to 30 minutes daily aerobic exercise. Can help maintain healthy blood sugar levels by burning off excess glucose. *Note:* May be particularly beneficial for Type 2 diabetics. |

# Additional Recommendations

The EZ Care Program consists of basic remedies that are commonly used for diabetes and have been found to work well in most cases. The remedies are most effective when combined, but can be used individually. The options stated below can supplement or replace EZ Care remedies and may be combined when suggested doses are followed.

## Diet

◆ **Avoid fasting.**

◆ **Drink** 6 to 8 glasses of pure water daily.

◆ **Eat generous amounts of raw garlic and onions**, which are considered to be blood and artery cleansers.

◆ **Eat smaller**, simpler meals throughout the day. Include protein at each meal to help balance sugar levels.
*Note:* If you have kidney disease, speak to a licensed healthcare professional before incorporating this diet.

◆ **Identify personal food sensitivities**. Avoid all common allergenic foods (e.g., dairy, eggs, wheat, corn, preservatives, sugar). Rotate moderately allergic foods on a four-day schedule (see Appendix C).

## Vitamins

♦ **B complex** – Dosage: 50 mg. daily of a natural, balanced B complex formula. *Note:* For highest assimilation, use a multi B complex which contains the vitamins in their coenzyme form and avoid mega-potency B complex products. B vitamins are crucial factors in carbohydrate metabolism and blood sugar balance.

♦ **C** (mineral ascorbates mixed with bioflavonoids) – Dosage: 1,000 mg., three to four times daily with meals. Essential for artery and blood vessel health.

♦ **E** (natural d-alpha tocopherol in a base of mixed tocopherols) – Dosage: 800 IU daily with meals. Protects from oxidation blood fats and pituitary and adrenal hormones involved in blood sugar regulation.

## Minerals

♦ **Magnesium** (elemental magnesium from amino acid chelate) – Dosage: 500 to 1,000 mg. daily in divided doses with meals and at bedtime. Activates enzymes important in carbohydrate metabolism.

♦ **Selenium** – Dosage: 200 mcg. daily from l-selenomethionine. Selenium and vitamin E are synergists; thus, they enhance each other's activity in the body.

♦ **Zinc** – (take only if over 14 years of age) Dosage: 25 to 50 mg. elemental zinc from amino acid chelate. Zinc is essential for normal storage and regulation of insulin.

## Herbs

♦ **Bilberry** (Vaccinium myrtillus) – Dosage: 50 mg., three times daily.
*Beneficial properties*: Powerful antioxidant that may protect the eyes and blood vessels from the damages of excessive sugar.

♦ **Fenugreek Seed** (Trigonella foenum-graecum) – Dosage: 2 capsules three times daily with meals.
*Beneficial properties*: May help balance blood sugar.
*Note:* Often used in conjunction with gymnema sylvestre.

♦ **Garlic** (Allium sativum) – Dosage: 1 to 2 capsules per meal of standardized allicin garlic or aged garlic extract. Fresh, raw garlic (a whole, living food) is preferable, but capsules should be considered if raw garlic is not taken consistently.
*Beneficial properties*: May improve circulation and reduce high blood pressure.
*Note:* Raw parsley taken with raw garlic helps prevent "garlic breath" and enhances garlic's blood-cleansing effects.

♦ **Gymnema Sylvestre** Dosage: 400 mg. daily.
*Beneficial properties*: An Indian herb that may stimulate the pancreas to produce more insulin as well as block sugar absorption.

## Homeopathy

See Appendix E for proper use and handling instruction prior to administering remedies described below.

♦ **Nat Sulph 6X** – Leading cell salt remedy for diabetes, perhaps because of its affinity for the liver. Depressed and tired of life; greenish or grayish coating on tongue; crave *or* have a strong aversion to foods such as yogurt; may have asthma in conjunction with diabetes. Dosage: Dissolve 5 pellets under the tongue, two to three times daily or as required.

## Miscellaneous

♦ **Coenzyme Q-10** – Dosage: 100 mg., two to three times daily with meals. Helps oxygenate heart cells and stimulates mitochondrial energy production.

♦ **Reduce** lifestyle **stress** and implement a relaxation program. Harmonizing practices (e.g., biofeedback, meditation, yoga, Tai Chi exercise) may prove beneficial.

# Diarrhea

Diarrhea is the passage of frequent or watery stools. It may occur from dietary intolerances, malabsorbtion, stress and anxiety, viral, fungal, bacterial, or parasitic infections. It can also occur as a side-effect to medications, such as antibiotics or chemotherapeutic agents. Diarrhea results when excess fluid remains in the intestines. Dehydration may occur secondary to excess loss of fluids, and electrolyte disturbances may result due to loss of essential minerals. If blood or mucus in the stools or fever accompany diarrhea, contact a healthcare professional immediately.

*Notes:* **(1)** Diarrhea can be life threatening if dehydration ensues, especially in infants, children, and the elderly. **(2)** Do not begin anti-diarrheal treatment in the first few hours of illness. Diarrhea is a mechanism that allows your body to rid itself of an infectious agent or some other unwanted entity. **(3)** *For children, always review any remedy with a pediatrician prior to use.*

Conventional treatments include adequate fluid intake with electrolyte-balanced formulas, and over-the-counter anti-diarrheal medications for adults.

| EZ Care Program | |
|---|---|
| Diet | **Drink** generous amounts of liquids, including water, herbal teas, broths, and diluted vegetable juices. Fluids help prevent dehydration, and also replace lost electrolytes and vitamins. <br> *Note:* Low-sugar fluid replacement drinks, such as Pedialyte, are very beneficial due to high amounts of electrolytes in them. |
| | **Food Intake** – If possible, avoid all foods except apples, natural applesauce, bananas, blueberries, and soft-cooked brown rice. Several times a day, serve unpeeled lightly steamed red apples. Option: with each serving, steam with 1 to 2 tbsp. blueberries. Some individuals do better with raw, unpeeled, red apples that have been pureed in a blender; however, blueberries are best served cooked. Soft-cooked brown rice is prepared by bringing 5 cups of water to a boil. Add 1 cup brown rice, lower the heat, and slowly simmer 2 to 3 hours. Serve separately from the apples and blueberries. |
| Miscellaneous | **Activated Charcoal** – Dosage: 1 tsp. Dissolved in 8 oz. water, or 2 capsules every three hours for up to five days. Then reduce dosage or as required. Absorbs diarrhea-producing toxins in the bowels. <br> *Note:* Long-term use of charcoal may impair nutrient absorption from the gut. |
| | **Colloidal (liquid) Bentonite Clay** – Dosage: 1 tsp. stirred in 8 oz. warm water two to three times daily. May help absorb excess fluids and infectious bacteria from the intestines. |
| | **L-Glutamine** – Dosage 500 mg., 2 to 3 times daily. Aids in support of intestinal mucosal lining. Useful for chronic diarrhea. |
| | **Probiotic Product** (friendly intestinal bacteria that aid digestion, nutrient assimilation, and toxin elimination) (L. acidophilus and bifidobacterium) – Use according to directions on label. Replaces friendly bacteria lost as result of diarrhea. |

## Additional Recommendations

The EZ Care Program consists of basic remedies that are commonly used for diarrhea and have been found to work well in most cases. The remedies are most effective when combined, but can be used individually. The options stated below can supplement or replace EZ Care remedies and may be combined when suggested doses are followed.

### Diet

- ♦ **Avoid** milk and milk products, raw vegetables, bran, sugary and spicy foods, caffeine and alcohol, most fruits (exceptions in EZ Care Program above), whole grain foods (except soft-cooked rice).

- ♦ **Consider Pedialyte** for children to replace lost electrolytes.

- ♦ **Eat** small, light meals as tolerated.

♦ **Identify personal food sensitivities** for chronic diarrhea. Avoid all common allergenic foods (e.g., dairy, eggs, wheat, corn, preservatives, sugar). Rotate moderately allergic foods on a four-day schedule (see Appendix C).

## Vitamins

♦ **Consider stopping intake of nutritional supplements**, especially vitamin C and magnesium, until diarrhea subsides. When diarrhea is present, supplements may be poorly absorbed and may worsen condition. After diarrhea subsides, reintroduce nutritional supplements gradually in accordance with bowel tolerance.

## Herbs

♦ **Goldenseal** (Hydrastis canadensis) – Dosage: 2-4 capsules or 40-50 drops liquid extract* three times daily for up to 14 days.
*Beneficial properties:* Traditionally used as an antibacterial and antibiotic. May be beneficial when diarrhea is accompanied by fever, which may indicate bacterial infection.
*Note:* Decrease dosage if diarrhea becomes worse.

♦ **Marshmallow Root** (Althea officinalis) – Dosage: 8 oz. warm tea prepared by decoction (see Appendix B) three to four times daily or as required. It is best to combine marshmallow root with raspberry leaf, white oak bark, witch hazel bark, or yarrow, because these astringent herbs add their drying effects to marshmallow root's demulcent, soothing effect.
*Beneficial properties:* Soothing to the lining of the bowel. Similar benefits to that of slippery elm. May be used in conjunction with, or in place of, slippery elm.

♦ **Raspberry Leaf** (Rubus idaeus) – Dosage: 8 oz. warm tea prepared by infusion (see Appendix B) three to four times daily or as required.
*Beneficial properties:* Raspberry leaves are astringent, soothing, and toning to the intestines.

♦ **Slippery Elm Bark** (Ulmus fulva) – Dosage: 8 oz. warm tea prepared by decoction (see Appendix B) three to four times daily or as required.
*Beneficial properties*: Soothing and healing to inflamed mucosal surfaces. Also absorbs gas and neutralizes acidity. Best to combine with raspberry leaf, white oak bark, witch hazel bark, or yarrow, because these astringent herbs add their drying effects to slippery elm's demulcent, soothing effect.

♦ **White Oak Bark** (Quercus alba) – Dosage: 6 oz. warm tea prepared by decoction (see Appendix B) every two to three hours daily or as required. Consider administering rectally (retain as long as possible) in small amounts (e.g., 8 oz. every 4 hours). If there is blood in the stools, add a pinch of cayenne pepper to each serving
*Beneficial properties*: Powerful astringent and cleanser for the mucous membranes of the g.i. tract. Especially relevant for bloody diarrhea or diarrhea due to parasite infestation.

♦ **Witch Hazel Bark** (Hamamelis virginiana) – Dosage: 6 oz. warm tea prepared by decoction (see Appendix B) every two to three hours daily or as required.

♦ **Yarrow** (Achillea millefolium) – 6 oz. warm tea prepared by infusion (see Appendix B) every two hours. Consider administering rectally (retain as long as possible) in small amounts (e.g., 8 oz. every four hours).
*Beneficial properties*: Acts as an astringent-tonic for the mucous membrane of the colon. Especially relevant for bloody diarrhea. Excellent in cases of chronic diarrhea and when diarrhea is accompanied by hemorrhoidal swelling and bleeding.

## Homeopathy

See Appendix E for proper use and handling instruction prior to administering remedies described below.

In addition to the appropriate remedy below, 5 pellets may be crushed and added to rectal injections of yarrow or white oak bark as described above.

♦ **Aconite 12C** – Diarrhea brought on by exposure to cold or as result of fright. Dosage: Dissolve 5 pellets under the tongue, two to four times daily or as required. For an infant, crush the pellets and dissolve in 4 oz. water. Administer 1 tsp. every two to four hours or as required.

♦ **Arsenicum 6C** – Diarrhea from food poisoning or stomach flu; frequent attacks of foul-smelling diarrhea; pain when passing stools, and discomfort afterward; may be accompanied by vomiting, burning sensation in stomach and of anus after passing stools; better with warmth and warm drinks; thirsty for small sips of water. Dosage: Take 5 pellets sublingually three to five times daily

♦ **Calcarea Carb 6C** – Sour, pale stools that lack pigment; crave eggs, sweets, ice cream, and salt; aversion and allergy to milk; diarrhea in teething infant. Dosage: Dissolve 5 pellets under the tongue, two to four times daily or as required. For an infant, crush the pellets and dissolve in 4 oz. water. Administer 1 tsp. every two to four hours or as required.

♦ **Chamomilla 6C** – Stool hot, green, watery, and foul-smelling, and resembles chopped spinach and eggs; distended abdomen very sensitive to touch; passing gas does not ease the pain; diarrhea in teething infant. Dosage: Dissolve 5 pellets under the tongue, two to four times daily or as required. For an infant, crush the pellets and dissolve in 4 oz. water. Administer 1 tsp. every two to four hours or as required.

♦ **Nux Vomica 12C** – Diarrhea from dietary, alcohol and drug indiscretion; diarrhea alternating with constipation; worse in the morning or after a large meal. Dosage: Dissolve 5 pellets under the tongue, two to four times daily or as required. For an infant, crush the pellets and dissolve in 4 oz. water. Administer 1 tsp. every two to four hours or as required.

♦ **Pulsatilla 6C** – Diarrhea from eating too much fruit, rich or greasy foods, from cold foods or drinks, or after exposure to cold; worse at night; watery, greenish diarrhea in infant; diarrhea with changeable nature of the stools. Dosage: Dissolve 5 pellets under the tongue, two to four times daily or as required. For an infant, crush the pellets and dissolve in 4 oz. water. Administer 1 tsp. every two to four hours or as required.

## Miscellaneous

♦ **Carob powder and cinnamon** – Dosage: Stir 1 tsp. carob powder into 8 oz. warm water. Add a pinch of cinnamon. Serve two to three times daily between meals.

♦ **Cold Sitz Bath** (see Appendix D) – Water should be as cold as can be comfortably tolerated and come up to just below navel. Keep feet out of water. Continue sitz bath for up to 10 minutes while continuously massaging the body with bare hands. Follow with vigorous towel-rubbing of the entire body. Perform one to two times daily or as required.

\* Most herbal extracts contain alcohol. Avoid use if alcohol sensitive or if there is a history of alcohol abuse. *Note:* Alcohol content can be reduced through evaporation by adding extract to very hot water (just below boiling point) and allowing to stand 5 to 7 minutes before drinking.

# Diverticulitis

Diverticula are spherical, protruding outpouches from the intestinal wall throughout the bowel. They occur in 50% of the western population over age 70. Diverticulitis is the infection or inflammation of one or several diverticula, potentially causing obstruction, perforation, or bleeding. Symptoms may include abdominal cramping (often in the lower left side), fever, nausea, and blood in the stools. Causes may include heredity, fiber deficiency, nutritional deficiency, stress, chronic constipation, and food sensitivities.

Conventional treatments include a high fiber diet, adequate fluid intake, and exercise. Additionally, antibiotics, bed rest, antispasmodic drugs, and painkillers can be prescribed. Surgery may be necessary in severe cases to remove the diseased section of colon, or to drain abcesses.

| EZ Care Program ||
|---|---|
| Diet | **Avoid** all caffeine, alcohol, refined sugars, dairy, red meat, spices, fried, and processed foods. |
| | **Chew** all foods to mush before swallowing. |
| | **Fiber Supplement** – Dosage: 1 to 3 tsp. psyllium seed and husk fiber in 8 oz. pure water, followed by another 8 oz. water, one to two times daily between meals. *Note:* Carefully read label; some brands require additional water. |
| | **Drink** 8 to 10 glasses of pure water daily. |

| EZ Care Program | |
|---|---|
| | **Flaxseed Tea** – To prepare: Add 2 tbsp. flaxseed to 2 cups cold water and bring to a boil. Simmer 15 minutes. Drink 1 cup of this gel two times daily on an empty stomach. After acute phase passes, add 1 tsp. unfiltered apple cider vinegar to each serving. Soothes the lining of the bowel and promotes bowel movements. Especially valuable if diverticulitis is accompanied by constipation. |
| | **Identify personal food sensitivities**. Avoid all common allergenic foods (e.g., dairy, eggs, wheat, corn, sugar, preservatives). Rotate moderately allergic foods on a four-day schedule (see Appendix C.) |
| | **Puree tough fruit skins** (e.g., apple peel) **and avoid fruits or vegetables with small seeds**, such as strawberries, tomatoes, cucumbers, watermelon, and figs. **Also avoid whole seeds,** such as sesame seed. Instead, use sesame seed or sunflower seed butter. |
| Herbs | **Aloe Vera Juice** (cold processed from organically grown, whole leaf aloe vera). Dosage: 2 to 3 tbsp. in 4 oz. warm water two to three times daily between meals. *Beneficial properties*: May help prevent constipation and colon problems. Reduce dose if diarrhea occurs. |
| Miscellaneous | **L-Glutamine** –1 to 2 grams 2 times daily between meals. An amino acid which reduces inflammation and supports regrowth of the intestinal mucosa. |
| | **Lactobacillus probiotic product** (friendly intestinal bacteria which aid digestion, nutrient assimilation and toxin elimination): L. acidophilus with bifidobacteria and fructo-oligosaccaharides (powder or capsules) – Use according to directions on label. |
| | **Omega-3 Fatty Acids** (Max EPA) – Dosage: 1000 to 4000 mg. twice daily with meals. *Beneficial properties:* Contains eicosapentaenoic acid (EPA) and docosahexanoic acid (DHA) which inhibit inflammatory processes. |

## Additional Recommendations

The EZ Care Program consists of basic remedies that are commonly used for diverticulitis and have been found to work well in most cases. The remedies are most effective when combined, but can be used individually. The options stated below can supplement or replace EZ Care remedies and may be combined when suggested doses are followed.

### Diet

♦   **A soft diet** is suggested during acute phase. Coarse roughage and raw vegetable fibers may aggravate diverticulitis. Try foods like soft-cooked steamed vegetables, stewed fruits, avocados, papayas, mashed ripe bananas, steamed carrots, baked yams, sweet potatoes, and tofu; carefully watch for any adverse reaction. Even after acute phase passes, limit intake of flesh foods, because they contain no fiber and may worsen constipation and bowel stasis.

♦   **Eat smaller meals** during acute phase, making sure to eat slowly and chew food well. Eating in a calm atmosphere also may be beneficial.

♦ A three-day **vegetable juice fast** is often helpful in reducing colon inflammation by avoiding mechanical irritation and bowel detoxification. It is preferable to work with a physician when fasting.

♦ **Raw, low salt sauerkraut** – Dosage: 1 to 2 tbsp. with meals two to three times daily. Use only raw sauerkraut found in refrigerated food section of health food stores. Only raw sauerkraut and its juice, which are rich in lactobacillus species, have therapeutic value. Sauerkraut should contain only raw cabbage and sea salt; no spices, vinegar, or preservatives. Avoid cooked or heavily salted sauerkraut. Be sure to keep raw sauerkraut refrigerated and use up before 7 to 10 days.

## Vitamins

♦ **A** (natural, from fish liver oil) – Dosage: 10,000 to 25,000 IU daily with meals. Required for maintenance and function of the mucosal lining of the gastrointestinal (GI) tract.
*Note:* Consult a physician before using higher doses of vitamin A. Avoid use if pregnant. Discontinue use if nausea, dry skin, sore lips, blurred vision, or other signs of vitamin A excess are experienced.

♦ **B complex** – Dosage: 50 mg. balanced B complex capsule. B complex vitamins are required for maintaining normal tone in the GI tract. The body's need for these vitamins increases during times of physiological stress.
*Note:* For highest assimilation, use a multi B complex which contains the vitamins in their coenzyme form and avoid mega-potency B complex products.

♦ **C** (mixed mineral ascorbates) – Dosage: 1,000 mg., three to four times daily with meals and at bedtime. Vitamin C stimulates immune system. Through antioxidant function, may help prevent infection and control inflammation.

♦ **E** (natural d-alpha tocopherol in a base of mixed tocopherols) – Dosage: 800 to 1200 IU daily with meals. Vitamin E may aid in healing inflamed, irritated, or ulcerated tissue.

♦ **Folic Acid** – Dosage: 800 mcg. two times daily with meals. Crucial for healthy intestinal mucosa. Normally manufactured by beneficial species of bowel bacteria that are frequently destroyed by infectious species.

## Minerals

♦ **Zinc** (take only if over 14 years of age) – Dosage: 50 mg. elemental zinc from amino acid chelate with meals. Supports immune function and wound healing; helps utilize and maintain body levels of vitamin A.

## Herbs

♦ **Chamomile Flowers** (Matricaria recutita) – Dosage: 2 to 3 capsules or 4 -6 oz. tea prepared by infusion (see Appendix B) three times daily.
*Beneficial properties*: Antispasmodic and soothing to the nerves.
*Note:* At bedtime, 1/2 tsp. raw unrefined honey can be added to warm tea to enhance sleeping.

♦ **Marshmallow Root** (Althea officinalis) – Dosage: 2 capsules three times daily with meals, or 6 oz. tea prepared by decoction (see Appendix B) two to three times daily between meals. If desired, serve aloe vera juice stirred into the marshmallow root tea servings.
*Beneficial properties:* Soothes lining of bowel. Similar benefits as slippery elm. May be used in conjunction with, or in place of, slippery elm.

♦ **Ginger Root** (Zingiber officinalis) – Dosage: 2 capsules three times daily, or 6-8 oz. dried ginger root tea prepared by decoction (see Appendix B) three times daily (Jamaican ginger root preferred). For enhanced effect, add a pinch of cayenne to each serving.
*Beneficial properties:* Especially beneficial if there is a great deal of flatulence.

♦ **Wild Yam Root** (Dioscorea villosa) – Dosage: 6 oz. tea prepared by decoction (see Appendix B), or 40-50 drops liquid extract* in 6 oz. warm water, or in 6 oz. of another herb tea listed above.
*Beneficial properties:* May soothe intestinal irritation and spasm through antispasmodic and anti-inflammatory action.

## Homeopathy

See Appendix E for proper use and handling instruction prior to administering remedies described below.

♦ **Capsicum 6C** – Diverticulitis with ineffective and painful straining at stools, and violent burning pain. Dosage: Dissolve 5 pellets under the tongue, two to three times daily or as required.

♦ **Phosphorus 6C** – Diverticulitis with stabbing, shooting pains, and burning sensation in anus. Dosage: Dissolve 5 pellets under the tongue, two to three times daily or as required.

## Miscellaneous

♦ **Black Currant Seed or Evening Primrose Oil** – Dosage: 1,000 to 2,000 mg., three times daily with meals. Contains GLA, which is a fatty acid that may promote healing and repair.

♦ **Cold Sitz Bath** – Dosage: 4 to 7 times weekly upon arising (see Appendix D). Be sure to rub abdomen vigorously with cold water. Always rub in a clockwise direction (i.e., right to left). May help reduce bowel inflammation and stimulate local healing processes.

♦ **Exercise** at least 30 minutes daily.

♦ **Gamma-oryzanol** – Dosage: 100 mg., three times daily with meals. A compound found in rice bran oil that may exert a healing effect on the colon.

♦ **Proteolytic Enzyme Formula** (Protein digesting enzymes that include pancreatic protease, bromelain, papain.). Use according to directions on label. As a digestive aid, take with meals. As an anti-inflammatory, take between meals.
*Note:* Avoid if there are stomach or duodenal ulcers; proteolytic enzymes may aggravate ulcers and induce bleeding.

♦ **Reduce** lifestyle **stress** and implement a relaxation program. Harmonizing practices (e.g., biofeedback, meditation, yoga, Tai Chi exercise) may prove beneficial.

# Ear Infections

Acute ear infections (otitis media) result from the growth of bacteria in the fluid of the middle ear. Children may present with crying, fever, tugging on the ear, poor feeding, or irritability. The buildup of fluid puts pressure on the eardrum, causing pain. If the buildup of fluid is great, the eardrum may rupture, resulting in a copius discharge from the ear. Ear infections are the number one reason for pediatric visits. External ear infections (otitis exterma) do not involve the middle ear, but affect the external skin and cartilage. The child may present with low-grade fever, redness, and pain. This condition is commonly referred to as swimmer's ear.

Conventional treatment of otitis media includes antibiotics, acetaminophen or ibuprofen for pain and fever, and nasal decongestants. Recurrent otitis media is treated with prophylactic antibiotics, or the surgical insertion of ventilation tubes into the child's ears. Antibacterial, anti-inflammatory, or antifungal medications are used in the management of otitis externa.

*Otitis media note:* Chronic ear infections may be caused by an underlying problem such as a food allergy. Consultation with a physician skilled in food allergy detection may be necessary to discover the cause of the problem. Chronic ear infections left untreated can cause permanent hearing damage.

| EZ Care Program | |
|---|---|
| Diet | **Identify personal food sensitivities.** Avoid all common allergenic foods (e.g., dairy, eggs, wheat, corn, sugar, preservatives). Rotate moderately allergic foods on a four-day schedule (see Appendix C). *Note:* In infants and children, milk and milk products are the most common allergenic foods and can be replaced by soy and rice products. Breast-feeding mothers should be careful to avoid any foods to which the child may be sensitive. |
| Vitamins | **C** (mineral ascorbates mixed with bioflavonoids) – Dosage: 250 mg., three times daily with meals. Children 5 years and older may tolerate 500 mg., three times daily with meals. If the child cannot swallow capsule or use chewables, empty capsule into water, stir well, and administer before the vitamin C precipitates out of solution. |

| EZ Care Program | |
|---|---|
| Herbs | **Garlic or Mullein** (Verbascum thaspus) **Oil** ear drops – Dosage: 2 drops warm (not hot) garlic or mullein oil in the ear three to four times daily for acute ear infection. Indicated when there is pain with sensation of ear feeling blocked-up. Mullein is particularly useful if ear canal is dry and scaly. *Beneficial properties:* May be used to help soothe pain and resolve infection. ***Note:*** *Do not use if the eardrum is perforated, or drainage is present.* |
| Miscellaneous | **Warm Application** – Add hot water to a hot water bottle. Wrap in a towel and place on a pillow. Have the child lay the painful ear upon the warm application. *Note*: It is best to treat both ears, even if only one is presenting with symptoms. |

# Additional Recommendations

The EZ Care Program consists of basic remedies that are commonly used for ear infections and have been found to work well in most cases. The remedies are most effective when combined, but can be used individually. The options stated below can supplement or replace EZ Care remedies and may be combined when suggested doses are followed.

## Diet

♦ **Avoid starchy foods in all babies under 14 months of age**. Infants have not yet begun producing starch-digesting enzymes. Starchy foods include grains and grain products, such as bread and pasta, potatoes, sweet potatoes, and yams.

♦ **Breast-feeding infants** for 6-12 months may help reduce occurrence of ear infections.

♦ **Feed** infant in a slightly **upright position** to help the fluid drain from the ear.

## Vitamins

♦ **A** – Dosage: 2,500 IU (for babies) to 10,000 IU (for older children) daily, preferably as Emulsified vitamin A drops dissolved in water. The need for vitamin A increases during fever and infection.
*Note: Consult a physician before using vitamin A with infants and babies.*

## Minerals

♦ **Zinc** –Dosage based on child's age, multiplied by 2.5 mg. elemental zinc from amino acid chelate daily. Supports immune function.
*Note:* Do not exceed 15 mg. daily.

## Herbs

♦ **Echinacea Root** (Echinacea purpurea) – Dosage: 10 to 25 drops (in accordance with age of child) of extract* in 2-4 oz. pure warm water three times daily. For baby, dissolve extract in two oz. water and administer 1 tbsp. every two hours. May be taken mixed with goldenseal extract.

*Beneficial Properties:* Traditionally used to fight infections and stimulate immune system.

> *Note:* Be certain to evaporate off the alcohol from the extract (see Appendix B).

♦ **Goldenseal Root** (Hydrastis canadensis) – Dosage: 5 to 10 drops of extract* (in accord with age of child) in 2-4 oz. pure warm water three times daily. For baby, dissolve extract in 2 oz. water and administer 1 tbsp. every two hours. May be taken mixed with echinacea extract.

*Beneficial Properties:* Traditionally used to fight infections and stimulate immune system.

> *Note:* Be certain to evaporate off the alcohol from the extract (see Appendix B).

## Homeopathy

See Appendix E for proper use and handling instruction prior to administering remedies described below.

*Note:* When treating young babies, crush the pellets and dissolve in 2 oz. pure water. Administer 1 tsp. every two hours or as required. Stir the medicated water before each successive dose. Always review remedies with the child's pediatrician prior to administering.

♦ **Aconitum 12C** – External ear hot and painful; great thirst; throbbing pain after exposure to cold; hypersensitivity to noise and music. Dosage: Dissolve 5 pellets under the tongue, two to four times daily at onset of earache.

♦ **Belladonna 12C** – Ear or ear canal red and face flushed; symptoms come on suddenly, pain throbbing, worse at night and with motion; may be a great deal of agitation, even delirium; usually right ear affected more than the left. Dosage: Dissolve 5 pellets under the tongue, two to three times daily or as required.

♦ **Chamomila 6X or 6C** – Great pain, impatience, irritability, sensitivity to touch, and child desires to be rocked or carried; frequently, the best remedy for ear infection during teething. Dosage: Dissolve 5 pellets under the tongue, two to three times daily or as required.

♦ **Hepar Sulph 6C** – Hypersensitivity; ears sensitive to touch; cold and ear symptoms relieved by warmth; irritability with temper tantrums; sharp, splinter-like pain in ears, with offensive-smelling discharge; may be accompanied by dry, croupy cough. Dosage: Dissolve 5 pellets under the tongue, two to three times daily or as required.

♦ **Pulsatilla 12C** – Earache begins after child wet or cold; pain worse at night and from warm bed, and ameliorated by cold applications; usually a little pain during day. Dosage: Dissolve 5 pellets under the tongue, two to three times daily or as required.

## Miscellaneous

♦ **Avoid** second-hand smoke, hair sprays, and gels; they are associated with increased risk of ear infections.

♦ **Craniosacral manipulation** from an osteopathic physician or other specialist may be extremely helpful in ending recurrent ear infections.

♦ **Warm Salt Compress** – Fashion a small bag from cotton cloth and fill it with coarse salt. Place the bag in a covered baking dish and heat in an oven at a low temperature—until thoroughly warm *but not hot*. Place against the ear. Consider heating 2 cotton bags of salt and treating both ears simultaneously.

\* *Note:* Most herbal extracts contain alcohol. Avoid usage if alcohol sensitive or if there is a history of alcohol abuse. Alcohol content can be reduced through evaporation by adding extract to very hot water (just below boiling point) and allow to stand 5 to 7 minutes before drinking.

# Eczema/Atopic Dermatitis

Eczema is a general term used to describe a superficial inflammation of the skin. Raised, red, swollen lesions that ooze and crust characterizes acute eczema. Later the skin may become scaly and thickened. This condition causes the skin to become itchy and red and may spread or become infected when scratched. Care should be taken to avoid scratching.

Conventional treatments include over-the-counter and prescription corticosteroid creams as well as oral anti-histamines. Oral corticosteroids may be prescribed for particularly stubborn cases.

| EZ Care Program | |
|---|---|
| Diet | **Identify personal food sensitivities**. Avoid all common allergenic foods (e.g., dairy, wheat, and citrus fruit). Rotate moderately allergic foods on a four-day schedule (see Appendix C). |
| Herbs | **Calendula Cream** – Apply externally 4 to 6 times daily to affected area. *Beneficial Properties*: May promote healing of tissue and soothe affected area. |
| | **Black Currant Oil** (Ribies nigrum) – Dosage: 500 to 1000 mg., two times daily. *Beneficial properties:* An excellent source of GLA, a fatty acid that supports the production of anti-inflammatory prostaglandin E1. |
| Aromatherapy | **Blue Chamomile** (Matricaria chamomilla) **essential oil** – Prepare a 2% solution as follows: 2 drops chamomile oil + 98 drops unrefined jojoba oil to a small amber glass dropper bottle. Shake well. Apply topically three to four times daily or as required. *Beneficial Properties*: Soothing, calming, anti-inflammatory. |
| Miscellaneous | **Fresh air** and **sunlight** may prove helpful for this condition. |
| | **Mud Mask Therapies**, particularly from the Dead Sea, may be very beneficial for this condition. Use according to directions on label. |

| EZ Care Program | |
|---|---|
| | **Limited hand washing** is a useful strategy to treat eczema of the hands and fingers. |
| | **Reduce lifestyle stress** and implement a relaxation program. Harmonizing practices (e.g., biofeedback, meditation, yoga, Tai Chi exercise) may prove beneficial because stress often plays a major role in skin problems. |

## Additional Recommendations

The EZ Care Program consists of basic remedies that are commonly used for eczema and have been found to work well in most cases. The remedies are most effective when combined, but can be used individually. The options stated below can supplement or replace EZ Care remedies and may be combined when suggested doses are followed.

### Diet

♦ **Avoid** all processed sugar, dairy, and white flour.

♦ **Flaxseed Oil** – Dosage: 1 to 2 tbsp. daily in divided doses with meals. Contains anti-inflammatory omega-3 fatty acids that are beneficial for good skin health.
*Note:* Use for a minimum of 3 months before determining effectiveness.

### Vitamins

♦ **A** (natural, from fish liver oil) – Dosage: 10,000 to 25,000 IU daily with meals. Crucial for maintaining skin health. Supplementation may be beneficial in treating skin conditions. Also may be used topically on rashes.
*Note:* Consult a physician before using higher doses of vitamin A. Avoid use if pregnant. Discontinue use if nausea, dry skin, sore lips, blurred vision, or other signs of vitamin A excess are experienced.

♦ **B complex** – Dosage: 50 mg. yeast-free balanced B complex capsule. Eczema is often a stress-related condition. The body's need for B vitamins increases during times of stress.
*Note:* For highest assimilation, use a multi B complex which contains the vitamins in their coenzyme form and avoid mega-potency B complex products.

♦ **Biotin** – Dosage: 1000 mg. twice daily. Biotin is a member of the B vitamin family essential for healthy nail and skin growth.

♦ **C** (mineral ascorbates mixed with bioflavonoids) – Dosage: 1,000 mg., three to four times daily with meals. A natural anti-inflammatory nutrient crucial for maintaining collagen, which is a protein necessary for forming connective tissue in skin.

♦ **E** (natural d-alpha tocopherol in a base of mixed tocopherols) – Dosage: 800 IU daily with meals. Exerts an antioxidant action that protects vitamin A, C, and the B vitamins, and may help heal and prevent premature aging of the skin. Also may be used topically (squeeze contents of a vitamin E capsule onto affected area) to counteract itching and scaling.

### Minerals

♦ **Selenium** – Dosage: 200 mcg. l-selenomethionine once daily with a meal. An antioxidant that may be useful in treating a variety of inflammatory disorders.
*Note:* Selenium and vitamin E are synergists; thus, they enhance each other's activity in the body.

♦ **Zinc** (take only if over 14 years of age) – Dosage: 25 to 50 mg. daily elemental zinc from amino acid chelate with meals. Helps utilize and maintain the body's level of vitamin A and supports healing of skin lesions.

### Herbs

♦ **Aloe Vera Gel** – Apply externally, 4 to 6 times daily.
*Beneficial Properties*: May soothe skin and promote healing of tissue.

♦ **Burdock Root** (Arctium lappa) – Dosage: 2 capsules with 8 oz. pure water or 8 oz. tea prepared by decoction (see Appendix B) three times daily between meals. Consider taking capsules in conjunction with Red Clover Tea or drinking a combination of 1 part **Burdock Root Tea** + 1 part **Chickweed Tea** + 1part **Red Clover Tea.** This combination tea also can be used as a topical wash. It may be more convenient to combine 1 part each of the 3 herbs and prepare together as a tea, by infusion.
*Beneficial properties:* May help in bowel detoxification. May act as blood and skin purifier.

♦ **Chickweed** (Stellaria media) – Dosage: 8 oz. of tea prepared by decoction (see Appendix B) three to four times daily between meals or as required. Also bathe the affected areas with the tea several times daily. Soothing and healing to inflamed skin. Another option: drinking a combination of 1 part **Burdock Root Tea** + 1 part **Chickweed Tea** + 1part **Red Clover Tea.** This combination tea also can be used as a topical wash. It may be more convenient to combine 1 part each of the 3 herbs and prepare together as a tea by infusion.

♦ **Licorice Root** (Glycyrrhiza uralensis or glabra) – Dosage: 2 capsules or 40 drops liquid extract 2-3 times daily with meals.
*Beneficial properties:* May exert a beneficial anti-inflammatory action.
*Note:* Avoid use if you have kidney or heart disease. If you have high blood pressure, consult a physician before using this herb because it may increase blood pressure via increased water retention. Chinese (uralensis) and deglycyrrhizinated licorice root are less problematic in this regard than the western variety (glabra).

♦ **Red Clover** (Trifolium pratense) – Dosage: 8 oz. of tea prepared by infusion (see Appendix B) three times daily between meals. Traditionally used as a blood-purifier in treating skin diseases. Consider taking red clover tea with burdock root capsules. Another option: drinking a combination of 1 part **Burdock Root Tea** + 1 part **Chickweed Tea** + 1part **Red Clover Tea.** This combination tea also can be used as a topical wash. It may be more convenient to combine 1 part each of the 3 herbs and prepare together as a tea by infusion.

♦ **Burdock Root** + **Yellow Dock** (Rumex crispus) + **Yarrow** (Achillea millefolium) + **Marshmallow Root** (Althea officinalis) **tea** – Combine equal parts of these herbs, then prepare a tea (see Appendix B) using 2 tsp. of herbs : 8 oz. pure water. Steep 30 minutes. Drink 4 oz. four to five times daily between meals. Also, bathe the affected areas with this tea several times daily.

### Aromatherapy

Select one of the essential oils listed below or use two in combination. Prepare a 2% dilution as follows:
2 drops essential oil for every 98 drops sweet almond or unrefined jojoba oil to an amber glass dropper bottle. Stopper, shake well, and store in a cool dark place. Rub into affected area several times daily or as required.

**Blue Chamomile**, **Lavender** (Lavendula vera), **Rose** (Rosa damascena)

### Homeopathy

See Appendix E for proper use and handling instruction prior to administering remedies described below.

♦ **Arsenicum 6C** – Eczema with burning and restlessness; with itching, burning, swelling and dry, rough, scaly skin; worse when cold and scratched; better from heat; eczema between fingers and on tips of fingers. Dosage: Dissolve 5 pellets under the tongue, two to three times daily before meals.

♦ **Graphites 6C** – Weeping eczema with thick, gluey, honey-like fluid discharge that comes out when eruption is scratched; eruptions on face, lips, hands, and behind ears. Dosage: Dissolve 5 pellets under the tongue, two to three times daily before meals.

♦ **Mezereum 6C** – Intolerable itching that is worse in bed and from touching; head covered with thick, leather-like crusts, under which, thick white pus collects; eczema of hairy parts of skin. Dosage: Dissolve 5 pellets under the tongue, two to three times daily before meals.

♦ **Petroleum 6C** – Eczema with bloody cracks in skin, but little or no discharge; eczema which disappears in summer but recurs in cold weather or winter; eruption may exude a thin watery discharge. Dosage: Dissolve 5 pellets under the tongue, two to three times daily before meals.

♦ **Sulphur 6C** – Eczema with intense burning and itching; skin rough, coarse, dry, and scaly; worse from warmth of bed, washing, or scratching. Dosage: Dissolve 5 pellets under the tongue, two to three times daily before meals.

### Miscellaneous

♦ **Lactobacillus Probiotic Product** (friendly intestinal bacteria that aids digestion, nutrient assimilation, and toxin elimination) (L. acidophilus with bifidobacterium) – Use according to directions on label. May be beneficial if antibiotics have been used, or if yeast infection is a contributing factor

♦ **Oatmeal Baths** – May relieve acute symptoms, such as itching. Prepare using one of the following methods; (1) Simmer 1 cup rolled oats in 2 qt. water for 1 hour. Strain off oats and pour liquid into a tub of warm water. (2) Grind 1 heaping cup rolled oats in a blender *to a fine powder* and add to tub water. Soak for approximately 20 minutes. Do not rinse after the bath; pat dry to allow demulcent substances from the oatmeal to remain on the skin. Repeat daily.

♦ **Omega-3 Fatty Acids** (Max EPA) – Dosage: 1000 to 4000 mg. twice daily with meals. *Beneficial properties:* Contains eicosapentaenoic acid (EPA) and docosahexanoic acid (DHA) which inhibit inflammatory processes and provide skin moisturization.

♦ **Reduced Glutathione** – Dosage: 100 mg., two times daily between meals for two months. A powerful antioxidant produced in the liver and used by the body to cleanse itself. May support skin health.

\* Most herbal extracts contain alcohol. Avoid use if alcohol sensitive or if there is a history of alcohol abuse. *Note:* Alcohol content can be reduced through evaporation by adding extract to very hot water (just below boiling point) and allowing to stand 5 to 7 minutes before drinking.

# Edema

Edema is the retention of excess fluid in the body. Symptoms usually include unexplained weight gain, swelling of feet and ankles, swelling around the eyes, swelling of the hands, and increased abdominal girth. Someone with edema may feel tightness in his or her shoes, rings, and waist from the fluid retention. In severe cases, fluid can accumulate in the lung, causing shortness of breath.

*Note:* Any number of very serious conditions could cause edema, and all treatments described below should be discussed with a physician prior to administration.

After a complete physical examination and workup, conventional therapy includes elevation of the effected extremity, wearing elastic stockings, prescription diuretics, weight monitoring, and dietary changes (low sodium, controlled fluid intake, and adequate electrolyte replacement).

| EZ Care Program | |
|---|---|
| Diet | **Avoid** caffeine, alcohol, and salt. *Note:* If salt is used at all, limit intake to small amounts and use only a brand of natural sea salt that contains an abundance of trace minerals. |

## EZ Care Program

| | |
|---|---|
| | Eat a diet consisting of large quantities of **fresh fruits and vegetables** and comparatively smaller quantities of whole grains, legumes, seeds, nuts, fish, and skinless chicken and turkey. Special emphasis should be on high fiber foods like raw cabbage, dark green, leafy vegetables, apples, whole grains, and legumes. Other beneficial foods include asparagus, beet, celery, fresh coconut, cucumber, grapes, green beans, leafy greens, okra, papaya, parsley, pineapple, potatoes, and sprouts. |
| | **Eat generous amounts of raw garlic and onions**, which are rich sources of silica, a trace mineral that is a natural diuretic. |
| | **Eat potassium-rich foods** such as green vegetables, millet, oats, watermelon, broccoli, bananas, most fruits, dandelion greens, pumpkin, onions, and squash. |
| | **Include flaxseed oil** – Dosage: 1 to 2 tbsp. daily. Contains anti-inflammatory omega-3 fatty acids. |
| | **Limit intake of animal proteins** such as eggs, meat, fish, and poultry to no more than once daily. Concentrate more on vegetable protein foods, especially almonds, adzuki beans, kidney beans, sesame seeds, and avocados. |
| Vitamins | **B6** (pyridoxal 5-phosphate) – Dosage: 50 mg., one to three times daily with meals or as required. In this form, B6 helps maintain the balance of sodium and potassium that regulate body fluids and serves as a natural diuretic. |
| Minerals | **Magnesium** (elemental magnesium from magnesium citrate or aspartate) – Dosage: 250 mg., four times daily. If loose stools occur, reduce dosage to three times daily. Helps promote absorption and metabolism of potassium and helps the body utilize vitamin C and B-complex vitamins. Particularly important in heart failure. Note: Speak to a healthcare practitioner prior to magnesium supplementation if you have kidney disease. |
| | **Potassium** – Dosage: 300 to 600 mg. daily with meals in addition to the potassium-rich diet mentioned above; a crucial element in the body's regulation of fluids. *Note:* Speak to a healthcare practitioner prior to potassium supplementation if you have kidney disease. |
| Herbs | **Dandelion Leaf** (Taraxacum officinalis) – Dosage: 8 oz. tea prepared by infusion (see Appendix B) two to three times daily between meals. *Beneficial properties:* Traditionally used as a diuretic. May help lower blood pressure and reduce fluid retention. *Note:* The leaf is preferred to the root because it acts as a much stronger diuretic. |
| Miscellaneous | **L-Taurine** Dosage 500 mg. three times daily away from meals. Taurine is an antioxidant amino acid that acts as a natural diuretic. |

## Additional Recommendations

The EZ Care Program consists of basic remedies that are commonly used for edema and have been found to work well in most cases. The remedies are most effective when combined, but can be used individually. The options stated below can supplement or replace EZ Care remedies and may be combined when suggested doses are followed.

## Diet

♦ **Drink allowable amounts of pure, room-temperature water** daily to help flush toxins from the body. Fluid intake levels should follow guidelines set by a healthcare practitioner. Weight measurements should be taken daily in patients with heart failure. A change in weight of over 2 pounds in one day or 10 pounds in one week should alert one to call their physician.

♦ **Fiber Supplement** – Dosage: 1 to 3 tsp. psyllium husk fiber in 8 oz. pure water one to two times daily between meals. Helps facilitate regular bowel movements. Constipation is an important factor in many cases of edema.
*Note:* Carefully read label; some brands require additional water.

♦ **Identify personal food sensitivities**. Avoid all common allergenic foods (e.g., dairy, eggs, wheat, corn, sugar, preservatives). Rotate moderately allergic foods on a four-day schedule (see Appendix C). Allergic reactions to food often entail fluid retention.

## Vitamins

♦ **B complex** – Dosage: 50 mg.
*Note:* For highest assimilation, use a multi B complex which contains some of the vitamins in their coenzyme form and avoid mega-potency B complex products. Always use a complete B complex formula in addition to vitamin B6, because high doses of one of the B vitamins may lead to imbalance in the body's pool of the other B vitamins.

♦ **C** (mixed mineral ascorbates) – Dosage: 2,000 to 5,000 mg. daily. Plays important roles in amino acid metabolism and absorption of other nutrients, including some B vitamins. Blood protein helps maintain fluid balance in the tissue; so poor protein assimilation is sometimes a factor in edema.

## Herbs

♦ **Black Cohosh Root** (Cimicifuga racemosa) + **Wild Yam Root** (Dioscorea villosa) + **Cayenne** (Capsicum annuum) **tea** – Prepare a tea by decoction (see Appendix B) using 1 tsp. each of black cohosh root and wild yam root to 2 cups pure water. Drink 6 oz. three to four times daily between meals. Add a pinch of cayenne pepper to each serving. May help reduce edema, especially if related to the menstrual cycle.

♦ **Burdock Root** (Arctium lappa) – Dosage: 2 capsules or 50 drops of extract* two to three times daily taken with dandelion tea.
*Beneficial properties:* Increases flow of urine, soothes the kidneys, and relieves congestion of lymphatics.

♦ **Horsetail** (Equisetum arvense) – 6 oz. of tea three to four times daily between meals. Place 2 tbsp. of dried herb in 16 oz. pure, cold water and soak for 2 hours; then bring to a boil, and simmer for 20 minutes. Let cool. Horsetail tea also can be mixed with dandelion tea and/or taken with burdock root.

*Beneficial properties:* Very rich in silica, which is a natural diuretic and promotes cleansing and elimination. Horsetail also promotes the flow of urine and is an excellent astringent diuretic; it should be considered whenever there is inflammation of the urinary tract.

*Note:* Restrict intake of this tea to the quantities described. Do not continue use for more than one week. Then wait one week, and begin again if edema is still ongoing. Horsetail contains crystals that can irritate the urinary tract if used to excess.

♦ **Juniper Berries** (Juniperus communis) – Dosage: 2 capsules or 50 drops of fluid extract* two to three times daily between meals. A good combination with horsetail or burdock root or dandelion leaf or all of these at the same time.

*Beneficial properties:* Helps heal the kidneys, bladder, and urinary passages. A stimulating diuretic that may help relieve passive congestion of the kidneys due to heart weakness.

## Homeopathy

See Appendix E for proper use and handling instruction prior to administering remedies described below.

♦ **Apis 6C** – Local and generalized edema; ascites (abdominal edema) with scanty urine; elevated level of albumin in the urine; edema from kidney disease or suppressed skin eruptions; puffiness and pitting of the skin; thirstless. Dosage: Dissolve 5 pellets under the tongue, two to four times daily between meals.

♦ **Arsenicum 6C** – Edema in heart disease; edema of the skin mostly about the face, eyes, and ankles; restlessness, anxiety, insomnia, and dryness of mouth; very chilly, with strong craving for heat. Dosage: Dissolve 5 pellets under the tongue, two to four times daily between meals.

♦ **Aurum Muriaticum 6C** – Edema related to heart, liver, or spleen disease, with elevated level of albumin in the urine and intermittent fever. Dosage: Dissolve 5 pellets under the tongue, two to four times daily between meals.

♦ **Kali Carb. 6X** – Edema caused by liver problems; one of the first remedies to consider in ascites (abdominal edema), especially if tongue is dry, sore, and whitish. Dosage: Dissolve 5 pellets under the tongue, three to four times daily between meals.

## Miscellaneous

♦ **Bromelain** (enzyme derived from pineapple) – Dosage: two to three 500 mg. capsules two to three times daily between meals. May help reduce inflammation and tissue congestion.

♦ **Coenzyme Q-10** – Dosage: 50 to 100 mg., two to three times daily with meals. Supports the energy respiration of all cells. Particularly valuable for the heart and maintenance of heart function.

- **Exercise** daily, incorporating 20 to 30 minutes of aerobic exercises, such as walking, hiking, or bicycle riding. Always consult a physician before beginning a new exercise program.

- **L-Carnitine** – Dosage 500 mg. two to three times daily. L-Carnitine is a fatty-acyl derivative that supports heart function. Especially useful in congestive heart failure.

- **Proteolytic Enzyme Formula** (protein digesting enzymes that include pancreatic protease, bromelain, papain) – Dosage: 2 to 3 or capsules two to three times daily. *Beneficial properties:* When taken *between* meals may decrease inflammation of tissues and related water retention. If taken *with* meals, the enzymes support the digestive process.

- **Pressure stockings**, worn daily, can decrease peripheral edema. Available in calf-high and thigh-high lengths.

# Fatigue

Fatigue is characterized by weakness, lack of energy, and exhaustion. Chronic Fatigue Syndrome, whose cause is unknown, is classified as fatigue that interferes with a person's ability to work and function normally, for a period of at least six months. One can suffer from fatigue for a number of reasons, some of which can be serious medical conditions such as anemia. Fatigue with unknown origins that does not go away on its own should be brought to the attention of a healthcare professional.

Conventional treatments include a thorough medical evaluation, including lab assay, dietary changes, vitamin and mineral supplementation, and exercise. When appropriate, anti-depressants may be prescribed.

| EZ Care Program | |
|---|---|
| Diet | **Drink** 6 to 8 glasses of pure water daily. |
| | **Eliminate** coffee and decaf, black tea, chocolate, soda, alcohol, and processed sugar, because extended use may decrease energy. Stimulants do not create more energy; they merely increase the rate of energy expenditure. Ultimately, they worsen the depletion of vital reserves and deepen chronic fatigue. |
| Vitamins | **Niacinamide** (A form of vitamin B3) – Dosage 500 mg. three times daily. Aids in glucose uptake into the cell and provides a substrate for the energy cofactor NADH. |
| Herbs | **Siberian Ginseng** (Eleutherococcus senticosus) – Dosage: 250 mg. standardized extract or 30 drops extract* in 4 oz. water three times daily. *Beneficial properties*: Traditionally used to support the adrenal (stress) |

| | EZ Care Program |
|---|---|
| | glands.<br>*Note:* Consult a healthcare practitioner prior to use if you suffer from hypertension. |
| Miscellaneous | **Get plenty of rest and sleep** and **keep a regular schedule**. This is the most important measure for overcoming fatigue. |
| | **DHEA** (dihydroepiandosterone) – Dosage 10 – 25 mg. daily. DHEA is a hormone naturally secreted by the adrenal gland. Useful for patients with adrenal weakness.<br>*Note:* Alternative medicine physicians can measure DHEA levels to determine baseline levels before instituting therapy. |
| | **Exercise** at least 30 minutes daily. Exercises such as swimming, walking, Tai Chi exercise and yoga are gentle and may be easier to incorporate into your lifestyle. May help increase energy production. |

## Additional Recommendations

The EZ Care Program consists of basic remedies that are commonly used for fatigue and have been found to work well in most cases. The remedies are most effective when combined, but can be used individually. The options stated below can supplement or replace EZ Care remedies and may be combined when suggested doses are followed.

### Diet

♦ **Identify personal food sensitivities**. Avoid all common allergenic foods (e.g., dairy, eggs, wheat, corn, sugar, preservatives). Rotate moderately allergic foods on a four-day schedule (see Appendix C). Food sensitivities may be an important factor in chronic fatigue.

### Vitamins

♦ **B5** (pantothenic acid) – Dosage: 500 mg. once to twice daily. Pantothenic acid supports the function of adrenal glands. Always use in conjunction with B complex.

♦ **B12** – Dosage: 1000 mcg. sublingual, twice daily. B12 is vital for energy regulation and aids in the production of healthy red blood cells. This vitamin is usually deficient in the elderly population.

♦ **B complex** – Dosage: 50 - 100mg. balanced B complex capsule. Helps the body deal with stress, and aids in energy production.<br>*Note.* For highest assimilation, use a multi B complex which contains the vitamins in their coenzyme form and avoid mega-potency B complex products.

♦ **C** (mineral ascorbates mixed with bioflavonoids) – Dosage: 1,000 mg., three to four times daily with meals. May help support the adrenal glands.

♦ **E** (natural d-alpha tocopherol in a base of mixed tocopherols) – Dosage: 400 IU two times daily. Teams up with coenzyme Q10 in the mitochondria ("powerhouse of the cell").

## Minerals

♦ **Calcium** (elemental calcium from amino acid chelate) – Dosage: 250 mg., two to three times daily with meals. Essential for regulating heart and muscle contraction and nerve conduction as well as utilization of iron.

♦ **Chromium** (as chromium polynicotinate) – Dosage: 200 mcg. two times daily with meals. Supports normal blood sugar regulation, thus preventing hypoglycemia.

♦ **Magnesium** (elemental magnesium from citrate or aspartate) – Dosage: 250 mg., two to three times daily with meals. Magnesium is required for synthesizing ATP, which is the primary cellular energy storage compound.

♦ **Potassium** (elemental potassium from citrate or aspartate) – Dosage: 99 mg., two to three times daily with meals. Fatigue and muscular weakness are two of the most common symptoms of potassium deficiency.

## Herbs

♦ **American Ginseng** (Panax quinquifolium) – Dosage: 1 to 2 capsules two times daily or 8 oz. ginseng tea prepared by decoction (see Appendix B), two times daily between meals. *Beneficial properties:* Traditionally used to support the adrenal (stress) glands.

♦ **Gotu Kola** (Hydrocotyle asiatica) – Dosage: 2 capsules or 30-60 drops extract* in 4 oz. water two to three times daily. *Beneficial properties:* May enhance mental function and ability to overcome fatigue.

♦ **Oat Seed Extract** (Avena sativa) – Dosage: 30-50 drops fluid extract* in 4 oz. pure water two times daily. *Beneficial properties:* May help strengthen and nourish the nervous system.

## Aromatherapy

All of the following essential oils may prove useful in resolving fatigue: **Clary Sage** (Salvia sclarea), **Lavender** (Lavendula vera), **Lemon** (citrus limonum), **Lemongrass** (Cymbopogon citratus) and **Rosemary** (rosmarinus officinalis).

Choose any 3 essential oils from the above list and use equal parts in combination as described here. Use a particular combination for one to two weeks, then blend a new combination using a different mix of oils.

*Suggested methods of application:*
**(1)** Add 6 drops of a given blend with baths described below
**(2)** Mix 6 drops of a given blend in 1 tsp. sweet almond oil. After showering in the morning, rub down with this mixture while the skin is still wet.
**(3)** Tap 3 to 4 drops of a given blend into the palm of one hand. Rub hands together. Inhale deeply 15 to 20 times from cupped palms, turning head to side when exhaling.
**(5)** Add several drops of a given blend to an aromatherapy diffuser and disperse into the air for two hours, two times daily.

## Homeopathy

See Appendix E for proper use and handling instruction prior to administering remedies described below.

*Note:* Fatigue is a symptom associated with many homeopathic remedies. The ones listed below represent some of the more prominent homeopathic responses.

♦ **Arnica 30C** – Acute fatigue due to overexertion, such as playing sports, or lifting heavy weights. Dosage: Dissolve 5 pellets under the tongue, one to two times only to help resolve acute fatigue. Take no further doses.

♦ **Carbo Vegetabalis 6C or 30C** – Debilitated or collapsed state, with weakness, coldness, and sluggishness; great indifference and apathy; great desire to be fanned; weak digestion with belching, bloating, indigestion, and intestinal flatulence. Dosage: Dissolve 5 pellets under the tongue, one to three times daily or weekly or as required.

♦ **Gelsemium 6C or 30C** – Great fatigue with mental, emotional, and physical weakness; heavy, drooping eyelids; forgetfulness and dullness of thought; worn out expression; desire to be quiet; loss of will power; fatigue from flu. Dosage: Dissolve 5 pellets under the tongue, one to three times daily or weekly or as required.

♦ **Sepia 30C** – Primarily a female remedy. Mental and physical sluggishness; irritability and indifference; any request by family is viewed as a burden; tearful and care-worn; feel overwhelmed by responsibilities; chilliness and depression. Dosage: Dissolve 5 pellets under the tongue, one time weekly or monthly or as required.

## Miscellaneous

♦ **Adrenal Glandular** – Dosage: 1 tablet hourly for 8 hours, three days consecutively. Then reduce to 1 to 2 tablets three times daily with meals. Supports the adrenal glands.

♦ **Apple Cider Vinegar and Honey Drink** – Dosage: 1 time daily between meals. Take 2 tsp. unfiltered apple cider vinegar + 1 tsp. raw honey in 8 oz. water. A pick-me-up. A rich source of potassium and enzymes.

♦ **Betaine HCL and Pepsin** – Dosage: one to two 700 mg. capsules at beginning of every meal with protein. Provides hydrochloric acid and pepsin to aid stomach phase of digestion. Many older people, or people with a chronic disorder do not produce adequate amounts of these two digestive substances. Certain crucial energy nutrients (including vitamin B12 ,iron, calcium) require hydrochloric acid for assimilation.
*Note:* Avoid if suffering from stomach or duodenal ulcers; discontinue use if a burning sensation in the stomach is experienced.

♦ **Coenzyme Q-10** – Dosage: 30 mg. gelcap, two to three times daily. Helps body cells (including heart cells) utilize oxygen.

♦ **L-carnitine** – Dosage: 500mg., two times daily with meals. An amino acid that may help increase endurance and counteract muscle fatigue.

♦ **Pancreatic Enzyme Formula** – Dosage: 1 to 2 tablets with each meal. Digestive aids help support the absorption of nutrients required for producing energy and reducing digestive stress that contributes to chronic fatigue.

\* Most herbal extracts contain alcohol. Avoid use if alcohol sensitive or if there is a history of alcohol abuse. *Note:* Alcohol content can be reduced through evaporation by adding extract to very hot water (just below boiling point) and allowing to stand 5 to 7 minutes before drinking.

# Fibrocystic Breast Disease

Lumps in the breast that are usually painless but that enlarge and become tender in the premenstrual period cause this condition. The lumps are usually benign, fluid filled sacs. However, breast cancer rates are higher in women with this condition, and monthly self-breast examination is strongly recommended. The condition is more common in younger women, and usually disappears at menopause, unless estrogen replacement is taken.

Conventional treatments include over-the-counter pain relievers, hormonal treatments, and needle aspiration or biopsy to drain or remove the lump. Alternative medicine physicians have reported success in shrinking breast lumps using a prescription formulation of potassium iodine.

*Note:* Women should perform self breast-exams monthly; women over age 50 should have a mammogram annually. Some physicians recommend screening starting at the age of 40. Those with a first-degree relative with a history of breast cancer should begin mammogram screening ten years before the age of diagnosis of the family member.

| EZ Care Program | |
|---|---|
| Diet | **Avoid** all foods containing estrogens and other hormones, including meats, poultry, eggs, and dairy products. Also avoid the use of plastic beverage containers, which release harmful chemical estrogens called xenoestrogens. <br> *Note:* Products organically produced and certified hormone-free may be acceptable. |
| | **Drink** 6 to 8 glasses of pure water daily. |
| | **Eat a high-water-content diet** consisting of large quantities of fresh fruits and vegetables and comparatively smaller quantities of whole grains, legumes, seeds, nuts, fish, skinless chicken and turkey. <br> *Note:* Limit flesh foods in the diet. Consume large amounts of broccoli, cabbage, kale, and brussel sprouts, which increase excess estrogen metabolism. |

| EZ Care Program | |
|---|---|
| | **Eliminate** all coffee and decaf, black tea, chocolate, and soda from the diet, because these contain substances (methylxanthines) that may worsen the condition. |
| Vitamins | **A** (from fish liver oil) – Dosage: 25,000 IU with meals. May relieve symptoms of fibrocystic breast disease. *Notes:* (1) Consult a physician before using higher doses of vitamin A. Avoid use if pregnant or if attempting pregnancy. (2)Vitamin A causes adverse reactions in some individuals. Reduce dosage or discontinue if headaches, blurred vision, or skin rashes are experienced. (3)The emulsified form is fat soluble and better absorbed. |
| | **E** (natural d-alpha tocopherol in a base of mixed tocopherols) – Dosage: 800 IU daily with meals. May help normalize hormones and relieve symptoms of fibrocystic breast disease. Also, squeeze vitamin E from a capsule and apply topically one to two times daily, in alternation with phytolacca oil and aromatherapy blends discussed below. |
| Herbs | **Dandelion Root** (Taraxacum officinalis) – Dosage: 1 capsule or 30 drops extract* in 4 oz. Water before each meal up to three times daily. *Beneficial properties*: A liver cleanser that may help remove excess estrogen from the body. |
| | **Evening Primrose Oil** (Oenothera biennis) – Dosage: four to eight 500 mg. capsules in divided dose with meals. *Beneficial properties*: Contains gamma-linoleic acid (GLA) that may inhibit inflammatory processes, support normal hormonal regulation, and reduce pre-menstrual breast swelling and tenderness. |
| Miscellaneous | **Kelp Tablets** – Dosage: 2 to 4 tablets daily in divided doses with meals. A rich source of natural iodine. May benefit fibrocystic breast disease, especially when hypothyroidism is a factor. |
| | **Natural Progesterone Cream** – Dosage: apply 2 times daily for last two weeks of each menstrual cycle. May normalize hormonal balance. Discontinue use at beginning of menstrual cycle. |

# Additional Recommendations

The EZ Care Program consists of basic remedies that are commonly used for fibrocystic breast disease and have been found to work well in most cases. The remedies are most effective when combined, but can be used individually. The options stated below can supplement or replace EZ Care remedies and may be combined when suggested doses are followed.

## Diet

- ♦ **Flaxseed Oil** – Dosage: 1 to 2 tbsp. daily. Contains anti-inflammatory omega-3 fatty acids.

## Vitamins

- ♦ **B6** (pyridoxal 5-phosphate) – Dosage: 50 mg., one to two times daily with meals. May normalize hormonal regulation and relieve premenstrual breast symptoms.

*Note:* Always use a complete B complex formula in addition to vitamin B6, because high doses of one of the B vitamins can lead to imbalance in the body's pool of the other B vitamins. *Note:* For highest assimilation, use a multi B complex which contains the vitamins in their coenzyme form and avoid mega-potency B complex products.

♦ **B complex** – Dosage: 50 mg. balanced B complex capsule once daily with meals.
*Note:* For highest assimilation, use a multi B complex which contains some of the vitamins in their coenzyme form and avoid mega-potency B complex products. B-vitamins are important for normal functioning of the neurohormonal system and the liver.

♦ **C** (mixed mineral ascorbates) – Dosage: 500 to 1,000 mg., two times daily. An essential nutrient for hormone metabolism. As an antioxidant, protects vitamins A, E and B from oxidation.

## Herbs

♦ **Chaste Tree Berries** (Vitex agnus castus) – Dosage: 2 capsules or 1 tsp. extract* upon arising, for at least 90 days.
*Beneficial properties:* May prove of value when hormonal imbalance contributes to breast disease.

♦ **Milk Thistle Seed Extract** (silybum marianum) – Dosage: 250 mg. daily of standardized extract or 30-60 drops liquid extract* in 4 oz. water three times daily with meals.
*Beneficial properties:* May help protect the liver, the body's major detoxification organ, from toxins.

♦ **Phytolacca Oil** (Phytolacca decandra)– Dosage: Massage onto breasts a small amount of this oil, one to two times daily. Use in alternation with topical applications of essential oils (described below under Aromatherapy) and/or alternate with vitamin E oil from opened capsule.
*Beneficial properties:* May help reduce breast cysts.

♦ **Blessed Thistle** (Carbenia benedicta) – Dosage: 40-50 drops liquid extract* in 4 oz. water two times daily.
*Beneficial properties:* May prevent breast swelling and tenderness.

♦ **Burdock Root** (Arctium lappa) – Dosage: 40-50 drops extract* in 4 oz. water three times daily.
*Beneficial properties:* May help in bowel detoxification; may be beneficial as blood purifier.

## Aromatherapy

Select one or more of the following essential oils: **Frankincense** (Boswellia carterii), or **Lavender** (Lavendula vera). Mix a total of 3 drops of one of these essential oils *or* a combination of the two oils into 1/2 tsp. aloe vera gel or natural vitamin E oil. Gently rub the solution into the skin of the breasts, two to three times daily or as required.

## Homeopathy

See Appendix E for proper use and handling instruction prior to administering remedies described below.

♦ **Belladonna 6C** – Tender swelling of the breast; great sensitivity to least movement; heat and spasmodic tearing, darting pains in breast. Dosage: Dissolve 5 pellets under the tongue, one to three times daily or as required.

♦ **Bryonia 6C** – Breast feels very hard and heavy; breast symptoms worse during period. Dosage: Dissolve 5 pellets under the tongue, one to three times daily or as required.

♦ **Conium 6C** – A leading remedy for marked tenderness in breast lumps before period and area feels hard. A remedy for lumps in right breast. Dosage: Dissolve 5 pellets under the tongue, one to three times daily or as required.

♦ **Phytolacca 6X** – Breast very hard, with swelling and soreness of lumps; very sensitive and painful; worse during menstrual period; lump in upper part of left breast; breast lumps in girls before puberty. Dosage: Dissolve 5 pellets under the tongue, one to three times daily or as required.

♦ **Pulsatilla 6C** – Breast lumps in girls before puberty. Dosage: Dissolve 5 pellets under the tongue, one to three times daily or as required.

## Miscellaneous

♦ **Fiber Supplement** – Dosage: 1 to 2 tsp. psyllium seed and husk fiber in 8 oz. pure water followed by another 8 oz. water, one to two times daily between meals. Constipation or sluggish bowel function may increase risk and severity of fibrocystic breast disease. *Note:* Carefully read label; some brands require additional water.

♦ **Hot Moist Compress**: hot, moist compress applied to each breast 3 to 4 times weekly. Heat a pot of water on stove. Be certain that water is tolerably hot but *not scalding*. Place 4 washcloths or small face towels in the water. Keep the water on low heat to maintain water temperature. Wring out 2 of the washcloths or towels and place one each over the breasts. Cover with dry towels. Whenever the underlying compress cools, replace with the washcloths or towels soaking in the hot water. Place the cooled cloths back into the hot water for reuse. Continue this procedure for 20 to 30 minutes; follow with a cool sponging of the breasts. Dry the breasts, then rub in the essential oil/aloe vera gel blend *or* the vitamin E oil blend (described above under Aromatherapy) *or* pure natural vitamin E squeezed from a capsule. May help limit cyst formation and symptoms.

♦ If using **oral contraceptives**, consult your physician about their possible link to fibrocystic breast disease.

♦ **Lactobacillus Probiotic Product** (friendly intestinal bacteria that aid digestion, nutrient assimilation, and toxin elimination) (L. acidophilus with bifidobacterium and fructo-oligosaccharides) – Mix with water and swish in mouth before swallowing. Supplementation may control fecal enzymes that resynthesize estrogens.

\*   Most herbal extracts contain alcohol. Avoid use if alcohol sensitive or if there is a history of alcohol abuse. *Note:* Alcohol content can be reduced through evaporation by adding extract to very hot water (just below boiling point) and allowing to stand 5 to 7 minutes before drinking.

# Food Allergies and Sensitivities

Food allergies are a hypersensitive reaction to the ingestion of certain foods. Mild reactions, such as rash, swollen lips, eczema, acne,  runny nose, abdominal pain, bloating, cramping, diarrhea, and constipation may occur. More extreme reactions, such as vomiting, fainting, and depression  are possible. Any of these reactions may be immediate, or may take several days to develop. The most severe form of food allergy is anaphylaxis, an immediate, life threatening condition that causes swelling and constriction of the throat.

Conventional treatments for anaphylaxis include allergy testing via skin or blood, and avoidance of suspected foods. Antihistamines are used to treat mild reactions. Epinephrine and intravenous steroids are used for severe reactions. However, many conventional physicians and allergists are not trained to diagnose or treat most cases of delayed-type, non-anaphylactic food allergies.

*Note:* Any reaction involving swelling of the tongue, lips, or throat requires immediate emergency treatment.

| EZ Care Program ||
|---|---|
| Diet | **Employ pulse-testing procedure** to help identify personal food sensitivities (see Appendix C). |
| | **Identify personal food sensitivities** – Avoid all common allergenic foods (e.g., dairy, eggs, wheat, corn, sugar, preservatives, peanuts). Rotate moderately allergic foods on a four-day schedule (see Appendix C). This is the key to preventing recurrent food intolerances. |
| Herbs | **Dandelion Root** (Taraxacum officinalis) – Dosage: 1 capsule or 30 drops extract\* in 4 oz. water up to three times daily before meals. *Beneficial properties*: A liver cleanser that also may help stimulate digestion. |
| Miscellaneous | **L-glutamine** – Dosage: 1,000 mg. with meals and at bedtime for up to two months. May restore integrity of the gastrointestinal lining. |

| **EZ Care Program** | |
|---|---|
| | **Probiotic Culture** (preferred strains include Lactobacillus acidophilus with bifidobacterium and fructo-oligosaccharides) – Dosage: 1 to 2 capsules Lactobacillus Acidophilus culture daily with a meal. |
| | **Quercetin** – Dosage: 500 mg., three times daily 30 minutes before meals. A bioflavonoid that may reduce allergic responses. It is a natural antihistamine. |

# Additional Recommendations

The EZ Care Program consists of basic remedies that are commonly used for food allergies and sensitivities and have been found to work well in most cases. The remedies are most effective when combined, but can be used individually. The options stated below can supplement or replace EZ Care remedies and may be combined when suggested doses are followed.

## Diet

♦ **Eat a high-water-content-diet** consisting of large quantities of non-allergic fresh fruits and vegetables and comparatively smaller quantities of whole grains, legumes, seeds, nuts, fish, skinless chicken and turkey.

## Vitamins

♦ **B complex** – Dosage: low potency (up to 50 mg.) yeast-free balanced B-complex capsule derived in part from rice bran.
*Note:* For highest assimilation, look for a multi-B vitamin in coenzyme form and avoid mega-potency B-complex products.

♦ **C** (mineral ascorbates mixed with bioflavonoids) – Dosage: 1,000 mg., three to four times daily with meals. May help lower allergenic responses. Blocks the release of histamine.

## Herbs

♦ **Ginger Root** (Zingiber officinalis) – Dosage: 2 capsules three times daily or 6-8 oz. dried ginger root tea three times daily (see Appendix B; Jamaican ginger root is preferred). For enhanced effect, add a pinch of cayenne to each serving.
*Beneficial properties*: May stimulate digestion.

♦ **Siberian Ginseng** (Eleutherococcus senticosus) – Dosage: 250 mg. standardized extract or 30 drops extract* in 4 oz. water three times daily.
*Beneficial properties*: Traditionally used to support the immune system.

## Miscellaneous

♦ **Mixed Essential Fatty Acid Formula** – Dosage: 1 tbsp. two times daily with meals. May help reduce inflammatory responses.

◆ **Proteolytic Enzyme Formula** (includes protease, bromelain, and papain) – May help with digestion. Take with meals as a digestive aid, and between meals as an anti-inflammatory agent.
*Note:* Avoid if there are stomach or duodenal ulcers. Proteolytic enzymes may aggravate ulcers and induce bleeding.

* Most herbal extracts contain alcohol. Avoid use if alcohol sensitive or if there is a history of alcohol abuse. *Note:* Alcohol content can be reduced through evaporation by adding extract to very hot water (just below boiling point) and allowing to stand 5 to 7 minutes before drinking.

# Gallstones

Gallstones are solid, round masses composed primarily of cholesterol. Gallstones begin small but can grow to the size of a marble or larger. The number of stones and their sizes vary from one large stone, to thousands of tiny ones. Gallstones can block the bile duct of the gallbladder, resulting in bloating, gas, pain, and nausea. The characteristic pain of a gallbladder attack starts in the right upper abdominal area and may radiate to the right shoulder. These symptoms, when present, are usually noticed after a fatty meal. Women are three times more likely than men to produce gallstones, especially 40 – 50 year-old women. Gallstones are more common in overweight people, and in those with high fat and/or high cholesterol diets, in addition to people who undergo rapid weight loss. Prevention of gallstones is very important, especially in the onset of rapid weight loss, because eliminating previously formed stones can be extremely difficult.

Conventional therapy consists of using urosdiol, a prescription medication used to dissolve sludge and small gallstones, along with the consumption of a low-fat diet. Careful monitoring by a physician is essential to good health maintenance. Lithotripsy, the use of ultrasound waves in the body can be effective in breaking gallstones into smaller, passable objects. Large stones that do not respond to the above therapies may require surgery to remove the entire gallbladder. Between 500,000 and 700,000 gallbladder removals, called cholecystecties, are performed annually in the United States. Many of these procedures are performed with small incisions and the use of a camera called a laparascope. However, more complex situations, or gallbladder infection, may necessitate standard abdominal surgery.

*Note:* Individuals with gallstones have been associated with a higher risk of gallbladder cancer.

| EZ Care Program | |
|---|---|
| Diet | **Avoid intake of refined sugars.** High sugar intake is associated with increased risk of gallstone formation. |
| | **Avoid rapid weight loss** (greater than two pounds during the first week and 1/2 to 1 pound per week thereafter) and avoid the total elimination of fat from the diet. Rapid weight loss may cause a predisposition to gallstones. |
| | **Be sure to eat breakfast daily.** Fasting periods of more than 14 hours increase the risk of gallbladder problems. |
| | **Identify personal food sensitivities.** Avoid all common allergenic foods, such as milk products and eggs. Rotate moderately allergic foods on a four-day schedule (see Appendix C). This is a very effective strategy to prevent gallbladder attacks. |
| | **Eat a low-fat diet.** May help prevent gallstone formation and reduce pain and inflammation of existing gallbladder conditions. |
| Herbs | **Dandelion Root** (Taraxacum officinalis) – Dosage: 2 capsules or 50 drops extract* in 4 oz. warm water before each meal up to three times daily. *Beneficial properties:* May help cleanse the liver and gallbladder |
| | **Milk Thistle Seed Extract** (Silybum marianum) – Dosage: 250 mg. daily of standardized extract or 30-60 drops liquid extract* in 4 oz. warm water three to four times daily. *Beneficial properties:* Assists with bile production and may protect the liver, the body's major detoxification organ, from toxins. |
| | **Wild Yam Root** (Dioscorea villosa) – Dosage: 1 to 2 capsules or 30-60 drops liquid extract* or 4 oz. of warm tea prepared by decoction (see Appendix B) four to six times daily or as required until the pain subsides. *Beneficial properties:* Antispasmodic herb that may benefit acute gallbladder pain. |
| Homeopathy | **Chelidonium 6C/China 6C** – Dosage: Days 1 through 14: **Chelidonium** 3 times daily after meals, **China** 2 times daily, morning and evening. Days 15 through 28: Reduce **China 6C** to 1 time daily, continuing combination of remedies. May promote the free flow of bile and passage of gallstones. |
| | **Mag Phos 6X** – May alleviate spasms during passage of gallstones. |
| Miscellaneous | **Lecithin** – Dosage: 2 tbsp. Granulated lecithin daily. May help emulsify (break down) gallstones. |
| | **Gallbladder flush** – This 7-day procedure can be useful in flushing gallstones from the gallbladder and should be used only under physician supervision. On days 1-5, consume only fresh organic apples and apple juice. Avoid all other foods. You may experience hunger, but it will subside. On days 6 and 7, consume apples and apple juice and take 1/3 cup of olive oil and the juice of 2 fresh lemons in the evening. Examine the morning stool for gallstones. Repeat if necessary. |

## Additional Recommendations

The EZ Care Program consists of basic remedies that are commonly used for gallstones and have been found to work well in most cases. The remedies are most effective when combined, but can be used individually. The options stated below can supplement or replace EZ Care remedies and may be combined when suggested doses are followed.

## Diet

♦ Eat a **high-water-content** diet consisting of large quantities of fresh fruits and vegetables and comparatively smaller quantities of whole grains, legumes, seeds, nuts, fish, skinless chicken and turkey.

♦ **Drink** 6 to 8 glasses of pure water daily.

♦ **Eliminate** coffee and decaf, black tea, chocolate, soda, alcohol, and processed sugar.

♦ **Eat foods** like apples, beets, carrots, leeks, radishes and artichokes. May help detoxify the liver.

♦ **Fiber Supplement** – Dosage: 1 to 3 tsp. psyllium husk fiber in 8 oz. pure water one to two times daily between meals to speed stool's transit time. In general, people with gallstones have slow stool transit times.
*Note:* Carefully read the label; some brands require additional water.

## Vitamins

♦ **C** (mineral ascorbates mixed with bioflavonoids) – Dosage: 1,000 mg., three to four times daily with meals. May reduce inflammation of the gallbladder and help with infection caused by stones.

## Herbs

♦ **Artichoke Leaf** (Cynara scolymus) – Dosage: 1 to 2 capsules three times daily for three months.
*Beneficial properties:* May reduce gallbladder inflammation and blood lipids.

## Homeopathy

See Appendix E for proper use and handling instruction prior to administering remedies described below.

♦ **Calc Phos 6X** – Dosage: 5 pellets under the tongue, three times daily. May prevent formation of new gallstones.

## Miscellaneous

♦ **Choline** – Dosage: 500 mg., two times daily with meals. May help reduce gallstone formation by making cholesterol more soluble.

♦ **L-Methionine** – Dosage: 500 mg., two times daily with meals. May normalize liver and gallbladder function.

\* Most herbal extracts contain alcohol. Avoid use if alcohol sensitive or if there is a history of alcohol abuse. *Note:* Alcohol content can be reduced through evaporation by adding extract to very hot water (just below boiling point) and allowing to stand 5 to 7 minutes before drinking.

# Gas (Flatulence)

Gas is common and produced by everyone on a daily basis. Occasional odorous gas is not a serious problem, and can be handled safely and easily. However, gas can be associated with abdominal discomfort and bloating. Flatulence may have several causes, including abnormal bowel flora, improper diet, poor digestion, yeast overgrowth, and constipation.

Conventional treatments include the prescription drug simethicone.

| EZ Care Program ||
|---|---|
| Diet | **Chew food** twenty to thirty times before swallowing, to allow for optimal digestion and assimilation with digestive enzymes. Avoid gas-producing foods such as milk, broccoli, and brussel sprouts for one week and reintroduce slowly into diet. **Avoid all carbonated beverages.** |
| Herbs | **Fennel Seed** (Foeniculum vulgare) – Dosage: 1 tsp. Ground fennel seed on food with each meal; or 90 minutes after each meal, drink 1 cup fennel seed tea (see Appendix B). *Beneficial properties:* May reduce or eliminate gas and bloating. |
|  | **Peppermint Leaf** (Mentha piperita) – Dosage: 1 cup peppermint tea, 90 minutes after each meal (see Appendix B). *Beneficial properties:* May aid in digestion, and alleviate gas. *Note:* Additional herbal teas that may help this condition include anise, chamomile, coriander, and caraway. |
| Miscellaneous | **Activated Charcoal** – Dosage: 1 to 2 capsules up to three times daily. *Beneficial properties:* May absorb toxic material in the colon. *Note:* Avoid long-term use to prevent the malabsorption of nutrients. |
|  | **Proteolytic Enzyme Formula** (including protease, bromelain, and papain) – May help with digestion of food. Take as directed on package. *Note:* Avoid if there is a history of stomach or duodenal ulcers; proteolytic enzymes may aggravate ulcers and induce bleeding. |
|  | **Lactobacillus Probiotic Product** (a friendly intestinal bacteria that aids in digestion, nutrient assimilation, and toxin elimination) (L. acidophilus with bifidobacteria and fructo-oligosaccharides in powder or capsule form) – Use according to directions on label. |

# Additional Recommendations

The EZ Care Program consists of basic remedies that are commonly used for gas and have been found to work well in most cases. The remedies are most effective when combined but can be used individually. The options stated below can supplement or replace EZ Care remedies and may be combined when suggested doses are followed.

## Diet

♦ **Eat a high-water-content diet** consisting of large quantities of fresh fruits and vegetables and comparatively smaller quantities of whole grains, legumes, seeds, nuts, fish, skinless chicken and turkey.

♦ A three-day **vegetable juice fast** is often helpful in detoxifying the colon. It is recommended to work with a physician when doing a fast.

♦ **Fiber Supplement** – Dosage: 1 to 3 tsp. psyllium husk fiber in 8 oz. pure water one to two times daily between meals to speed up the stool's transit time.
*Note:* Carefully read the label; some brands require additional water.

## Herbs

♦ **Gentian Root** (Gentiana lutea) – Dosage: 30-60 drops extract* in 4 oz. water 1/2 hour before meals three times daily.
*Beneficial properties:* Tonic bitter; traditionally used to aid digestion and elimination and as a liver cleanser.
*Note:* Extract is preferable in this case, because actual perception of gentian's bitter taste may enhance the body's response.

## Homeopathy

See Appendix E for proper use and handling instruction prior to administering remedies described below.

♦ **Mag Phos 6X** – Flatulence with spasmodic pain; belching gives no relief. Dosage: 5 pellets under the tongue, every 15 minutes, with a sip of warm water until relief is obtained.

♦ **Nat Phos 6X** – Flatulence with acid stomach and sour reflux. Dosage: 5 pellets under the tongue, three times daily 1 hour after meals, or every 15 minutes, or as required in acute cases.

## Miscellaneous

♦ **Alfalfa Tablets** – Take 4 tablets three times daily for three to four weeks.
*Beneficial properties:* May help improve colon function.

♦  **Cool Sitz Bath** – Daily on rising, fill tub with cool water so water reaches to just below the level of your navel. Lean backward in the tub, keeping feet out of the water. Rub your abdomen with one hand, making clockwise circles from right to left. Remain in the tub up to 5 minutes; then dry well. This remedy can be extremely effective for chronic flatulence.

♦  **Exercise daily,** incorporating aerobic exercise. May help promote elimination and enhance digestion.

♦  In painful **acute cases**, lie face down with abdomen on a half-full hot water bottle that is resting on a pillow. May provide additional relief.

\*  Most herbal extracts contain alcohol. Avoid use if alcohol sensitive or if there is a history of alcohol abuse. *Note:* Alcohol content can be reduced through evaporation by adding extract to very hot water (just below boiling point) and allowing to stand 5 to 7 minutes before drinking.

# Gout

Gout is a type of arthritis typically caused either by an overproduction or inability to excrete uric acid. The substance may crystallize in joint tissues, causing great pain. Gout is most commonly seen in the great toe, although other joints may be affected. The joint becomes red, swollen, warm, and very painful to touch. Symptoms often disappear gradually, only to return again. Untreated chronic gout may lead to permanent joint deformity. Elevated levels of uric acid in the blood also can lead to more serious problems, such as kidney stones or kidney failure.

Conventional treatments include a thorough history, physical, lab assay, and x-ray to evaluate the problem. Acute therapy may entail use of medications such as nonsteroidal anti-inflammatory agents or colchicine. Chronic prevention may involve dietary changes with a reduction in protein consumption and use of prescription agents such as allopurinol or methotrexate.

| EZ Care Program | |
|---|---|
| Diet | Avoid all **alcohol** intake, because this substance may increase the formation of uric acid. |
| | **Eat** foods rich in anthocyanidins, such as fresh **cherries** and **blueberries**, because they may help lower uric acid in the body. |
| | **Eliminate** coffee and decaf, black tea, chocolate, soda, and processed sugar. |

| EZ Care Program | |
| --- | --- |
| | **Eliminate purine-rich foods**, such as meats, shellfish, yeast, herring, mackerel, sardines, and anchovies; and reduce other moderately high-purine rich foods, such as poultry, legumes, spinach, asparagus, fish, and mushrooms. |
| Vitamins | **C** (mineral ascorbates mixed with bioflavonoids) – Dosage: 1,000 mg., three to four times daily with meals. May help remove uric acid from body tissues. |
| | **Folic Acid** – Dosage: 800 to 1200 mcg. one to two times daily with meals. Green, leafy vegetables are also an excellent source. It is not coincidental that the words *folic* and *foliage* derive from the same root. May be beneficial in reducing uric acid in joints and tissues. |
| Herbs | **Devil's Claw** (Harpagophytum procumbens) – Dosage: 2 to 4 capsules or 50 drops liquid extract* three times daily with meals. *Beneficial properties:* Anti-inflammatory that may help during acute stages of gout. |
| Raw Juices | **Black Cherry Juice Concentrate** – Dosage: 1 tbsp. in 8 oz. warm water. Drink two times daily between meals. |
| Homeopathy | **Colchicum 6C** – Use when there is swelling and tearing pain in feet, legs, and toes; pain becomes worse with movement and at night; there may be nausea, weakness, feelings of dejection, and/or irritability. Dosage: Dissolve 5 pellets under the tongue, three to four times daily or as required. When acute phase passes, switch to Colchicum 12C and decrease to two doses daily until gout symptoms are gone. |
| | **Arnica 6C or 30C** – Dosage: Dissolve 5 pellets under the tongue, one to three times daily for the first day or two after pain begins. May help reduce swelling and pain. Arnica cream can also be directly applied to swollen area. |
| Miscellaneous | In acute attacks, **keep affected limb elevated and at rest** as much as possible**.** |

# Additional Recommendations

The EZ Care Program consists of basic remedies that are commonly used for gout and have been found to work well in most cases. The remedies are most effective when combined but can be used individually. The options stated below can supplement or replace EZ Care remedies and may be combined when suggested doses are followed.

## Diet

♦ **Drink 8 glasses pure, room-temperature water** daily upon arising and between meals. Water helps flush uric acid from the body.

♦ **Identify personal food sensitivities.** Avoid all common allergenic foods (e.g., dairy, eggs, wheat, corn, sugar, preservatives (see Appendix C).

♦ **Maintain a normal weight** – Excessive body weight places abnormal stress on the skeletal system, including joints. Body tissues can heal only when the stress on them is reduced to normal levels.

## Vitamins

♦ **B complex** – Dosage: 50 mg. balanced, yeast-free B complex capsule.
  *Note:* For highest assimilation, use a multi B complex which contains the vitamins in their coenzyme form and avoid mega-potency B complex products.

♦ **E** (emulsified or "dry" forms natural d-alpha tocopherol in a base of mixed tocopherols) – Dosage: 400 IU two times daily with meals.

## Herbs

♦ **Comfrey** (Symphytum officinale) **Poultice** – Blend dried comfrey leaves with sufficient warm water to make a thick paste. Spread the paste on a square of linen. Apply paste side down to affected area. Keep in place two hours. Repeat two to three times daily as desired.
  *Beneficial properties:* May help ameliorate local inflammation and pain.

♦ **Juniper Berries** (Juniperus communis) or **Horsetail** (Equisetum arvense) – Dosage: 6 oz. tea (see Appendix B) three times daily between meals. If these two herbs are used in combination, use equal parts of each herb.
  *Beneficial properties:* May help reduce retention of uric acid.

♦ **Stinging Nettle** (Urtica urens) – Dosage: 2 capsules or 50 drops liquid extract* three times daily. Devil's claw and stinging nettle extracts can be used together: 25 drops of each.
  *Beneficial properties:* May help reduce uric acid load and dredge the kidneys.

## Miscellaneous

♦ **Activated Charcoal** – Dosage: 1 to 2 capsules up to three times daily.
  *Note:* Avoid long-term use, because it may prevent absorption of nutrients.

♦ **Alternating Foot Baths** – may be useful in treating gout (see Appendix D).

♦ **Proteolytic Enzyme Formula** (including protease, bromelain, and papain) – Take as directed on package. May help improve digestion.
  *Note:* Avoid if stomach or duodenal ulcers; proteolytic enzymes may aggravate ulcers and induce bleeding.

\* Most herbal extracts contain alcohol. Avoid use if alcohol sensitive or if there is a history of alcohol abuse. *Note:* Alcohol content can be reduced through evaporation by adding extract to very hot water (just below boiling point) and allowing to stand 5 to 7 minutes before drinking.

# Gum Disease (Gingivitis)

Gum disease or gingivitis causes gums to redden, swell, and easily bleed. It may be caused by a buildup of plaque at the base of the teeth. Gingivitis also may be associated with diabetes, leukemia, or poor dental hygiene. It is the beginning of periodontal disease, and if left untreated, can cause tooth loss and nerve damage. Proper nutrition and routine oral hygiene can be very effective in both prevention and treatment of this problem. This includes good brushing techniques, daily flossing, and regular visits to the dentist for checkups and cleaning.

Conventional treatments includes scraping plaque and tartar off the teeth, improving nutrition, and reducing intake of junk food, especially foods high in starch or refined sugar.

| EZ Care Program | |
|---|---|
| Diet | Eat a **high-water-content** diet consisting of large quantities of fresh fruits and vegetables and comparatively smaller quantities of whole grains, legumes, seeds, nuts, fish, skinless chicken and turkey. |
| Vitamins | **C** (mineral ascorbates mixed with bioflavonoids) – Dosage: 1,000 mg., three to four times daily with meals.  Strengthens gum tissue and is essential for gum health. |
| | **Folic Acid** – Dosage: 1 mg., two times daily with meals. May reduce gum inflammation. Also consider folate mouthwash (0.1% folic acid solution), which may bind toxins secreted by plaque; rinse mouth two times daily after brushing teeth. |
| Herbs | **Myrrh  Mouth Rinse** (Commiphora myrrha) – Mix 30 drops myrrh tincture into 4 oz. warm water, or 1 tsp. powdered myrrh into 2 tbsp. warm water. Swish around gums for 1 minute, then swallow. Repeat two to three times daily or as required. *Beneficial properties:* Cleansing tonic for gum tissue. |
| Miscellaneous | **Coenzyme Q-10** – Dosage: 30 mg., two to three times daily with meals. An important nutrient for maintaining healthy gums. |

## Additional Recommendations

The EZ Care Program consists of basic remedies that are commonly used for gingivitis and have been found to work well in most cases. The remedies are most effective when combined but can be used individually. The options stated below can supplement or replace EZ Care remedies and may be combined when suggested doses are followed.

## Diet

♦ **Avoid** all processed sugar, because this may promote the growth of bacteria that can exacerbate the condition.

♦ **Eat** foods rich in anthocyanidins, such as fresh **cherries** and **blueberries**, because they help strengthen the gums.

## Vitamins

♦ **Beta-Carotene** – Dosage: 25,000 IU three times daily with meals. Helps maintain integrity of gum tissue.

♦ **E** (natural d-alpha tocopherol in a base of mixed tocopherols) – Dosage: 800 IU one to two times daily with meals. Beneficial for tissue health.

## Minerals

♦ **Zinc** (take only if over 14 years of age) – Dosage: 15 mg. elemental zinc from amino acid chelate two times daily with meals. An important nutrient for preventing periodontal disease; a beta-carotene synergist.

## Herbs

♦ **Brush** with toothpaste containing **Myrrh.**
*Beneficial properties:* May reduce plaque buildup and development of gum disease.

♦ **Grape Seed Extract** – Dosage: 50 to 100 mg., three times daily.
*Beneficial properties:* Rich source of antioxidants that may help prevent and treat gingivitis by strengthening the gums.

## Homeopathy

See Appendix E for proper use and handling instruction prior to administering remedies described below.

♦ **Merc Sol 12C** – Chronic case; gums inflamed and bleeding, pocketing around teeth. Dosage: Dissolve 5 pellets under the tongue, two times daily for up to 30 days, then reduce dosage as required.

## Miscellaneous

♦ **Avoid** use of all **tobacco** products.

♦ Investigate possibility that **mercury amalgam fillings** are causing or worsening gum disease.

# Hayfever

Hayfever is the acute seasonal form of allergic rhinitis. It can be caused by an allergic reaction to environmental agents, such as grass, pollen, ragweed, and dust. The allergic reaction is characterized by inflammation of the membrane lining of the nose and throat, sometimes extending to the eyes. The symptoms include sneezing, headaches, sinus pressure, nasal discharge, nasal obstruction, hoarseness, itching, tearing eyes, and a dry cough.

Conventional treatments include use of antihistamines, inhalers and vaporizers, and removal from or desensitization to known allergens. It may also be recommended to remove curtains, drapery, and carpeting from a room, to wash all bedding in hot water, and encase mattresses and pillows with dust mite covers.

| EZ Care Program | |
|---|---|
| Diet | **Identify personal food sensitivities**. Avoid all common allergenic foods, such as milk products and eggs. Rotate moderately allergic foods on a four-day schedule (see Appendix C). Elimination of food allergies will reduce the burden of environmental allergies. |
| | **Drink** 6 to 8 glasses of pure water daily. |
| Vitamins | **C** (mineral ascorbates mixed with bioflavonoids) – Dosage: 1,000 mg., three to four times daily with meals. May strengthen immune system and decrease severity of allergic reactions. |
| Herbs | **Goldenseal Root** (Hydrastis canadensis) **irrigation** – Add 1-1/2 tsp. goldenseal powder to a pint of boiling water. Shake the solution well. Let stand two hours, shaking occasionally. Blow nose completely clear of mucus, then use the prepared solution as with the nasal irrigation described just below. |
| | **Stinging Nettle** (Urtica dioica) – Dosage: 2 freeze-dried capsules every two to four hours as needed. *Beneficial properties:* May help relieve symptoms of hayfever. |
| Homeopathy | **Allium Cepa 6C** – Use for frequent sneezing; extensive, irritating, watery dripping from nose that burns the skin; profuse, burning tearing from the eyes. Dosage: Dissolve 5 pellets three times daily or as required. |
| Miscellaneous | **Quercitin** – Dosage: 250 mg., two to four times daily in divided doses among meals. A bioflavonoid that acts as a natural antihistamine. *Note:* Begin taking 2 to 4 weeks prior to the beginning of the allergy season; continue throughout duration of the season. |
| | **Evening Primrose Oil** (Oenothera biennis) – Dosage: 1300 mg., two times daily with meals. *Beneficial properties*: Contains gamma-linoleic acid (GLA) that may inhibit inflammatory processes. |

| | **EZ Care Program** |
|---|---|
| | **Nasal Irrigation** to flush the sinuses. Dosage: 1/2 tsp. Kosher salt (or less if not tolerated) in 1 cup warm water. First gargle with a part of the solution, then blow the nose completely clear of mucus. Pour the balance of the solution into cupped hands and inhale; or tilt the head back and squirt the solution gently into one nostril at a time using a rubber bulb syringe; or sniff the solution into one nostril at a time. Keep the opposite nostril closed with hand. After each flush, gently blow the nose with tissue. Flush several times daily for acute conditions. *Note:* May be performed daily as a preventive measure. |

# Additional Recommendations

The EZ Care Program consists of basic remedies that are commonly used for hayfever and have been found to work well in most cases. The remedies are most effective when combined but can be used individually. The options stated below can supplement or replace EZ Care remedies and may be combined when suggested doses are followed.

## Diet

◆ **Avoid milk** and all milk products, because they increase mucus formation. Consider dairy alternatives such as soy, or nut milks and cheeses.

◆ **Avoid all processed sugar**, because it may suppress immunity.

◆ Eat a **high-water-content** diet consisting of large quantities of fresh fruits and vegetables and comparatively smaller quantities of whole grains, legumes, seeds, nuts, fish, skinless chicken and turkey.
*Note:* Higher quantities of dark green, leafy vegetables, deep yellow, and orange vegetables should be consumed.

◆ **Consume ground flaxseeds**, or use 1 tbsp. flaxseed oil over salads. Contains alpha-linolenic acid, which promotes anti-inflammatory prostaglandin production.

## Vitamins

◆ **A** (natural, from fish liver oil) – Dosage: 10,000 to 25,000 IU daily with meals.
*Note:* Consult a physician before using higher doses of vitamin A. Avoid use if pregnant. Discontinue use if nausea, dry skin, sore lips, blurred vision, or other signs of vitamin A toxicity are experienced.

◆ **B6** (pyridoxal 5-phosphate) – Dosage: 25 mg., two times daily with meals. May be beneficial in reducing respiratory spasm.
*Note:* Always use a complete 25 mg. to 50 mg. B complex formula in addition to B6, because high doses of one of the B vitamins may lead to imbalance in the body's pool of the other B vitamins.

### Minerals

◆ **Zinc** (take only if over 14 years of age) – Dosage: 25 mg. elemental zinc from amino acid chelate two times daily with meals. May strengthen immune system.
*Note:* Zinc and vitamin A are synergistic and work well together in this context.

### Herbs

◆ **Eyebright** (Euphrasia officinalis) – Dosage: 1 to 2 capsules three times daily.
*Beneficial properties:* May help alleviate symptoms of allergies, particularly of the eyes.

### Homeopathy

See Appendix E for proper use and handling instruction prior to administering remedies described below.

◆ **Dulcamara 6C** – Eyes swell and water, nose runs and is stuffy, constant sneezing; symptoms worse in dampness and in open air. Dosage: Dissolve 5 pellets three times daily or as required.

◆ **Gelsemium 6C** – Eyes hot and heavy, violent sneezing, tingling of nose; nose runs constantly in morning; discharge acrid, and irritates nostrils. Dosage: Dissolve 5 pellets three times daily or as required.

# Headache

There are many types of headache, each with its own cause. To correctly treat a headache, first diagnose which type you have. Some common headaches include:

*Tension headache* – The most common type of headache in adults. Usually begins in the afternoon or early evening. A band-like area of pain comes up the neck and back of head. Usually caused by stress and tension in the ligaments of the neck.

*Eyestrain headache* – Steady pain occurs in the forehead and around the eyes. Usually caused by excessive reading, use of computers, or poor vision.

*Sinus Headache* –Pain and pressure in the cheeks, often accompanied by dizziness. Usually caused by sinus infection or allergies.

*Migraine headache* – Throbbing, often on one side of the head, often preceded by nausea or an aura such as seeing flashing lights. May be hereditary; or brought on by stress, hormonal imbalance, birth control pills, bright lights, changes in the weather, food sensitivities, and/or allergies.

Conventional treatments vary according to the type of headache. In general, treatments include over-the-counter pain relievers, stress reduction techniques, various prescription medications, and in some cases, surgery.

Migraines can be more complex. Conventional therapy of migraines begins with rest, a dark quiet environment, and various pharmacological agents, including analgesics, beta-blockers, and occasionally an anti-convulsant. Hypnosis, biofeedback, and yoga also may be recommended.

Headaches are very complex, and only briefly covered in this section. If your headaches last for more than three days, if they get more frequent and severe, or if they appear following a head injury, contact a physician immediately.

**Prolotherapy injections**, are performed by physicians, and can be useful to permanently stop headaches. The injections are given into the facet joints in the neck, causing tissue rebuilding. This technique helps to alleviate pressure and pain in the neck. Once the area has healed, headaches (especially of the tension variety) will be reduced or eliminated. See Appendix F for more information.

| EZ Care Program | |
|---|---|
| Diet | **Identify personal food sensitivities**. Avoid all common allergenic foods for period of 4 weeks to see if frequency reduces. Add back one food at a time and note if headaches return. Most common offending foods include caffeine, wheat, alcohol, sugar, chocolate, dairy products, wine, monosodium glutamate (MSG), and other preservatives (see Appendix C). |
| | **Eliminate caffeine and chocolate** – These substances have been correlated with headache prevalence. Chocolate contains caffeine and is associated with migraines. |
| Minerals | **Magnesium** (elemental magnesium from amino acid chelate) – Dosage: 500 to 1,000 mg. daily in divided doses with meals and at bedtime. Essential for relaxing the nervous system. Stabilizes blood vessel spasm, which is useful to prevent migraines. *Note:* If headaches occur at consistent times, take two hours before expected time of onset. |
| Herbs | **Feverfew** (Tanacetum parthenium) – Dosage: 1 to 2 capsules two times daily or as required. *Beneficial properties:* Traditionally used for pain relief in ways similar to aspirin, but without aspirin's stomach-irritant property. Particularly beneficial for migraines and may be used long-term as a prevention method. *Note:* Take for a minimum of 90 days for preventive measures. |

| EZ Care Program | |
|---|---|
| Miscellaneous | **Avoid** all forms of tobacco. |
| | **Apple Cider Vinegar Head Vapor** – Add equal parts of pure water and unfiltered apple cider vinegar to a small pan; cover and bring to a boil. Remove cover, place towel over head, lean over pan and inhale rising vapor. Inhale deeply at least 80 times. Be careful not to scald face. |
| | **Breathing Exercise** – Following is a yoga breathing exercise to calm the mind: Inhale through the nose for a count of 4, hold for a count of 7, exhale through the mouth for a count of 8. Practice two times daily, four to eight repetitions each time. *Note:* To enhance concentration and be certain the exercise is performed properly, you might lie down, place a lightweight book on your abdomen, then peacefully observe the book's rise-and-fall motion as you breathe deeply. |
| | **Reduce** lifestyle **stress** and implement a relaxation program. Harmonizing practices (e.g., biofeedback, meditation, yoga, Tai Chi exercise) may prove beneficial. |

## Additional Recommendations

The EZ Care Program consists of basic remedies that are commonly used for headaches and have been found to work well in most cases. The remedies are most effective when combined but can be used individually. The options stated below can supplement or replace EZ Care remedies and may be combined when suggested doses are followed.

### Diet

+   **Avoid overly rich, heavy foods**; they give rise to headaches, especially when combined with sedentary lifestyle habits.

+   **Flaxseed oil** – add to salads, or into yogurt. Provides a source of omega-3 fatty acids that are essential for membrane stability. Keep refrigerated, and open 1 capsule of vitamin E into oil container during storage to prevent rancidity.

### Vitamins

+   **B complex** – Dosage: 50 - 100mg. balanced B complex capsule daily. Helps support the nervous system.
    *Note:* For highest assimilation, use a multi B complex which contains the vitamins in their coenzyme form and avoid mega-potency B complex products.

+   **DLPA** (d,l-phenylalanine) 500 mg. twice daily. DLPA contains the amino acid phenylalanine, which helps with neurotransmitter production and pain reduction.

+   **GABA** (gamma-aminobutyric acid) 500 mg. twice daily. GABA is a neurotransmitter directly involved in inhibition of pain transmission.

## Minerals

◆ **Calcium** (elemental calcium from amino acid chelate) – Dosage: 500 to 1,000 mg. daily in divided doses with meals and at bedtime. Essential for the relaxation of the nervous system. Considered a "lullaby mineral"
*Note:* If headaches occur at consistent times, take two hours before expected time.

## Herbs

◆ **Burdock Root** (Arcium lappa) – Dosage: 1 to 2 capsules or 30-60 drops extract* in 4 oz. water, three times daily.
*Beneficial properties:* May help in bowel detoxification; may be beneficial as a blood purifier.

◆ **Chaste Tree Berries** (Vitex agnus castus) – Dosage: 2 capsules or 1 tsp. extract* upon arising, for at least 90 days.
*Beneficial properties:* May assist hormonal harmonization in women; may be specific for headaches made worse by hormonal imbalance.

◆ **Dandelion Root** (Taraxacum officinalis) – Dosage: 1 to 2 capsules with each meal.
*Beneficial properties:* Liver tonic that may help stimulate digestion.

◆ **Gentian Root** (Gentiana lutea) – Dosage: 1 to 2 capsules or 30-60 drops extract* in 4 oz. water, three times daily.
*Beneficial properties:* Tonic bitter; traditionally used to aid digestion and elimination and as a liver cleanser.
*Note:* Extract may be preferable in this case, because actual perception of its bitter taste will enhance the body's response.

◆ **Ginger Root** (Zingiber officinalis) – Dosage: 2 capsules three times daily, or 6-8 oz. dried ginger root tea three times daily (see Appendix B; Jamaican ginger root is preferred). For enhanced effect, add a pinch of cayenne to each serving.
*Beneficial properties:* May aid digestion.

◆ **Milk Thistle Seed Extract** (silybum marianum) – Dosage: 250 mg. daily standardized extract or 30-60 drops liquid extract* in 4 oz. water three times daily with meals.
*Beneficial properties:* May help protect the liver, the body's major detoxification organ, from toxins.

◆ **Valerian Root** (Valeriana officinalis) – Dosage: 2 capsules or 30-60 drops liquid extract* in 4 oz. water two to three times daily.
*Beneficial properties:* Calms nerves and acts as sedative. Traditionally used for excitability and nervous tension.

## Homeopathy

See Appendix E for proper use and handling instruction prior to administering remedies described below.

♦ **Aconite 12C** – Sudden, violent headaches; feels like skull will burst through forehead, or skull feels constricted with a tight band. Dosage: Dissolve 5 pellets under the tongue, every hour until pain begins to subside.

♦ **Arnica 12C** – Headaches caused by a blow to head, or other form of head trauma. Dosage: Dissolve 5 pellets under the tongue, every hour until pain begins to subside.

♦ **Belladonna 12C** – Throbbing headaches with violent shooting pains, flushed face, and dilated pupils; pain often right-sided and may "drive you wild"; helped by applying pressure and bending head backward. Dosage: Dissolve 5 pellets under the tongue, every hour until pain begins to subside.

♦ **Nux Vomica 12C** – A splitting headache, feels like a nail driven into skull, often accompanied by nausea and vomiting; overindulgence in alcohol and/or rich food; pain usually begins on waking or after eating. Dosage: Dissolve 5 pellets under the tongue, every hour until pain begins to subside.

## Miscellaneous

♦ **Have vision checked** if headaches occur after reading, working at the computer, or other activities that may strain the eyes.

♦ **Hot Foot Bath with Mustard** – This therapy is most suitable for congestive headaches, with fullness and sensation of heat in the head. Fill a bucket with hot water and add 1 tbsp. mustard powder. While soaking feet, drink 1 to 2 cups hot peppermint tea, or hot water with juice of 1/2 lemon.

♦ **Regular exercise** may help relieve headaches caused by muscular and mental tension.

♦ **Proteolytic Enzyme Formula** (including protease, bromelain, and papain). Dosage: Take as directed on package. May help with digestion of food.
*Note:* Avoid if stomach or duodenal ulcers; proteolytic enzymes may aggravate ulcers and induce bleeding.

♦ **Consider** acupuncture or spinal manipulation from a qualified professional.

* Most herbal extracts contain alcohol. Avoid use if alcohol sensitive or if there is a history of alcohol abuse. *Note:* Alcohol content can be reduced through evaporation by adding extract to very hot water (just below boiling point) and allowing to stand 5 to 7 minutes before drinking.

# Heartburn

Heartburn, or gastro-esophageal reflux (GERD), occurs when a weakened lower esophageal sphincter allows acid from the stomach to enter into the esophagus. It usually causes a burning sensation in the throat and chest.

Heartburn is a clear sign that the stomach is aggravated by one of many things, some of which may include tobacco, alcohol, hormones, medications, overconsumption of food, or eating while stressed.

Conventional treatments include avoiding many of the above-mentioned irritants, elevating the head of the bed at night, and use of over-the-counter antacids. Medications may be prescribed to suppress the secretion of stomach acid, tighten the lower esophageal sphincter, and speed the passage of food from the stomach to the small intestine. Surgery may be required in severe cases.

*Note:* Chronic heartburn can cause esophageal scarring if left untreated. This condition, known as *Barrett's Esophagus*, is a precancerous condition. Also, chronic acid suppression can lead to malabsorbtion of nutrients, minerals, and vitamins. Do not take acid suppressing drugs for longer than is recommended.

| EZ Care Program | |
|---|---|
| Diet | **Avoid** all foods that upset your stomach. Most common offenders include coffee, alcohol, milk, and spicy, and acidic foods. |
| | Eat a **high-water-content** diet consisting of large quantities of fresh fruits and vegetables with comparatively smaller quantities of whole grains, legumes, seeds, nuts, fish, skinless chicken and turkey. Special emphasis should be on high fiber foods, such as raw cabbage, dark green, leafy vegetables, broccoli, apples, whole grains, and legumes. |
| | **Eat smaller and simpler meals**, which make digestion easier. |
| Minerals | **Calcium** (elemental calcium from amino acid chelate) – Dosage: 500 to 1,000 mg. daily in divided doses with meals and at bedtime. A natural antacid that may benefit heartburn. |
| Herbs | **Licorice Root** (Glycyrrhiza uralensis or glabra) – Dosage: 1 to 2 capsules or 40-50 drops liquid extract * before each meal.<br>*Beneficial properties:* May soothe and nourish the stomach.<br>*Note:* Avoid use if you have kidney or heart disease. If you have high blood pressure, consult a physician before using this herb because it may elevate blood pressure by increasing water retention. Chinese (uralensis) and de-glycerinated licorice root (DGL) are less problematic in this regard than the western variety (glabra). |
| | **Peppermint** (Mentha piperita) or **Spearmint** (Mentha specter) – Prepare as an infusion (see Appendix B). Dosage: 6 oz. of tea 1 hour after each meal or as required.<br>*Beneficial properties:* May aid in digestion and soothe the stomach. |
| Homeopathy | **Nat Phos 6X** – For an acid stomach with sour reflux, loss of appetite, and creamy yellow coating at back of tongue; sour taste in mouth, severe pain beginning two hours after eating; gastric ulcers; parasite infestation. Dosage: Dissolve 5 pellets under the tongue, every 15 minutes until relief is obtained. |
| Miscellaneous | **Avoid** all forms of **tobacco**, because it is a stomach irritant. |

| EZ Care Program |
| --- |
| **Activated Charcoal Capsules** – Dosage: 1 to 2 capsules with 6 oz. warm water every hour until relief is obtained. |
| **Betaine Hydrochloride Capsules** – Poor stomach digestion, resulting in chronic heartburn, is frequently related to deficient hydrochloric acid secretion by the stomach. Dosage: 1 to 2 capsules at beginning of each meal. If causes burning sensation in the stomach, discontinue use. *Note:* Do not use with a history of gastric ulcers or gastritis. |

# Additional Recommendations

The EZ Care Program consists of basic remedies that are commonly used for heartburn and have been found to work well in most cases. The remedies are most effective when combined but can be used individually. The options stated below can supplement or replace EZ Care remedies and may be combined when suggested doses are followed.

## Diet

♦   **Drink** 6 to 8 glasses of pure water daily.

## Herbs

♦   **Gentian Root** (Gentiana lutea)  – Dosage: 1 to 2 capsules or 30-60 drops extract* in 4 oz. water two times daily 30 minutes before a meal.
    *Beneficial properties:* Tonic bitter; traditionally used to aid digestion and elimination and as a liver cleanser.
    *Note:* Extract may be preferable in this case, because actual perception of its bitter taste will enhance the body's response.

♦   **Ginger Root** (Zingiber officinalis) – Dosage: 6 oz. Ginger Tea prepared by infusion (see Appendix B) at end of meals or as required.

♦   **Meadowsweet** (Filipendula ulmaria) – Dosage: 6 oz. meadowsweet tea prepared by infusion (see Appendix B) 1 hour after meals or as required.

♦   **Slippery Elm** (Ulmus fulva) – Dosage: 1 to 2 capsules or 6 oz. tea prepared by decoction (see Appendix B), at end of meals.
    *Beneficial properties:* May soothe the stomach and assist in digestion.

## Homeopathy

See Appendix E for proper use and handling instruction prior to administering remedies described below.

♦   **Argentum Nitricum 6C** – Heartburn with white-coated tongue, flatulence, and constipation. Dosage: Dissolve 5 pellets under the tongue, every two hours until relief is obtained.

♦ **Capsicum 3C** – Heartburn with acid stomach and burning sensation. Dosage: Dissolve 5 pellets under the tongue, every 15 minutes until relief is obtained.

♦ **Lycopodium 12C** – Heartburn feels like fire rising from stomach to throat. Dosage: Dissolve 5 pellets under the tongue, every hour until relief is obtained.

## Miscellaneous

♦ **Lecithin Granules** – Dosage 1 tsp. with each meal. Lecithin aids in the absorption of fats, and also provides a source of phosphatidyl choline, which is essential for normal gastrointestinal function.

♦ **Breathing Exercises** – Following is a yoga breathing exercise that helps the body deal with stress: Inhale through the nose for a count of 4, hold for a count of 7, exhale through the mouth for a count of 8. Practice two times daily, four to eight repetitions each time.
*Note:* To enhance concentration and be certain the exercise is performed properly, you might lie down, place a lightweight book on your abdomen, then peacefully observe the book's rise-and-fall-motion as you breathe deeply.

♦ **Proteolytic Enzyme Formula** (including protease, bromelain, and papain) – May help with digestion of food. Take as directed on package.
*Note:* Avoid if stomach or duodenal ulcers; proteolytic enzymes may aggravate ulcers and induce bleeding.

♦ **Rolled Oats** – Dosage: 1 to 2 tsp. dry rolled oats. Chew well to help neutralize stomach acidity.

* Most herbal extracts contain alcohol. Avoid use if alcohol sensitive or if there is a history of alcohol abuse. *Note:* Alcohol content can be reduced through evaporation by adding extract to very hot water (just below boiling point) and allowing to stand 5 to 7 minutes before drinking.

# Hemorrhoids

Hemorrhoids occur when the veins in the rectum and anus swell and distend. At times, they may burst, causing bleeding. Some symptoms include rectal pain, bleeding, itching, and burning. The primary cause of the condition is straining during bowel movements, usually due to constipation. Other possible factors include lack of exercise, poor diet, prolonged sitting or standing, rectal surgery, and pregnancy.

Conventional treatments include icing affected area, warm sitz baths, anesthetic suppositories, and topical corticosteroids. Hemorrhoids also may be injected with a sclerosing solution, ligated with rubber bands, or surgically removed.

| EZ Care Program | |
|---|---|
| Diet | **Avoid** coffee, alcohol, tomatoes, peanuts, soda, sugar, spicy foods, and citrus fruit, because these may irritate hemorrhoids. |
| | **Drink 8 glasses of pure, room-temperature water** daily. |
| | Eat a **high-water-content** diet consisting of large quantities of fresh fruits and vegetables and comparatively smaller quantities of whole grains, legumes, seeds, nuts, fish, skinless chicken and turkey. Special emphasis on high fiber foods, such as raw cabbage, dark green, leafy vegetables, broccoli, apples, whole grains, and legumes. |
| | **Fiber Supplement** – Dosage: 1 to 3 tsp. Psyllium Husk fiber in 8 oz. pure water 1 to 2 times daily between meals. *Note:* Carefully read label; some brands require additional water. |
| Vitamins | **Bioflavonoids** – Dosage: 500 mg., two times daily taken with vitamin C. Supports collagen formation and elasticity of blood vessels. |
| | **C** (mineral ascorbates) – Dosage: 1,000 mg., three to four times daily with meals. May strengthen veins. |
| Herbs | **Butcher's Broom** (Ruscus aculeatus) – Dosage: 100 mg., three times daily. *Beneficial properties:* May help constrict blood vessels, reduce inflammation, and increase circulation. |
| | **Witch Hazel** (Hamamelis virginiana) and **Catnip** (Nepeta cataria) – Prepare a strong infusion (see Appendix B) using 1 tbsp. witch hazel bark and 1 tsp. catnip. Steep in 1 cup boiling water for 20 minutes. *For external hemorrhoids,* dip a small piece of cotton in this tea and bathe the affected area. *For internal hemorrhoids,* inject 2 tbsp. of the infusion rectally with a bulb syringe. The infusion should be administered after it has cooled, and should be retained as long as possible. *Beneficial properties:* May soothe and reduce inflammation, shrink swollen hemorrhoids, and reduce bleeding. *Note:* Avoid use on broken skin; may cause burning sensation. |
| Miscellaneous | **Address constipation**. Do not strain when having a bowel movement. Straining increases pressure on the veins of the rectal area, causing them to swell. |
| | **Aloe Vera Gel with Essential Oil of Cypress** (Cupressus semipervirens) – Dosage: A small amount of aloe gel mixed with 2 to 3 drops cypress oil. Apply to hemorrhoids two to three times daily; use a cotton swab to apply to internal hemorrhoids. *Beneficial properties:* May soothe discomfort and promote healing of tissue. |
| | **Avoid standing** for long periods of time. |
| | **Avoid** using **tobacco**. |
| | **Cool or Warm Sitz Baths** – May enhance circulation in rectal area and remove congestion from swollen hemorrhoidal tissue. Some cases respond better to cold, others to warmth. Whether the cool or warm sitz bath is preferable in a given case can be determined only by personal experimentation. *To perform:* Fill a tub with either cool (approx. 80°F) or warm (approx. 100°-105°F) water, high enough to cover the anus. Sit in tub 15 minutes. Repeat two to three times daily. |

| **EZ Care Program** | |
|---|---|
| | Exercise regularly to help tone the blood vessels, increase circulation, and prevent constipation. |
| | Consider purchasing a **doughnut seat cushion**. Use at work, home, and during travel. |

## Additional Recommendations

The EZ Care Program consists of basic remedies that are commonly used for hemorrhoids and have been found to work well in most cases. The remedies are most effective when combined but can be used individually. The options stated below can supplement or replace EZ Care remedies and may be combined when suggested doses are followed.

### Diet

♦ **Eat flavonoid-rich foods**, such as apricots, cherries, blackberries, blueberries, grapes, grapefruits, and lemons. Flavonoids exert antioxidant and anti-inflammatory effects.

### Vitamins

♦ **E** (natural d-alpha tocopherol in a base of mixed tocopherols) – Dosage: 800 IU daily with meals. Can also be useful for hemorrhoids when applied as a rectal suppository.

### Minerals

♦ **Calcium** (elemental calcium from amino acid chelate) – Dosage: 250 mg., two to three times daily with meals. Deficiency contributes to poor bowel tone and disposes to hemorrhagic disorders.

♦ **Magnesium** (elemental magnesium from amino acid chelate) – Dosage: 250 mg., two to three times daily with meals. Deficiency contributes to chronic constipation and poor bowel tone.

### Herbs

♦ **Collinsonia Root** (Collinsonia canadensis) – Dosage: 2 capsules or 30 drops extract* in 4 oz. water three times daily.
*Beneficial properties:* May help shrink hemorrhoid tissue.

♦ **Horse Chestnut** (Aesculus hippocastanum) – Dosage: 2 capsules or 30 drops extract* in 4 oz. water three times daily.
*Beneficial properties:* May help shrink hemorrhoid tissue.

♦ **White Oak Bark** (Quercus alba) – Dosage: Prepare an infusion using 2 tsp. white oak bark steeped in 1 cup boiling water for 30 minutes. Administer in same fashion as witch hazel/catnip infusion described above.

### Homeopathy

See Appendix E for proper use and handling instruction prior to administering remedies described below.

♦ **Aesculus Hip. 3X** – Hemorrhoids produce discomfort in rectum; low back pain with constipation; general absence of bleeding; worse when walking. Dosage: Dissolve 5 pellets under the tongue, three times daily.

♦ **Aloe 6C** – Prolapsed hemorrhoids that protrude like a bunch of grapes and produce heat, chafing, and soreness; feelings of insecurity in rectum; constipation. Dosage: Dissolve 5 pellets under the tongue, three times daily.

♦ **Hamamelis 6C** – Bleeding hemorrhoids with loose bowels. Dosage: Dissolve 5 pellets under the tongue, three times daily.

\* Most herbal extracts contain alcohol. Avoid use if alcohol sensitive or if there is a history of alcohol abuse. *Note:* Alcohol content can be reduced through evaporation by adding extract to very hot water (just below boiling point) and allowing to stand 5 to 7 minutes before drinking.

# High Blood Pressure (Hypertension)

High Blood Pressure is defined as three consecutive measurements of a blood pressure reading of 140/90 or above. The diagnosis can be made on elevation of either systolic (top number) or diastolic (bottom number) pressures. It is essential, when blood pressure readings are taken, that the patient sit in a comfortable chair and have the arm supported at the level of the heart. The person performing the blood pressure reading should insure proper fit of the cuff and slowly release the cuff pressure during examination to obtain an accurate reading. A variation from any of the above procedures could influence blood pressure readings by up to 10 mm Hg.

Regular doctor visits are important for treating this condition, because high blood pressure does not always have symptoms, yet nevertheless can be deadly. Although symptoms are rare, they include dizziness, blurred vision, nose bleeds, palpitations, confusion, blood in the urine, and headaches. High blood pressure can shorten lifespan by 10 to 20 years, so it is important not to let this problem go unchecked. Possible risk factors include family history, race, gender, emotional stress, sedentary lifestyle, aging, obesity, excessive alcohol consumption, tobacco use, high sodium diet, and kidney disease.

Conventional treatments include lifestyle and dietary changes, stress management, and exercise. Prescription medications also may be used, including diuretics, alpha-blockers, beta-blockers, calcium channel blockers, ACE inhibitors, and vasodilators.

*Note:* A change in diet, lifestyle, and supplementation could reduce or eliminate the level of medication needed and should be reviewed regularly with a healthcare professional. *Never discontinue any medications without consulting a healthcare professional.*

| EZ Care Program | |
|---|---|
| Diet | **Avoid** all stimulants, especially those that contain caffeine, including coffee and decaf, black tea, alcohol, soda, chocolate, and processed sugars. |
| | **Eat potassium-rich foods**, such as green vegetables, cantaloupe, avocado, prunes, raisins, millet, oats, watermelon, broccoli, bananas, fruit, dandelion greens, pumpkin, onions, raw goats' milk, and squash. |
| | **Eat generous amounts of raw garlic and onions**, which have antioxidant qualities to maintain normal blood pressure. |
| | **Eat fish**, such as mackerel, herring, trout, and salmon, because they contain the same omega-3 fatty acids that help protect the arteries and decrease resistance to blood flow. |
| | **Flaxseed oil** – Dosage: 1 to 2 tbsp. daily. Contains anti-inflammatory omega-3 fatty acids. |
| Minerals | **Magnesium** (elemental magnesium from amino acid chelate) –- Dosage: 500 to 1,000 mg. daily of elemental magnesium from amino acid chelate in divided doses with meals and at bedtime. Magnesium is an antispasmodic and essential for normal cardiac muscle function. Lowers blood pressure from dilation of blood vessels. Acts as a natural calcium channel blocker. |
| | **Garlic** (Allium sativum) – Dosage: 1 to 2 capsules per meal of standardized allicin garlic, or aged garlic extract. Fresh, raw garlic (a whole, living food) is preferable, but capsules should be considered if use of raw garlic is inconsistent. <br> *Beneficial properties:* May improve circulation, purify blood, reduce plaque in arteries and reduce high blood pressure. <br> *Garlic Note:* Raw parsley taken with raw garlic will help prevent "garlic breath" and enhance garlic's blood-cleansing effects. |
| Herbs | **Hawthorn leaves** (Crataegus oxycantha) – Dosage: 250 mg. of a standardized extract, three 3 times daily. <br> *Beneficial properties:* May strengthen the heart. |
| | **Avoid** all forms of **tobacco**, which is known to raise blood pressure and cause heart and lung disease. |

| EZ Care Program | |
| --- | --- |
| Miscellaneous | **Exercise** regularly, incorporating an aerobic exercise, such as walking 20 to 30 minutes daily. |
| | **Maintain** body weight within 5 to 10 pounds of your recommended weight. Obesity plays a major role in high blood pressure. Even reductions of 10-20% of current body weight is beneficial to lower blood pressure. |
| | **Reduce** lifestyle **stress** and implement a relaxation program. Harmonizing practices (e.g., such as biofeedback, meditation, yoga, and Tai Chi exercise) exercise may prove beneficial. |

## Additional Recommendations

The EZ Care Program consists of basic remedies that are commonly used for high blood pressure and have been found to work well in most cases. The remedies are most effective when combined but can be used individually. The options stated below can supplement or replace EZ Care remedies and may be combined when suggested doses are followed.

### Diet

◆ **Drink** the appropriate level of pure, room-temperature **water** as suggested by a healthcare practitioner. Water should be consumed upon arising and between meals.

◆ **Eat celery** regularly, because this may help eliminate fluid from the body.

◆ **Eat high fiber foods**, such as whole grains, legumes, broccoli, raw cabbage, and dark green, leafy vegetables.

◆ **Fiber Supplement** – Dosage: 1 to 3 tsp. psyllium husk fiber in 8 oz. pure water one to two times daily between meals.
*Note:* Carefully read the label; some brands require additional water.

◆ **Identify personal food sensitivities**. Avoid all common allergenic foods (e.g., dairy, eggs, wheat, corn, preservatives, sugar). Rotate moderately allergic foods on a four-day schedule (see Appendix C).

◆ **Limit or eliminate salt** intake; salt may increase blood pressure in salt-sensitive individuals. If salt is tolerated, use only an unrefined sea salt noted for containing an abundance of beneficial trace minerals.

### Vitamins

◆ **B complex** – Dosage: 50 mg. balanced B complex capsule. Helps support the nervous system.
*Note:* For highest assimilation, use a multi B complex which contains the vitamins in their coenzyme form and avoid mega-potency B complex products.

♦ **C** (mineral ascorbates mixed with bioflavonoids) – Dosage: 1,000 mg., three to four times daily with meals. Causes the release of nitric oxide, a natural blood vessel dilator.

## Herbs

♦ **Dandelion Leaf** (Taraxacum officinalis) – Dosage: 1 capsule or 30 drops extract* in 4 oz. water three times daily.
*Beneficial properties:* Traditionally used as a diuretic to help lower blood pressure and reduce fluid retention.
*Note:* The leaf is preferred over the root, because it acts as a much stronger diuretic.

♦ **Forskolin** (Coleus forskolii) – Dosage: 1 capsule, twice daily. Increases the production of C-GMP, allowing for blood vessel dilation.

♦ **Ginkgo Biloba** – Dosage: 1 to 2 capsules (40-80 mg.) 24% standardized extract or 30-60 drops extract* in 4 oz. water three times daily.
*Beneficial properties:* May improve general circulation and blood flow to the heart.

♦ **Mistletoe** (Viscum album) – Dosage: 1 to 2 capsules or 35 drops liquid extract* three to four times daily.
*Beneficial properties:* Traditionally used as an anti-hypertensive medicine.

♦ **Valerian Root** (Valeriana officinalis) – Dosage: 2 capsules or 30-60 drops liquid extract* in 4 oz. water two to three times daily.
*Beneficial properties:* Calms nerves and acts as a sedative. May be helpful if stress is a major factor in high blood pressure.

## Homeopathy

See Appendix E for proper use and handling instruction prior to administering remedies described below.

♦ **Aconite 6C** – High blood pressure with full, strong, hard pulse, anxiety, and restlessness. Dosage: Dissolve 5 pellets under the tongue, two times daily until symptoms subside.

♦ **Aurum Met 12C** – Suppressed anger or resentment, oversensitivity, roaring in head, dizziness, violent headaches, fear of death, hopelessness, despondency. Dosage: Dissolve 5 pellets under the tongue, one time daily until symptoms subside.

♦ **Belladonna 6C** – Violent palpitations, echoing sound in head, labored breathing. Dosage: Dissolve 5 pellets under the tongue, two times daily until symptoms subside.

♦ **Lachesis 12C** – Blood pressure worse on waking, feelings of restlessness, cannot bear tight clothing. Dosage: Dissolve 5 pellets under the tongue, two times daily until symptoms subside.

## Miscellaneous

♦ **Coenzyme Q-10** – Dosage: 100 mg., one to three times daily with meals.

♦ **L-Arginine** – Dosage: 1000 to 2000 mg. twice to three times daily, taken on an empty stomach or away from protein. L-Arginine supports cardiac function and causes the release of nitric oxide, a blood vessel dilator.
*Note:* Because L-arginine works via the nitric oxide pathway, do not use if taking long acting nitrate medications such as isosorbide dinitrate, nitroglycerine patches or if using nitroglycerine pills.

* Most herbal extracts contain alcohol. Avoid use if alcohol sensitive or if there is a history of alcohol abuse. *Note:* Alcohol content can be reduced through evaporation by adding extract to very hot water (just below boiling point) and allowing to stand 5 to 7 minutes before drinking.

# Hyperactivity and Attention Deficit Disorder

Attention Deficit Disorder (ADD) and Attention Deficit Hyperactivity Disorder (ADHD) are recently-defined disorders that pertain to the inability to focus on tasks that need to be done. The disorder has been focused mostly on children who experience problems with learning and behavior, often classified as learning disabled (LD); however, adults also are affected. Symptoms include lack of concentration, restlessness, temper tantrums, impulsivity, sleep disturbances, and behavior problems at school or work. Many people have more than one symptom.

Conventional treatments include a full medical evaluation and lab assay. The drug methylphenidate hydrochloride (Ritalin) is commonly used, as well as counseling and therapy. Ritalin has many documented side-effects and can be addictive. Dietary changes and behavior modification also may be useful in treating the disorder.

Many different factors are thought to contribute to the disorder, including heredity, problems during pregnancy, artificial food additives, antibiotic overuse and yeast overgrowth, food allergies, diet, environmental pollutants, and heavy metal toxicity. These causes can be fully evaluated by physicians specialized in holistic and environmental medicine.

| EZ Care Program | |
|---|---|
| Diet | **Avoid** processed sugar, white flour, pasta, cheese, milk, and wheat. Simple carbohydrates cause spikes in blood sugar, resulting in both hyperactivity and difficulty in concentration. |

| EZ Care Program | |
|---|---|
| | **Avoid** all preservatives, chemicals, additives, food coloring, and artificial flavors. |
| | **Avoid** stimulating foods, such as caffeine, chocolate, and soda. |
| | **Eat** a high-water-content diet consisting of large quantities of fresh fruits and vegetables and comparatively smaller quantities of whole grains, legumes, seeds, nuts, fish, skinless chicken and turkey. |
| | **Identify personal food sensitivities**. Avoid all common allergenic foods (e.g., dairy, eggs, wheat, corn, sugar, preservatives). Rotate moderately allergic foods on a four-day schedule (see Appendix C). |
| Minerals | **Calcium** (elemental calcium from amino acid chelate) – Dosage: 600 mg. daily in divided doses with meals and at bedtime. Essential for relaxing the nervous system. Considered a "lullaby" mineral. |
| | **Magnesium** (elemental magnesium from amino acid chelate) – Dosage: 400 mg. daily in divided doses with meals and at bedtime. Essential for relaxing the nervous system. Considered a "lullaby" mineral. |
| | **Zinc** (elemental zinc from amino acid chelate) (take only if over 14 years of age) – Dosage: 25 mg. taken with meals separately from calcium. Essential for proper brain functioning and the metabolism of essential fatty acids. |
| Herbs | **Evening Primrose Oil** (Oenothera biennis) – Dosage: 1300 mg., two times daily with meals. *Beneficial properties*: Contains gamma-linoleic acid (GLA), an essential fatty acid necessary for proper brain function. |
| | **Passion Flower** (Passiflora incarnata) + **Catnip** (Nepeta cataria) + **Chamomile** (Matricaria chamomilla) – Prepare a strong infusion (see Appendix B) using 1 part each of these three herbs. Do not sweeten. Serve 6 oz. three times daily between meals. *Beneficial properties:* May calm the nervous system. |
| Miscellaneous | **Review Homeopathy** section for appropriate remedies. |

# Additional Recommendations

The EZ Care Program consists of basic remedies that are commonly used for hyperactivity and ADD and have been found to work well in most cases. The remedies are most effective when combined but can be used individually. The options stated below can supplement or replace EZ Care remedies and may be combined when suggested doses are followed.

## Diet

♦ **Flaxseed Oil** – Dosage: for children ages two to five, 1/2 tbsp. daily; for children over age five, 1 tbsp. daily. Contains omega-3 fatty acids, which are needed for brain formation and function.

## Vitamins

♦ **B3** (niacin) – Available in 500 mg. as inositol nicotinate that does not cause uncomfortable flushing. Dosage: 2 times daily with meals.

*Note: Always work with a licensed healthcare professional before administering these supplements to children.* Always use both Niacin and B6 in conjunction with a complete 25 to 50 mg. B complex formula, because high doses of one of the B vitamins may lead to imbalance in the body's pool of the other B vitamins.

◆  **B6** (pyridoxal 5-phosphate is preferred) – Dosage: 25 mg. daily with meals.
*Note: Always work with a licensed healthcare professional before administering these supplements to children.* Always use both niacin and B6 in conjunction with a complete 25 to 50 mg. B complex formula, because high doses of one of the B vitamins may lead to imbalance in the body's pool of the other B vitamins.

◆  **C** (mixed mineral ascorbates) – Dosage: 500 mg., two times daily with meals. Helps in chelation of heavy metals and prevents oxidation of some crucial B complex vitamins.

◆  **GABA** (gamma-aminobutyric acid) 500 mg. twice daily. GABA is an inhibitory neurotransmitter, which has a calming effect.

◆  **Phosphatidylserine** (PS) – Dosage: 100 mg. daily. Phosphatidylserine, also containing phosphatidylcholine from lecithin, provides phospholipids that aid in cell to cell communication in the brain. Can help improve concentration.

## Herbs

**Note:** *Always consult a healthcare practitioner before administering any herbal remedies to children.*

◆  **Grape Seed Extract** *or* **Pine Bark Extract** (Pycnogenol) – Dosage: 25 mg., two times daily taken with vitamin C.
*Beneficial properties:* May help improve brain function and help body cope with allergies to chemical additives in foods.

◆  **Ginkgo Biloba** – Dosage: 40 mg. encapsulated 24% standardized extract one to two times daily between meals.
*Beneficial properties:* May improve general circulation and blood flow to the brain, and improve memory.

## Homeopathy

See Appendix E for proper use and handling instruction prior to administering remedies described below.

***Please note****:* Homeopathic prescribing is highly individual and usually requires the services of an experienced, professional homeopath. However, to provide some insight into the individualization of ADD cases, a few remedies frequently used to treat this disorder are described below.

◆  **Cina 30C** – Extremely irritable, cannot stand to be touched or looked at; child often pinches, scratches, or strikes parent when frustrated; this anger can lead to violent tantrums and even convulsions; child tends to be a "hard case" with no tolerance for being reprimanded by a parental authority; child grinds teeth during sleep and is often infested with parasites, especially pinworms. Dosage: Dissolve 5 pellets under the tongue, once weekly or monthly or as required.

♦ **Hyoscyamus 30C or 200C** – Poor control over impulses; talk, joke, or throw tantrums at most inappropriate times; prone to tremendous jealousy, often provoke fights; child must be watched carefully because capable of wreaking great harm on younger siblings; can be coldly malicious and detached; precocious sexual behavior, secretive sexual play, and exhibitionism; cursing is strongly characteristic, often for the sake of its shock value; play malicious practical jokes, shameless, always feel self is the injured party. Dosage: Dissolve 5 pellets under the tongue, once weekly or monthly or as required.

♦ **Nux Vomica 30C or 200C** – Over-excitable, rebellious, tend to throw temper tantrums at home and in public, vigorously resist any attempt at being restrained; great sensitivity to pain, touch, noise, odors, music, food, prescription drugs; tend to be a light sleeper, get angry at being wakened. Dosage: Dissolve 5 pellets under the tongue, once weekly or monthly or as required.

♦ **Stramonium 30C or 200C** – Prone to impulsive and uncontrolled rage without malicious forethought; troubles often begin after a strong fright, such as a car accident, violent attack, sexual abuse, or witnessing a very violent act; very strong fears, including water, death, and darkness; fear of being alone and of animals; often stammer and a dreamy, sleepy look; strong tendency to terror and, in some cases, religious fanaticism. Dosage: Dissolve 5 pellets under the tongue, once weekly or monthly or as required.

♦ **Tuberculinum 30C or 200C** – Restless, loud, demanding, and irrational; can be coldly malicious and deliberately destructive; a great intolerance of contradiction, tendency to strike others, indifference to reprimand and corporal punishment; often great obstinacy, ritualistic behavior, desire to travel, strong sense of unfulfillment, and fear of cats; may have a strong milk allergy, recurring upper respiratory infections, and eczema; child often has long, fine eyelashes, and is sexually hyperactive. Dosage: Dissolve 5 pellets under the tongue, once weekly or monthly or as required.

## Miscellaneous

♦ **Acetyl-L-Carnitine** – Dosage 500 mg. twice daily. Acetyl-L-carnitine, a derivative of carnitine, can assist with memory, and learning and speech abilities. Increases fatty acid transport into brain tissue.

♦ **Consider counseling** from a qualified professional.

♦ **Decrease** the amount of **stimulation** and provide a quiet place to study, as well as to calm the nerves.

♦ A professional should test for the following: **high levels of aluminum** or **lead** in the system, hearing and/or vision problems, learning disorder, and depression.

# Impotence

Impotence is the inability for a man to maintain a complete erection during sexual intercourse.  Causes of impotence include depression, decreased penile blood flow, often due to advanced diabetes, hormonal imbalance such as low testosterone, neurological injury, chronic kidney failure, vascular disease, prostate surgery or radiation, fatigue, anxiety, and stress. Alcohol, narcotics, and certain drugs such as many high blood-pressure medications also can cause impotence. If you are on any prescription medication, please review the side effects for it to see if that might be the cause of your symptoms.

Most cases are organic (physiological) in nature; however, men who have impotence from psychological reasons are still able to have spontaneous morning erections. Another method to distinguish between psychological and organic origins of impotence is the stamp test. To perform the stamp test, paste a ring of stamps around your penis prior to going to sleep. If the ring is broken in the morning, your problem may be psychological. Stress and anxiety management would be indicated.

Conventional treatments include a history, physical, nocturnal tumescence testing, and abnormal/psychological evaluation, as necessary. Therapy depends on the underlying cause. Pharmacological therapy with sildenafil citrate (Viagra) has been used successfully on many men; be cautious, however, because cardiovascular-related disease and death have occurred with use of this drug in some men. Careful cardiovascular screening by a physician is essential prior to the use of Viagra. Other treatments include prescription injections into the penis, and the use of surgically implantable pumps. These treatments can be discussed in full with a urologic surgeon.

| EZ Care Program | |
|---|---|
| Diet | **Avoid** all caffeine, soda, alcohol and sugar, because they may interfere with penile blood flow and may affect the nervous system, which are responsible for triggering the erection. |
| Herbs | **Ginkgo Biloba** – Dosage: 80 mg. encapsulated 24% standardized extract two to three times daily between meals. <br> *Beneficial properties:* May improve general circulation and penile blood flow. |
| | **Ginseng Root** (Panax ginseng) – Dosage: 1,000 mg. extract two times daily with meals. <br> *Beneficial properties:* A renowned energy and reproductive organ tonic. Also strengthens the body's stress mechanism. |
| | **Saw Palmetto Berry** (Serenoa repens) – Dosage: 160 mg. standardized |

| EZ Care Program | |
|---|---|
| | extract (standardized to contain 85% total fatty acids and 0.15% phyto-sterols) two times daily between meals. Can be taken at same time as ginkgo biloba.<br>*Beneficial properties:* May tone and improve genito-urinary function. |
| Homeopathy | **Yohimbinum 12C** – Use for impotency due to nervous exhaustion. Dosage: Dissolve 5 pellets under the tongue, two times daily for one week. Then use 5 pellets under the tongue, daily for two weeks. Thereafter, 5 pellets under the tongue, two to three times weekly or as required.<br>*Note:* Does not pose the risk of side effects as the herbal form. |
| Miscellaneous | **Avoid** all forms of **tobacco,** because it may interfere with penile blood flow. |
| | **L-Arginine** – Dosage 4000 to 6000 mg. used one-half hour before attempting intercourse. Causes the release of nitric oxide in blood vessels allowing for increased circulation. Do not use with a history of cardiovascular disease. At this dosage, hypotension (low blood pressure) is a possible side effect. For safety, start at lower doses and increase as tolerated. |
| | **Pumpkin Seed Oil** – Dosage: 1,000 mg., two times daily for two months.<br>*Beneficial properties:* May provide nutrients necessary for improved sexual function. |
| | **Reduce** lifestyle **stress** and implement a relaxation program. Harmonizing practices (e.g., biofeedback, meditation, yoga, Tai Chi exercise) may prove beneficial. |
| | **Regular exercise** supports blood circulation and tissue oxygenation. Exercises such as swimming, walking, Tai Chi exercise, and yoga should be considered. |

## Additional Recommendations

The EZ Care Program consists of basic remedies that are commonly used for impotence and have been found to work well in most cases. The remedies are most effective when combined but can be used individually. The options stated below can supplement or replace EZ Care remedies and may be combined when suggested doses are followed.

### Diet

♦ **Avoid** intake of **red meats**, **fried foods,** and **partially hydrogenated oils** (e.g., margarine)

♦ **Drink** 8 glasses of pure, room-temperature water daily.

♦ Eat a **high-water-content** diet consisting of large quantities of fresh fruits and vegetables and comparatively smaller quantities of whole grains, legumes, seeds, nuts, fish, skinless chicken and turkey.

♦ **Eat generous amounts of raw garlic and onions**, which aid in blood vessel dilation.

♦ **Eat fish**, such as mackerel, herring, trout, and salmon, because they contain omega-3 fatty acids that help protect the arteries and decrease resistance to blood flow.

♦ **Flaxseed Oil** – Dosage: 1 to 2 tbsp. daily. Contains anti-inflammatory omega-3 fatty acids.

## Vitamins

♦ **B6** (pyridoxal 5-phosphate is preferred) – Dosage: 25 mg. daily with meals. Can be helpful for impotence caused by minor nerve damage.
*Note:* Always use a 50 mg. complete B complex formula (preferably in coenzyme form) in addition to vitamin B6, because high doses of one of the B vitamins may lead to imbalance in the body's pool of the other B vitamins.

♦ **B12** – Dosage: 2,000 mcg. sublingual tablet two to three times weekly. Crucial for the vitality of both blood and nerves. Frequently deficient in older individuals.
*Note:* Always use a 25-50 mg. complete B complex formula (preferably in coenzyme form) in addition to vitamin B12, because high doses of one of the B vitamins may lead to imbalance in the body's pool of the other B vitamins.

♦ **C** (mixed mineral ascorbates) – Dosage: 1,000 mg., two times daily with meals. Plays a role in cholesterol metabolism and hormone synthesis. Also helps prevent oxidation of crucial B vitamins and vitamin E.

♦ **E** (natural d-alpha tocopherol in a base of mixed tocopherols) – Dosage: 600 IU two times daily with meals. Vitamin E prevents oxidation of both pituitary and adrenal hormones, and promotes proper functioning of essential fatty acids.

♦ **Tocotrienols** – Dosage: 200 – 800 IU divided twice daily. Tocotrienols are members of the vitamin E family and are found in rice bran oil. Tocotrienols inhibit the cholesterol forming enzyme HMG-CoA reductase, and may aid in plaque removal from arteries.

## Minerals

♦ **Zinc** (elemental zinc from amino acid chelate) – Dosage: 25 mg., two times daily with meals. Required for developing and maintaining the reproductive organs and crucial for a healthy prostate gland.

## Herbs

♦ **Hawthorn Leaf** (Crataegus oxyacantha) – Dosage: 500 mg. standardized extract two times daily with meals.
*Beneficial properties:* A cardiotonic that provides nutritional support for the proper functioning of the cardiovascular system. Helps improve blood circulation and has an anabolic (i.e., tissue building) effect on the metabolism.

♦ **Siberian Ginseng** (Eleutherococcus senticosus) – Dosage: 1,000 mg. capsule three times daily with meals.

*Beneficial properties*: Adaptogen (i.e., buffers the body's alarm reaction and builds up the body's ability to resist stress effects) which may help counteract a decrease of libido as a result of worry and stress.

## Aromatherapy

The following essential oils may prove useful in helping to alleviate impotence, especially if used in combination: **Jasmine** (Jasmine grandiflora), and **Sandalwood** (Santalum album). *Blend as follows:* 14 drops each of jasmine, and sandalwood; Mix 5 drops of the blend with 15 drops of sweet almond oil. After a cool sitz bath (see Appendix D), 1 time daily rub into abdomen just above pubic bone and into kidney region. Discontinue use if local skin irritation occurs. Also, consider dispersing scent into air during sexual intercourse; in this case, add 8 to 10 drops of undiluted blend to an aromatherapy diffuser.

## Homeopathy

See Appendix E for proper use and handling instruction prior to administering remedies described below.

♦ **Damiana 6X** – General impotence remedy. Dosage: Dissolve 5 pellets under the tongue, two times daily for one week. Then 5 pellets daily for two weeks. Thereafter, 5 pellets two to three times weekly or as required.

♦ **Lycopodium 1M** – For impotence of long-standing or old age. Dosage: Dissolve 5 pellets under the tongue, once every other month.

♦ **Nux Vomica 12C** – For impotence accompanied by general nervous depletion, irritability, digestive disorders, and constipation. Dosage: Dissolve 5 pellets under the tongue, two times daily for one week. Then 5 pellets daily for two weeks. Thereafter, 5 pellets two to three times weekly or as required.

## Miscellaneous

♦ **Coenzyme Q-10** – Dosage: 100 mg., two times daily with meals. An important factor in cardiovascular health and cellular production of energy.

♦ **Rescue Remedy** – A Bach flower remedy that may be helpful for emotional disturbances. Dosage: 5 drops under the tongue, three times daily. Hold drops in mouth for 1 minute before swallowing. For performance anxiety, take every 15 to 30 minutes until acute phase subsides.

*Note:* Because of toxicity and potential side-effects, the popular herbal remedy yohimbe is not recommended.

# Indigestion

Indigestion is a general term that describes complaints such as cramps, bloating, regurgitation, abdominal pain, belching and nausea. Possible causes are stress, deficiency of digestive enzymes, improperly chewed food, rushed eating, and food allergies. It could also be the underlying symptom of a more serious illness, such as an ulcer. If you suffer from chronic indigestion, seek medical advice.

Conventional treatments include a thorough evaluation of possible causes and the use of antacids, proton pump inhibitors and histamine antagonists to reduce stomach acids.

| EZ Care Program | |
|---|---|
| Diet | **Avoid** fried, spicy and salty foods, sugars, caffeine, alcohol, coffee, black tea, chocolate, cheese, and milk. |
| | **Eat** a high-water content diet consisting of large quantities of fresh fruits and vegetables and comparatively smaller quantities of whole grains, legumes, seeds, nuts, fish, skinless chicken, and turkey. |
| | **Identify personal food sensitivities.** Avoid all common allergenic foods (e.g., dairy, eggs, wheat, corn, preservatives, sugar) and rotate moderately allergic foods on a four-day schedule (see *Appendix C*). |
| Herbs | **Ginger Root** (Zingiber officinalis) - Dosage: 2 capsules or 4 oz. dried ginger root tea before each meal (see *Appendix B*; - Jamaican ginger root is preferred). For enhanced effect, add a pinch of cayenne to each serving. *Beneficial properties:* May aid digestion and reduce gas and bloating. |
| | **Peppermint Leaf** (Mentha piperita) - Take 1 cup of peppermint tea (see *Appendix B*) after each meal. *Beneficial properties:* May aid digestion and soothe the stomach. |
| Homeopathy | **Nat Phos 6X -** Use for acid, and rising sour taste in mouth, and trapped gas that is worse after eating; creamy yellow coating at the back of the tongue. Dosage: Dissolve 5 pellets under the tongue, every 30 minutes until symptoms subside. |
| Miscellaneous | **Avoid all forms of tobacco.** This can exacerbate indigestion. |
| | **Avoid stressful discussions, environments, television shows, etc., while eating.** Stress stimulates the "fight or flight" mechanism which, as part of the body's stress response, inhibits the process of digestion by shifting blood from the gut to the muscles and brain. |
| | **Eat slowly,** taking the time to chew your food at least 10 to 15 times per bite. Hasty eating and inadequate chewing are a primary cause of indigestion. Also, do not eat after 8 PM, or at least 2 hours before retiring. |
| | Review various **digestive aides** under the Miscellaneous section. |

# Additional Recommendations

The EZ Care Program consists of basic remedies that are commonly used for indigestion and have been found to work well in most cases. The remedies are most effective when combined, but can also be used individually. The options stated below can supplement or replace EZ Care remedies and may be combined when suggested doses are followed.

## Diet

♦ **Avoid** all preservatives, artificial sweeteners, colorings, and flavorings.

## Minerals

♦ **Calcium** (elemental calcium from amino acid chelate) - Dosage: 500 to 1,000 mg daily in divided doses with meals and at bedtime. Essential for the relaxation of the nervous system. Considered a "lullaby" mineral.

♦ **Magnesium** (elemental magnesium from amino acid chelate) - Dosage: 500 to 1,000 mg daily in divided doses with meals and at bedtime. Essential for the relaxation of the nervous system.

## Herbs

♦ **Chamomile Flowers** (Matricaria chamomilla) – Dosage: 6 oz. of tea three times daily between meals. *To prepare tea:* Place 1 heaping tsp. of herb in a non-aluminum cooking pot (preferably glass). Pour 8 oz. boiling pure water over the herb. Cover and steep for 20 minutes; strain and drink while warm.
*Beneficial properties:* May benefit stress-related indigestion. Antispasmodic and soothing to nerves.

♦ **Gentian Root** (Gentiana lutea) – Dosage: 2 capsules or 40 drops extract* in 4 oz. water three times daily just before eating.
*Beneficial properties:* Tonic bitter; traditionally used to stimulate production of digestive enzymes.
*Note:* Extract may be preferable in this case, because actual perception of its bitter taste will enhance the body's response.

♦ **Licorice Root** (Glycyrrhiza uralensis or glabra) – Dosage: 1 to 2 capsules or 40-50 drops liquid extract * before each meal.
*Beneficial properties:* May soothe and nourish the stomach.
*Note:* Avoid use if you have kidney or heart disease. If you have high blood pressure, consult a physician before using this herb, because it may elevate blood pressure by increasing water retention. Chinese (uralensis) and de-glycerinated licorice root (DGL) are less problematic in this regard than the western variety (glabra).

♦ **Dandelion Root** (Taraxacum officinalis) – Dosage: 2 capsules after breakfast and dinner.
*Beneficial properties:* May stimulate the liver and assist in digestion of fats
*Note:* Root is the preferred form because the leaf acts as more of a diuretic.

## Homeopathy

See Appendix E for proper use and handling instruction prior to administering remedies described below.

◆ **Arsenicum Album 12C** – Burning pain in stomach soon after eating; relieved by warm drinks. Dosage: Dissolve 5 pellets under the tongue, hourly until symptoms subside.

◆ **Carbo Vegetabalis 6C** – Pain and tenderness in pit of stomach 30 minutes after eating. Dosage: Dissolve 5 pellets under the tongue, hourly until symptoms subside.

◆ **Nux Vomica 12C** – Heartburn and gas from overindulgence in coffee, tobacco, and alcohol. Dosage: Dissolve 5 pellets under the tongue, hourly until symptoms diminish.

◆ **Pulsatilla 6C** – Bloating with sensation of having eaten too much and needing to loosen clothing; thickly coated, moist, white tongue; worse after eating fatty food; lack of thirst, and weepy. Dosage: Dissolve 5 pellets under the tongue, hourly until symptoms subside.

## Miscellaneous

◆ **Bile Salts and Whole Beet Concentrate** – May help with problems of fat digestion, especially if gallbladder surgically removed. Dosage: 1 to 2 tablets per meal or as required.

◆ **Do not overeat.** Choose foods wisely, and eat small portions. Overeating taxes the digestive system and reduces its efficiency.

◆ **Hydrochloric Acid and Pepsin** – Dosage: Begin with 1 tablet (700 mg. hydrochloric acid and 10 mg. pepsin) daily with meals. Increase dose to 2 tablets per meal. If a burning sensation in the stomach occurs, reduce the dosage. Aids in the complete breakdown of foods.
*Note:* Very useful in cases of low stomach acid (hypochlorhydria). This condition is frequently mistaken for excess gastric acidity; however, the acidity is due to acid fermentation resulting from poor digestion and increased time of acid excretion due to diminished potency.

◆ **Probiotic Culture** (friendly intestinal bacteria that aid digestion, nutrient assimilation, and toxin elimination) (L. acidophilus with bifidobacteria, powder or capsules) – Dosage: according to directions on label.

◆ **Proteolytic Enzyme Formula** (including protease, bromelain, and papain) – May aid digestion. Dosage: according to directions on label. A combination of plant enzymes and glandular extracts is preferred for maximal potency.

◆ **Unfiltered Apple Cider Vinegar** – Dosage: 2 drops apple cider vinegar in 1 tbsp. pure water 5 minutes before eating. Hold in the mouth 15 seconds, then swallow. Increases salivary flow and secretion of digestive fluids in stomach.

\* Most herbal extracts contain alcohol. Avoid use if alcohol sensitive or if there is a history of alcohol abuse. *Note:* Alcohol content can be reduced through evaporation by adding extract to very hot water (just below boiling point) and allowing to stand 5 to 7 minutes before drinking.

# Insomnia

Insomnia is defined as either difficulty falling asleep, or frequent waking with difficulty falling back asleep. It also can be a combination of the two. The quality of sleep is restless and unsatisfying. Causes include anxiety, tension, noise, emotions, sleep phobia, sleep apnea, restless legs syndrome, hypoglycemia, depression, side effects from medications, pain, stimulant use, or alcohol ingestion. Insomnia also can occur from nutritional deficiencies.

Conventional treatments include sleep medications (both prescription and over-the-counter), counseling, evaluation by a sleep clinic, and the use of CPAP (continuous positive airway pressure) machines for obstructive sleep apnea. Careful reviewing of medication also is standard protocol.

| EZ Care Program | |
|---|---|
| Diet | **Avoid** alcohol. |
| | **Avoid** all stimulants, especially those with caffeine, including coffee and decaf, black tea, soda, and chocolate. |
| | **Do not skip dinner.** While low blood sugar causes fatigue, the brain requires adequate blood sugar to produce normal sleep. |
| | **Eat judiciously at dinner**. Avoid overeating and avoid rich, difficult-to-digest foods. Indigestion is a common cause of sleeplessness. |
| Vitamins | **B complex** – Dosage: 100 mg., daily with meals. Helps the body cope with stress. *Note:* For highest assimilation, use a multi B complex which contains the vitamins in their coenzyme form and avoid mega-potency B complex products. |
| Minerals | **Calcium** (elemental calcium from amino acid chelate) – Dosage: 1,000 mg. at bedtime. Essential for relaxing the nervous system. Considered a "lullaby" mineral. |
| | **Magnesium** (elemental magnesium from amino acid chelate) – Dosage: 1,000 mg. at bedtime. Essential for relaxing the nervous system. |
| Herbs | **See Herbs** section below for appropriate remedy. |
| Miscellaneous | **Avoid working late** and going directly to bed. Allow at least 1 hour before bed for the mind to relax. |
| | **Avoid watching** frightening, violent, or otherwise disturbing television programs in the evening. |

| | |
|---|---|
| **EZ Care Program** ||

| | |
|---|---|
| | **Exercise regularly,** including 20 to 30 minutes of aerobic exercise. *Note:* Make sure all exercise is completed at least two hours before bedtime. |
| | **Incorporate skilled relaxation**, such as deep breathing, meditation, and visualization into daily routine. Can be very helpful in calming the mind and relaxing the body. Soothing music also may help. |
| | **L-5HTP** (5-hydroxytryptophan) – Dosage: 100 mg. at bedtime. L-5HTP stimulates the production of serotonin, and is useful for insomnia caused by anxiety. |
| | **Melatonin** – Dosage: .5 - 3 mg., 30 minutes before bed. A natural hormone produced in the brain to help with sleep and reset the body's internal clock. Not recommended for patients under age 30. |

# Additional Recommendations

The EZ Care Program consists of basic remedies that are commonly used for insomnia and have been found to work well in most cases. The remedies are most effective when combined, but can be used individually. The options stated below can supplement or replace EZ Care remedies and may be combined when suggested doses are followed.

## Diet

♦ **Eat** foods high in **tryptophan**, such as bananas, walnuts, pineapple, and turkey. May induce feelings of sleepiness.

♦ **Eat** a dinner consisting primarily of steamed and raw vegetables, complex carbohydrates like brown rice, millet, or baked potato, and a smaller amount of a vegetable protein food such as lentils or tofu. Avoid a dinner consisting primarily of animal protein like red meat or chicken. Protein foods, especially those derived from animal sources, are stimulating; whereas, complex carbohydrates tend to cause comfortable satiation and relaxation.

## Vitamins

♦ **B6** (pyridoxal 5-phosphate is preferred) – Dosage: 25 to 50 mg. daily with breakfast. *Note:* Always use a *complete B complex formula* in addition to vitamin B6, because high doses of one of the B vitamins can lead to imbalance in the body's pool of the other B vitamins.

♦ **B complex** – Dosage: 25 to 50 mg. Daily with a meal. *Note*: For highest assimilation, use a multi B complex which contains the vitamins in their coenzyme form and avoid mega-potency B complex products.

## Herbs

♦ **Chamomile Flowers** (Matricaria recutita) – Dosage: 4 to 8 oz. of tea 30 minutes before bedtime. Also, 1/2 tsp. raw honey can be added to enhance sleep-aid effect. *Beneficial properties:* Soothes nerves (see Appendix B).

*Note:* Chamomile is best suited for people who are prone to irritability and restlessness. Chamomile is safe for usage in children.

♦   **Hops** (Humulus lupus) – Dosage: 50 drops liquid extract* in 4 oz. water 30 minutes before bedtime.
    *Beneficial properties:* Of particular benefit for insomnia due to poor digestion, or agitation due to excessive sexual excitement. Can be used in combination with valerian root.
    *Note:* In Europe, sleeping on a small pillow stuffed with dried hops is a well-known folk remedy for insomnia.

♦   **Kava Kava** (Piper methysticum) – Dosage: 2 capsules standardized extract or 30 drops liquid extract* in 4 oz. water 30 minutes before bedtime. A good combination with oat seed extract.
    *Beneficial properties:* Significant relaxant properties. May benefit an overactive mind.

♦   **Oats** (Avena sativa) – Dosage: 50 drops liquid extract* of oat seeds in 4 oz. warm water 30 minutes before bedtime. A good combination with kava kava.
    *Beneficial properties:* A gentle nervine tonic useful for insomnia due to mental overactivity, or preoccupation with worries and responsibilities.

♦   **Valerian Root** (Valeriana officinalis) – Dosage: 2 capsules or 30-60 drops liquid extract* in 4 oz. water 30 minutes before bedtime.
    *Beneficial properties:* Sedative and sleep aid. Traditionally used for excitability, nervous tension, and insomnia.

## Aromatherapy

Essential oils that may prove of value for sleeplessness in people prone to fears or fearful dreams at night and/or who waken from the slightest noise: **Melissa** (Melissa officinalis) or **Lavender** (lavendula vera)

Essential oils that may prove of value for sleeplessness in people who are physically underactive, chronically fatigued and enervated, yet prone to mental overactivity and preoccupation with worries and responsibilities: **Neroli** (Citrus aurantium- flowers), and **Lavender** (Lavendula vera)

In either case, use each of the essential oils listed. Dosage: mix 5 drops of each with 18 drops sweet almond oil. At bedtime, rub into chest, throat, and inside surface of forearms. Also, 3 drops each of the essential oils selected can be added to an aromatherapy diffuser, and dispersed into the air throughout the night.

## Homeopathy

See Appendix E for proper use and handling instruction prior to administering remedies described below.

- **Argentum Nitricum 6C** – Perpetually agitated, particularly before bedtime; tend to act hurriedly, impulsively; driven; prone to frightening dreams; difficulty falling asleep if room too warm. Dosage: Dissolve 5 pellets under the tongue, in the evening or as required.

- **Chamomilla 6X** – Difficulty falling asleep due to irritability or pain. Dosage: Dissolve 5 pellets under the tongue, 30 minutes before bedtime and hourly thereafter or as required.

- **Coffea 12C** – Wide-awake, unable to close eyes due to physical excitement over happiness, pleasant surprise, prolonged anticipation or waiting. Dosage: Dissolve 5 pellets under the tongue, 30 minutes before bedtime and every two hours thereafter or as required.

- **Nux Vomica 12C** – Sleeplessness due to alcohol, coffee, black tea, tobacco, prescription medication, or rich food; worried and irritable, dream about work or quarrels, sensitive to and irritated by slightest noise, wake at three a.m. to four a.m., difficulty falling back asleep. Dosage: Dissolve 5 pellets under the tongue, one to two times daily or as required.

### Miscellaneous

- **Neutral Bath** – Quiets sensory nerves and, thus, is quite sedative. Very useful before sleep for hypersensitive, light sleeper. Water and skin approximately equivalent temperature

* Most herbal extracts contain alcohol. Avoid use if alcohol sensitive or if there is a history of alcohol abuse. *Note:* Alcohol content can be reduced through evaporation by adding extract to very hot water (just below boiling point) and allowing to stand 5 to 7 minutes before drinking.

# Irritable Bowel Syndrome (IBS)

Irritable bowel syndrome presents most commonly with abdominal pain, alternating constipation and diarrhea, mucus in stools, bloating, and cramping. An individual may display one or more of these symptoms. Stress and anxiety often exacerbate this condition, but are seldom the primary cause. Possible causes include food sensitivities, antibiotic use, bowel flora imbalances, intestinal infections, alcohol use, and gluten intolerance.

Conventional treatments include stress management, altering diet and lifestyle, psychological counseling, fecal softening agents, and antispasmodic drugs. Holistic-oriented physicians may recommend specialized stool studies, evaluating for bacterial and yeast overgrowth, in conjunction with food allergy testing, and intestinal permeability studies.

*Special note:* If you have been on numerous antibiotics in the past, a yeast overgrowth is likely to contribute to IBS. Please see section on candidiasis for remedies to combat yeast overgrowth.

| EZ Care Program | |
|---|---|
| Diet | **Chew food slowly, and very well.** Hasty eating and inadequate chewing are primary causes of indigestion. |
| | **Do not overeat.** Be judicious regarding food selection and quantity. |
| | **Drink** 6 to 8 glasses of pure water daily. |
| | **Eliminate** coffee and decaf, caffeine, alcohol, artificial sweeteners, and refined sugars, because they may irritate the digestive tract. |
| | **Fiber Supplement** – Dosage: 1 to 3 tsp. Psyllium Husk fiber in 8 oz. pure water one to two times daily between meals. *Note:* Carefully read label; some brands require additional water. |
| | **Identify personal food sensitivities.** Avoid all common allergenic foods (e.g., dairy, eggs, wheat, corn, sugar, preservatives). Rotate moderately allergic foods on a four-day schedule (see Appendix C). Food allergy testing is paramount to discover cause of IBS. |
| Herbs | **Chamomile Flowers** (Matricaria recutita) – Dosage: 4 to 8 oz. of tea several times daily. *Beneficial properties:* Soothes nerves. Beneficial when IBS is stress-related (see Appendix B). |
| | **Ginger Root** (Zingiber officinalis) – Dosage: 2 capsules three times daily, or 6 to 8 oz. dried ginger root tea before each meal (see Appendix B; Jamaican ginger root is preferred). For enhanced effect, add a pinch of cayenne to each serving. *Beneficial properties:* May aid digestion; may reduce gas and bloating. |
| | **Peppermint Oil** (enteric coated capsules) – Dosage: two 0.2 ml. capsules two to three times daily between meals. *Beneficial properties:* Soothes bowel; may aid in digestion and reduce spasm and gas in intestine. *Note:* It is important that these capsules be *enteric-coated*, because this prevents the oil from being released in the stomach. For the active compounds in peppermint oil to benefit symptoms of IBS, they must be released in the colon. |
| Miscellaneous | **Avoid stressful discussions, environments, television shows, etc., while eating.** Stress stimulates the "fight or flight" mechanism, which as part of the body's stress response, inhibits digestion by shifting blood from the gut to the muscles and brain. Also, overstimulation of the stress response can induce gastrointestinal spasms. |
| | **Avoid** all forms of **tobacco**, because it may irritate the bowels. |
| | **Butyrate** (calcium and magnesium butyrate in 2:1 ratio) – Dosage: 300 to 600 mg., two to three times daily with meals. A short-chain fatty acid that maintains the structure and function of the mucosal cells of the colon. |

| EZ Care Program | |
| --- | --- |
| | **Lactobacillus Probiotic** (friendly intestinal bacteria that aid digestion, nutrient assimilation, and toxin elimination) (L. acidophilus with bifidobacteria) – Dosage: according to directions on label. Keep refrigerated. |
| | **L-Glutamine** – Dosage: 1,000 to 2,000 mg., two times daily for one to two months; then adjust accordingly. An amino acid that is a major energy source for intestinal cells. It carries potentially toxic ammonia to the kidneys for excretion. The gastrointestinal tract uses very large amounts of glutamine during times of stress and inflammatory bowel conditions. |
| | **Proteolytic Enzyme Formula** (protein digesting enzyme that includes protease, bromelain, and papain) – Dosage: Take as directed on package. *Note:* Avoid if stomach or duodenal ulcers are present; proteolytic enzymes may aggravate ulcers and induce bleeding. |

## Additional Recommendations

The EZ Care Program consists of basic remedies that are commonly used for irritable bowel and have been found to work well in most cases. The remedies are most effective when combined, but can be used individually. The options stated below can supplement or replace EZ Care remedies and may be combined when suggested doses are followed.

### Diet

♦ A three-day **vegetable juice fast** is often helpful. It is preferable to work with a physician when doing a fast.

♦ **Eat high fiber foods**, such as whole grains, legumes, broccoli, raw cabbage, and dark green, leafy vegetables.

♦ **Flaxseed Oil** – Dosage: 1 to 2 tbsp. daily. Contains anti-inflammatory omega-3 fatty acids that help promote a healthy colon.

### Vitamins

♦ **A** (natural, from fish liver oil) – Dosage: 10,000 to 25,000 IU daily with meals. May have beneficial effect on lining of intestinal tract.
*Note:* Consult a physician before using higher doses of vitamin A. Avoid use if pregnant. Discontinue use if nausea, dry skin, sore lips, blurred vision, or other signs of vitamin A toxicity are experienced.

♦ **B complex** – Dosage: 50 mg. balanced B complex capsule. May help the body handle stress.
*Note:* For highest assimilation, use a multi B complex which contains some of the vitamins in their coenzyme form and avoid mega-potency B complex products.

♦ **E** (natural d-alpha tocopherol in a base of mixed tocopherols) – Dosage: 800 IU daily with a meal.

## Minerals

♦ **Zinc** (take only if over 14 years of age) – Dosage: 50 mg. elemental zinc from amino acid chelate with meals.
*Note:* Zinc and vitamin A are synergistic and work well together in this context.

## Herbs

♦ **Gentian Root** (Gentiana lutea) – Dosage: 1 to 2 capsules or 30-60 drops extract* in 4 oz. water before each meal.
*Beneficial properties:* Tonic bitter; traditionally used to aid digestion and elimination.
*Note:* Extract may be preferable in this case, because actual perception of its bitter taste will enhance the body's response.

## Homeopathy

See Appendix E for proper use and handling instruction prior to administering remedies described below.

♦ **Argentum Nitricum 30C** – Warm-blooded, impulsive, anxious, hurried, highly emotional; rumbling and flatulence; loud explosive belching; flatulence worse from sugar and in the morning; passing flatus does not relieve distention; noisy diarrhea that is worse from drinking water and eating sweets; fluids "go right through"; diarrhea before a panic attack or from nervous anticipation; offensive-smelling stool, like chopped green spinach with shreds of mucus. Dissolve 5 pellets under the tongue, once weekly or every two weeks, or monthly, as required.

♦ **Colocynthis 30C** – Pent-up emotions, especially anger or grief; abdominal pains relieved by pressure, bending double, and by lying face down; severe cutting and cramping pains in abdomen often centered around the navel (sometimes radiating to pubic region), worsened or triggered by anger, indignation, excitement; intestinal colic, with cramps in calves; pain worse before diarrhea and from drinking; diarrhea and cramping worse from eating, especially fruit, and from strong emotions; diarrhea relieved by drinking coffee; jelly-like stools that may have a musty odor. Dissolve 5 pellets under the tongue, once or twice weekly or once every two weeks, or monthly, as required.

♦ **Lycopodium 30C** – Marked feelings of inferiority; extreme lack of self-confidence, yet compensate with haughtiness; loud rumbling in abdomen, with bloating and distention, better with belching and passing flatus, worse when even a small amount of food is eaten; stool hard, difficult, small, incomplete, or begins hard and difficult to pass, and then becomes soft or loose; symptoms worse when eating oysters, onion family, or cabbage family vegetables; crave sweets; worse with cold drinks; symptoms may worsen between four p.m. and eight p.m. Dissolve 5 pellets under the tongue, once weekly or every two weeks, or monthly, or as required.

♦ **Nat. Carb 30C** – Gentle, refined, dignified, unselfish, devoted; weak digestion and extensive food sensitivities; pronounced intolerance of dairy foods, which give rise to great flatus and diarrhea; sudden urging for stool; stool shoots out like a torrent; sputtering diarrhea with much gas; chronic belching and heartburn; aversion to milk;

crave potatoes. Dissolve 5 pellets under the tongue, once weekly or every two weeks, or monthly, as required.

◆ **Nux Vomica 30C** – Ambitious, independent, type "A" personality; crave spicy and fatty foods, alcohol, and coffee; constipation with constant, ineffectual urging for stool; constipation from sedentary habits; pass small amount of stool which provides temporary relief, however, urging returns shortly thereafter; constant uneasiness in rectum; diarrhea alternating with constipation; diarrhea worse when cold and with alcohol, better with warmth of bed. Dissolve 5 pellets under the tongue, once weekly or every two weeks, or monthly, as required.

## Miscellaneous

◆ **Bile Salts and Whole Beet Concentrate** – May prove of value with fat digestion problems, especially if gallbladder surgically removed. Dosage: 1 to 2 tablets per meal or as required.

◆ **Cold Sitz Bath** – Morning, 3 to 5 times weekly upon arising (see Appendix D for details). Be sure to rub the abdomen vigorously with the cold water. Always rub in a clockwise direction (right to left).

◆ **Fructo-oligosaccharides** (FOS) – A natural carbohydrate that helps provide the proper growth medium for beneficial intestinal bacteria like Lactobacillus. Dosage: 1 gram one to two times daily in water, or sprinkled on food as desired.

◆ **Hydrochloric Acid and Pepsin** – Very useful in cases of hypochlorhydria (low stomach acid). Hypochlorhydria is frequently mistaken for excess gastric acidity; however, the acidity is often due to acid fermentation resulting from poor digestion and increased time of acid secretion due to diminished potency. Dosage: Begin with 1 tablet (700 mg. hydrochloric acid and 10 mg. pepsin) daily with a meal. Increase up to 1 to 2 tablets per meal, as long as burning sensation in stomach is not experienced, in which case reduce dosage.

◆ **N-Acetyl-D-Glucosamine** – Dosage: 250 to 500 mg., two to three times daily with meals. A type of glycosaminoglycan, which are substances that build and maintain the matrix of connective tissue, and form the protective mucous secreted by intestinal cells.

◆ **Reduce** lifestyle **stress** and implement a relaxation program. Harmonizing practices (e.g., biofeedback, meditation, yoga, Tai Chi exercise) may prove beneficial.

◆ **Sialic Acid** – Dosage: 500 mg., three times daily with meals. A proteoglycan extracted from mucin, the chief constituent of protective mucous.

\* Most herbal extracts contain alcohol. Avoid use if alcohol sensitive or if there is a history of alcohol abuse. *Note:* Alcohol content can be reduced through evaporation by adding extract to very hot water (just below boiling point) and allowing to stand 5 to 7 minutes before drinking.

# Jet Lag

Jet lag is fatigue that occurs after traveling across time zones. It is also partially due to the stress of airline travel.

Conventional treatment includes rest, adequate fluid intake, and analgesics such as aspirin or ibuprofen if headache occurs.

| EZ Care Program | |
|---|---|
| Diet | **Avoid** all coffee, soda, salty foods, and alcohol, because they may increase dehydration. |
| | **Maintain** adequate **water intake** by consuming 8oz. of bottled water every two hours while flying to prevent dehydration. |
| Herbs | **Siberian Ginseng** (Eleutherococcus senticosus) – Dosage: 250 mg. standardized extract or 30 drops extract* in 4 oz. water three times daily. Begin taking at least 4 days prior to flight and continue 5 days after flight.<br>*Beneficial properties:* Traditionally used to support the adrenal (stress) glands. |
| Homeopathy | **Arnica 12C** – Most commonly used homeopathic remedy for jet lag. Dosage: Dissolve 5 pellets under the tongue, 2 times daily for two days prior to flight, 3 times on day of flight, and 2 times daily for two days after flight. |
| Miscellaneous | **Consider using a "personal air purifier"** (see Resource Guide). This small (about 2/3 the size of a pack of playing cards) battery powered, air purifier is worn about the neck like a pendant. It produces a continuous flow of pure air past the nose and mouth and offsets the deleterious effects of recirculated, chemical-laden air found in airplanes. Commonly recommended by allergists to patients with environmental allergies. |
| | **Melatonin** – Dosage: 3 mg., 30 minutes before bedtime for as long as required. A natural hormone produced in the brain that helps with sleep and resets the circadium rhythm. |
| | Consider remedies from the **Aromatherapy** section below. |

## Additional Recommendations

The EZ Care Program consists of basic remedies that are commonly used for jet lag and have been found to work well in most cases. The remedies are most effective when combined, but can be used individually. The options stated below can supplement or replace EZ Care remedies and may be combined when suggested doses are followed.

### Vitamins

♦ **B complex** – Dosage: 50 mg. balanced B complex capsule to help the body cope with the stress of flying.
*Note:* For highest assimilation, use a multi B complex which contains the vitamins in their coenzyme form and avoid mega-potency B complex products.

♦ **C** (mineral ascorbate mixed with bioflavonoids) – Dosage: 1,000 mg., three to four times daily with meals. May strengthen immune system to resist effects of exposure to airborne germs circulating in an airplane.

### Herbs

♦ **Echinacea** (Echinacea purpurea) – Dosage: 2 to 4 capsules or 50 drops liquid extract* three times daily. Begin treatment one week prior to flight, and continue for one week after.
*Beneficial properties:* May strengthen immune system to resist effects of exposure to the airborne germs circulating in an airplane.

### Aromatherapy

Take 9 drops of the essential oil of **ginger** (Zingiber officinalis). Mix with 48 drops sweet almond oil. For 2 days prior to flight, rub a small amount of this blend into chest, inside of arms, neck, throat, and temples two times daily (*avoid getting into eyes*). During flight, tap 3 drops of the undiluted oil (i.e., without sweet almond oil) into the palm of a hand. Rub palms together, then breathe in deeply from cupped palms 10 to 15 times, turning head to side as exhale. Repeat every 2 to 3 hours during the flight.

### Homeopathy

See Appendix E for proper use and handling instruction prior to administering remedies described below.

♦ **Cocculus 12C** – Feeling spacey, confused, or dizzy as a result of jet lag. Dosage: Dissolve 5 pellets two to three times daily or as required.

♦ **Gelsemium 12C** – Feeling anxious, nervous, exhausted, and shaky as a result of jet lag. Dosage: Dissolve 5 pellets two to three times daily or as required.

### Miscellaneous

♦ **Consider using a "light box."** When used properly, this compact source of bright light can help reset the body's circadium rhythm when traveling across time zones. Dosage: according to manufacturer's recommendations.

♦ **Rescue Remedy** – A Bach flower remedy that may be helpful for stressful situations. Dosage: 5 drops under the tongue, three times daily. Hold the drops in the mouth for 1 minute before swallowing. During stressful situations like flying, can take every 15 to 30 minutes until stressful situation ends.

* Most herbal extracts contain alcohol. Avoid use if alcohol sensitive or if there is a history of alcohol abuse. *Note:* Alcohol content can be reduced through evaporation by adding extract to very hot water (just below boiling point) and allowing to stand 5 to 7 minutes before drinking.

# Kidney Stones

Kidney stones are most commonly caused by a buildup of either calcium phosphates, oxalates, or uric acid. Prevention of stones is much easier than actual treatment. The treatment of active stones should be under a physician's supervision. There are several factors involved with the formation of stones: dehydration, use of diuretic substances like coffee, refined carbohydrates, and an increase in calcium loss due to eating acid-forming foods (not necessarily acidic foods). Kidney stones can cause back and flank pain, blood in the urine, and infection. They require medical attention for early evaluation.

Conventional treatments include adequate oral and sometimes intravenous hydration as well as antibiotics and even surgery with vascular stents for severe cases. The patient is required to strain the urine and collect the stones that pass, because treatment guidelines vary with the composition of stones (calcium or uric acid). Analgesics such as acetaminophen (Tylenol) or ibuprofen may be recommended, because these attacks can be quite painful.

| EZ Care Program | |
|---|---|
| Diet | **Avoid foods high in purine and oxalates**, including dairy products, beans (legumes), cocoa, parsley, red beet tops, tomato, nuts, rhubarb, spinach, and black tea. |
| | **Add** 1 tbsp. **unfiltered apple cider vinegar** to raw vegetable salads. |
| | **Drink** 2 to 4 glasses unsweetened **cranberry juice** daily. May help kidney and urinary tract inflammations. If it is not palatable, take 500 mg. of an encapsulated cranberry concentrate three times daily. |
| | **Eliminate** sugar, white flour, soda, alcohol, coffee, caffeine, chocolate, and junk food. |
| | **Reduce or eliminate intake of meat and other animal foods**. Vegetarians have a decreased risk of developing kidney stones. Reduction of protein intake while increasing consumption of fresh fruits and vegetables may help prevent kidney stone formation. |
| Vitamins | **B6** (pyridoxal 5-phosphate is preferred) – Dosage: 50 mg. daily with morning meal. May reduce production and urinary excretion of oxalate stones. *Note:* Always use B6 in conjunction with a complete B complex formula, because high doses of one of the B vitamins may lead to imbalance in other B vitamins. |

| EZ Care Program | |
|---|---|
| Minerals | **Magnesium** (elemental magnesium from amino acid chelate or magnesium citrate) – Dosage: 200 mg., three to four times daily with meals and at bedtime. May inhibit calcium oxalate stone formation. |
| Miscellaneous | **Review Homeopathy** and **Miscellaneous** sections below for appropriate remedies. |

# Additional Recommendations

The EZ Care Program consists of basic remedies that are commonly used for kidney stones and have been found to work well in most cases. The remedies are most effective when combined, but can be used individually. The options stated below can supplement or replace EZ Care remedies and may be combined when suggested doses are followed.

## Diet

♦ **Drink** 8 glasses of pure, room-temperature **water** daily. This may help flush current stones and prevent the formation of new ones.

## Vitamins

♦ **A** (from fish liver oil) – Dosage: 25,000 IU daily with meals. Deficiency may contribute to the development of kidney stones.
   **Note:** Consult a physician before using higher doses of vitamin A. Avoid use if pregnant. Discontinue use if it nausea, dry skin, sore lips, blurred vision, or other signs of vitamin A toxicity are experienced.

♦ **C** (mineral ascorbate mixed with bioflavonoids) – Dosage: 1,000 mg., three to four times daily with meals. Vitamin C increases uric acid excretion. Although thought in conventional circles to cause kidney stones, numerous studies have proven otherwise. Vitamin C deficiency also may contribute to developing kidney stones.

## Minerals

♦ **Potassium Citrate** – Dosage: 100 to 200 mg. daily. May help prevent kidney stone recurrence because some people who are prone to stones have abnormally low levels of citrate in the urine.

♦ **Restrict Calcium supplementation** in the diet. Avoid calcium carbonate and other non-chelated forms of calcium.

♦ **Zinc** (take only if over 14 years of age) – Dosage: 50 mg. elemental zinc from amino acid chelate with meals for two months. May help prevent formation of stones in the urine.

## Herbs

♦ **Bearberry or Uva ursi** (Arctostaphylos uva ursi) – Dosage: 2 capsules three times daily. *Beneficial properties:* Traditionally used as an antiseptic for the urinary tract.

♦ **Rose Hips (Rosa canina)** – Dosage: 8 to 12 oz. warm tea (see Appendix B) daily in divided amounts between meals.
*Beneficial properties:* May reduce formation of kidney stones.

♦ **Valerian Root** (Valeriana officinalis) – Dosage: 4 to 8 oz. warm tea three to four times daily or hourly, as required until pain is relieved. To enhance the effects, combine with equal parts of **peppermint leaves** (Mentha piperita) and **carrot seeds** (Daucus carota).
*Beneficial properties:* May exert antispasmodic effect that can help relieve acute pain during passage of kidney stones. Dosage: 1-1/2 heaping tsp. valerian *or* 1/2 tsp. each of the 3 above mentioned herbs together (see Appendix B).

## Homeopathy

See Appendix E for proper use and handling instruction prior to administering remedies described below.

♦ **Belladonna 6C** – Shooting pain from kidney along urethra through which stone is passing. Dosage: Dissolve 5 pellets under the tongue, every 15 minutes until pain is relieved.

♦ **Berberis 6C** – Leading homeopathic remedy for acute pain of kidney stones, especially when pain is on left side and extends from kidney to urethra with strong urge to urinate. Dosage: Dissolve 5 pellets under the tongue, every 15 minutes until pain is relieved.

♦ **Causticum 6C** – Excruciating pain that radiates from kidney to testicles; attack comes on while sleeping, and urine is passed drop by drop. Dosage: Dissolve 5 pellets under the tongue, every 15 minutes until pain is relieved.

♦ **Dioscorea 6C** – Writhing, with crampy pains, with passing kidney stones; spasmodic stricture of urethra, with pain around navel; cannot keep still. Dosage: Dissolve 5 pellets under the tongue, every 15 minutes until pain is relieved.

## Miscellaneous

♦ **Hot compresses**, alternating with ice pack and cold compress. For acute kidney stone attacks. Begin with very hot compress (as hot as can be tolerated) over the kidneys to dilate urinary passages and relax painful tissue. Keep compress hot with hot water bottle. Keep head cool with a cold compress. Hot compress application 5 to 10 minutes. Follow with less than 1 minute of ice pack. Follow with 5 minutes of cold compress. Repeat cycle 2 or 3 more times or as required.

♦ **Hot bath with light careful massage** – Sit in a hot bath with water level reaching to just above kidneys; intermittently administer a light careful massage from the kidney region downward. This may help move a kidney stone from the urethra to the bladder.
*Note:* Avoid if frail or have a heart condition, and hot baths are not recommended.

# Memory Problems

Poor memory is a problem for both the elderly and non-elderly. It can be caused by medications, poor circulation to the brain, stress, age, nutritional deficiencies, hormonal imbalance, sleep deprivation, free-radical damage, strokes, dementia and menopause. If symptoms of memory loss develop, bring this to the attention of a healthcare practitioner. A complete mental status examination should be performed.

Conventional treatments include possible determination of underlying causes, replacement of necessary nutrients or hormones, and prescribing drugs based on the diagnosis. Holistically oriented physicians will also perform blood screening for heavy-metal toxicity.

| EZ Care Program | |
|---|---|
| Diet | **Avoid** intake of processed sugar, white flour, fried foods, and partially hydrogenated oils (e.g., margarine). |
| | **Eat fish**, such as mackerel, herring, trout, and salmon, because they contain omega-3 fatty acids, important for brain function. |
| | **Flaxseed Oil** – Dosage: 1 to 2 tbsp. daily. Contains omega-3 fatty acids and other nutrients that are essential for proper brain functioning. |
| Herbs | **Ginkgo Biloba** – Dosage: 1 to 2 capsules (40-80 mg.) of 24% standardized extract or 30-60 drops extract* in 4 oz. water three times daily. *Beneficial properties:* May improve circulation and nutrient flow to the brain. *Note:* Avoid use with history of cerebral hemmorhage, easy bleeding, or if using anticoagulant drugs such as warfarin sodium (Coumadin). Also use with caution with ginger, garlic, and ginseng. |
| Miscellaneous | **Coenzyme Q-1O** – Dosage: 50 mg., two to three times daily. Improves cellular oxidative metabolism. |
| | **L. Glutamine** – Dosage: 500 mg., one to two times daily with meals. Known as brain fuel that can pass the blood-brain barrier; a precursor for neurotransmitters L-glutamic acid and GABA. |
| | **Lecithin** – Dosage: 1 tbsp. lecithin granules three times daily added to food. Contains phosphatidylcholine, the precursor to the neurotransmitter acetylcholine that is required for transmitting brain signals. |
| | **Test** for **heavy metals** like **lead, cadmium, mercury,** and **aluminum.** Heavy metals may interfere with brain functioning. Speak to a holistic physician about obtaining a blood or urine analysis (see Resource Guide). |

# Additional Recommendations

The EZ Care Program consists of basic remedies that are commonly used for memory enhancement and have been found to work well in most cases. The remedies are most effective when combined, but can be used individually. The options stated below can supplement or replace EZ Care remedies and may be combined when suggested doses are followed.

## Diet

♦ **Avoid** caffeine and alcohol, because they may decrease blood flow to the brain.

♦ **Eat a high-water-content diet** consisting of large quantities of fresh fruits and vegetables with comparatively smaller quantities of whole grains, legumes, seeds, nuts, fish, skinless chicken and turkey.

♦ **Eat generous amounts of raw garlic and onions**; may help circulation and blood flow to the brain.

♦ **Drink** 6 to 8 glasses of pure **water** daily.

## Vitamins

♦ **B12** – Dosage: 500 to 1,000 mcg. daily for 30 days; then every other day for two months. Vitamin B12 supplements are poorly absorbed from the gut, so sublingual tablets are preferable.
*Notes:* (1) Always use a *complete B complex formula* in addition to vitamin B12, because high doses of one of the B vitamins may lead to imbalance in the body's pool of the other B vitamins. (2) In cases of frank B12 deficiency, intramuscular vitamin B12 injections, administered by a physician, are the primary and most effective option. (3) Vitamin B12 is a cofactor in producing red blood cells and is commonly deficient in elderly individuals.

♦ **B Complex** - Dosage: 50 to 100 mg daily with a meal.
*Note:* For highest assimilation, use a multi B complex which contains the vitamins in their coenzyme form and avoid mega-potency B complex products.

♦ **C** (mineral ascorbates mixed with bioflavonoids) – Dosage: 1,000 to 3,000 mg. daily. Vitamin C deficiency is common among elderly individuals with symptoms of senility. Converts folic acid to its active form and protects B vitamins from oxidation. Also counteracts effects of heavy metal toxicity.

♦ **Folic Acid** – Dosage: 800 mcg. one to two times daily with meals. Commonly given with vitamin B12, because they are intimately related regarding red blood cell production. Green, leafy vegetables are an excellent source of folic acid. It is not coincidental that the word *folic* and *foliage* derive from the same root.

### Herbs

♦ **Siberian Ginseng** (Eleutherococcus senticosus) (0.4% eleutherosides) – Dosage: 250 mg. standardized extract or 30 drops extract* in 4 oz. water three times daily. *Beneficial properties:* May improve mental alertness and decrease cortisol release during stress.

### Miscellaneous

♦ **Acetyl-l-carnitine** – Dosage: 500 mg., two times daily. May increase cerebral blood flow, stimulate acetylcholine formation, and transport fatty acids into nerve cells. Useful to enhahce mental concentration.

♦ **Avoid aluminum** and **silicon,** which may play a role in causing poor mental function. They are commonly found in antacids, antiperspirants, aluminum pots, baking pans, and water supplies.

♦ **Avoid** all **tobacco** products, because these may restrict blood flow to the brain.

♦ **Get** adequate amounts of **rest** and **sleep**. Sleep deprivation is a common factor in decreased memory function.

♦ **Phosphatidylserine** – Dosage: 100 mg., one to two times daily with meals. Supplies phospholipids, important for mental performance and memory function to brain cells.

♦ **Vinpocetine** – Dosage 5 mg. once daily. Similar in function to ginkgo biloba, vinpocetine improves cerebral circulation.

* Most herbal extracts contain alcohol. Avoid use if alcohol sensitive or if there is a history of alcohol abuse. *Note:* Alcohol content can be reduced through evaporation by adding extract to very hot water (just below boiling point) and allowing to stand 5 to 7 minutes before drinking.

# Menopause

Menopause is the time in a woman's life when her menstruation periods become erratic, and eventually stop. This is commonly known as the "change of life." Menopause may be natural, or surgically produced by removal of the ovaries. In menopause, the ovaries reduce production of estrogen and progesterone, producing symptoms such as hot flashes, irregular menses, fatigue, depression, anxiety, vaginal dryness, insomnia, urinary incontinence, and memory impairment. It is also common for women to gain ten pounds during menopause. A lack of progesterone may be responsible for an increase in bone loss.

Conventional treatments are a combination of estrogen/progesterone replacements, and calcium and vitamin D supplementation. Weight bearing exercises are also used to help prevent osteoporosis. Estrogen replacement was once thought to prevent heart attacks in postmenopausal women. However, recent studies bring this issue to be questioned. Synthetic estrogen replacement should be avoided in patients with a history of breast and endometrial cancer. Consult your gynecologist prior to being placed on conventional estrogen replacement therapy. Holistic physicians employ specific hormonal analysis and replacement, using plant-based estrogens.

| EZ Care Program | |
|---|---|
| Diet | **Eat** generous amounts of soy products, such as soybeans, soy nuts, soy milk, tofu, and miso. Soy contains plant-like estrogens known as phytoestrogens that may greatly reduce symptoms of hot flashes. In Japan, a word to describe menopause does not exist because of a high soy protein intake. |
| | **Eat a high-water-content diet** consisting of large quantities of fresh fruits and vegetables along with comparatively smaller quantities of whole grains, legumes, seeds, nuts, fish, skinless chicken and turkey. |
| Vitamins | **B complex** – Dosage: 50 mg. balanced B complex capsule daily with a meal. *Note:* For highest assimilation, use a multi B complex which contains the vitamins in their coenzyme form and avoid mega-potency B complex products. |
| | **C** (mixed mineral ascorbates) – Dosage: 1,000 to 3,000 mg. daily. Vitamin C plays a role in hormone synthesis and protects certain B vitamins from oxidation. |
| | **E** (natural d-alpha tocopherol in a base of mixed tocopherols) – Dosage: 800 IU daily with a meal. Essential for normal functioning of reproductive organs. Protects crucial hormones from oxidation and may help alleviate hot flashes. |
| Minerals | **Calcium** (elemental calcium from amino acid chelate or citrate) Dosage: 200 mg., four times daily with meals and at bedtime. May help with hot flashes, insomnia, and prevention of osteoporosis. |
| | **Magnesium** (elemental magnesium from amino acid chelate or citrate) – Dosage: 200 mg., four times daily with meals and at bedtime. May help with hot flashes, insomnia, and prevention of osteoporosis. |
| Herbs | **Black Cohosh Root** (Cimicifuga racemosa) – Dosage: 25 mg. of a 4:1 extract three times a day. *Beneficial properties:* May help reduce hot flashes and ease symptoms of menopause. |
| | **Evening Primrose Oil** (Oenothera biennis) – Dosage: 1300 mg., two times daily with meals. *Beneficial properties:* Contains gamma-linoleic acid (GLA), that may inhibit menopausal symptoms. |

| EZ Care Program | |
|---|---|
| Miscellaneous | **DHEA** (dihydroepiandosterone) – Dosage: 10 mg. daily. Associated with increased emotional well being. DHEA is an adrenal hormone that can increase estrogen levels. DHEA production declines with age.<br>*Note:* Check with a physician before starting use of this or any hormonal product. |
| | **Natural Progesterone** skin cream (3% progesterone) for perimenopausal symptoms or natural 1:1:8 estrogen skin cream for postmenopausal maintenance. May help with depression, anxiety, and osteoporosis. Use as directed on label.<br>*Note:* Check with a physician before starting use of this or any hormonal product. |
| | **Review homeopathy** section for appropriate remedies. |

# Additional Recommendations

The EZ Care Program consists of basic remedies that are commonly used for menopause and have been found to work well in most cases. The remedies are most effective when combined, but can be used individually. The options stated below can supplement or replace EZ Care remedies and may be combined when suggested doses are followed.

## Diet

- **Avoid** hot sauces, spicy foods, and hot drinks when hot flashes are a persistent problem.

- **Eat high fiber foods**, such as whole grains, legumes, broccoli, raw cabbage, and dark green, leafy vegetables.

- **Eliminate or reduce alcohol**, caffeine, coffee, dairy products, white flour, and sugar, because they put stress on the adrenals and liver.

## Vitamins

- **Bioflavonoids** – Dosage: 1 to 3 grams citrus bioflavonoids daily in divided doses taken with vitamin C. May help stabilize mast cells that are partially responsible for hot flashes.

- **PABA** – Dosage: 50 mg. one to two times daily with B complex. A B vitamin which may relieve nervous irritability.

## Herbs

- **Chaste Tree Berries** (Vitex agnus castus) – Dosage: 2 capsules or 1 tsp. extract* on waking for at least 90 days.
  *Beneficial properties:* May assist hormonal harmonization in women.

- **Dong Quai** (Angelica sinensis) – Dosage: 2 capsules two to three times daily with meals.
  *Beneficial properties:* A Chinese herb traditionally used for hot flashes, insomnia, and depression associated with menopause.

## Homeopathy

See Appendix E for proper use and handling instruction prior to administering remedies described below.

- **Lachesis 12C** – Hot flashes, depression, and irritability; external pressure of clothing intolerable; a severe headache that begins at back of head and passes over front of head; symptoms predominantly left-sided and worse after waking. Dosage: Dissolve 5 pellets under the tongue, one to two times daily or as required.

- **Pulsatilla 6C** – Irritable and changeable temperament; hot perspiration in closed, warm rooms; prone to weeping when discussing condition. Dosage: Dissolve 5 pellets under the tongue, one to two times daily or as required.

- **Sepia 15C** – Vaginal discharge, low back pain, bitter, disgruntled; easily depressed; may have dark complexion and fine delicate skin; sudden hot flashes with sweat, weakness, and tendency to faint. Dosage: Dissolve 5 pellets under the tongue, one to two times daily or as required.

## Miscellaneous

- **Breathing exercise** – Following is a yoga breathing exercise for calming the mind, and may reduce hot flashes: Inhale through the nose for a count of 4, hold for a count of 7, exhale through the mouth for a count of 8. Practice two times daily, four to eight sets each time, being sure to inhale deep into belly.
  *Note:* To enhance concentration and be certain the exercise is performed properly, you might lie down, place a lightweight book on your abdomen, then peacefully observe the book's rise-and-fall-motion as you breathe deeply.

- **Di-indolymethane** (DIMM) – Dosage: 60 mg., two times daily with meals. A phyto-chemical extracted from cruciferous vegetables, which promotes the healthy metabolism of estrogen. Early research shows benefit in patients with breast and uterine cancer.
  *Note:* Check with a physician before starting use of this or any hormonal product.

- **Pregnenolone** – Dosage: 10 to 20 mg. daily. A natural hormone made from cholesterol in the body; the basic precursor for estrogen and progesterone.
  *Note:* Check with a physician before starting use of this or any hormonal product.

# Menstrual Cramps

Menstrual cramps occur from excessively strong uterine contractions, or when clots are passed during the menstruation period. The pain may be in the entire abdomen or only in the lower quadrants, and often radiates to the lower back. Hormonal imbalance is often the reason for this condition, but dietary sensitivities or intolerances also can play a large role.

Conventional medical treatments include analgesic pain relievers, such as acetaminophen and non-steroidal anti-inflammatory drugs (NSAIDs) like ibuprofen or naproxen sodium. Warm compresses and baths, with a regular exercise program, are also recommended. Hormonal treatments may be used, such as oral contraceptives, to balance the menstrual cycle.

| EZ Care Program | |
|---|---|
| Diet | **Eat a high-water-content diet** consisting of large quantities of fresh fruits and vegetables along with comparatively smaller quantities of whole grains, legumes, seeds, nuts, fish, skinless chicken and turkey. |
| | **Eat fish**, such as mackerel, herring, trout, and salmon, because they contain omega-3 fatty acids. |
| | **Eliminate** chocolate, soda, coffee, tea, and all other forms of caffeine. |
| | **Flaxseed Oil** – Dosage: 1 to 2 tbsp. daily. Contains anti-inflammatory omega-3 fatty acids. |
| Vitamins | **B complex** – Dosage: 50 mg. balanced B complex capsule. B complex vitamins, especially B6 and niacin, may relieve abnormal menstrual symptoms, including cramping. <br> *Note:* For highest assimilation, use a multi B complex which contains the vitamins in their coenzyme form and avoid mega-potency B complex products. |
| Minerals | **Calcium** (elemental calcium from amino acid chelate) – Dosage: 1,000 mg. daily in divided doses, with meals and at bedtime. Essential for the normal contraction of muscle, and relaxation of the nervous system. Considered a "lullaby" mineral. |
| | **Magnesium** (elemental magnesium from amino acid chelate) – Dosage: 1,000 mg. daily in divided doses with meals and at bedtime. Essential for relaxing the muscular and nervous system. A natural antispasmodic. |
| Herbs | **Cramp Bark** (Viburnum opulus) – Dosage: 2 capsules three to four times daily or as required. For more dynamic effect, take with 4 oz. Of warm raspberry leaf, chamomile, catnip (Nepeta cataria), or peppermint (Mentha piperita) tea (see Appendix B). <br> *Beneficial properties:* An antispasmodic herb that may help relax the uterus and ameliorate cramping. |
| | **Evening Primrose Oil** (Oenothera biennis) – Dosage: 1300 mg., two to three times daily with meals for at least 6 to 8 weeks. Then reduce to 1 to 2 capsules daily or as required. <br> *Beneficial properties:* Contains gamma-linolenic acid (GLA), which is a natural anti-inflammatory substance and can reduce cramping. |
| Homeopathy | **Mag Phos 6X** – Use for painful menstruation or pain preceding the flow; warmth tends to decrease pain, and motion tends to increase it. Dosage: Dissolve 5 pellets four times daily or as required, or every 15 minutes during episode of acute cramping. |
| Miscellaneous | **Avoid sexual stimulation**, because this may worsen pelvic congestion. |
| | **Hot water bottle applied to abdomen**. Continue application until relief is obtained. For greater effect, prior to applying hot water bottle, massage in an aromatherapy blend as described below. |

| EZ Care Program | |
| --- | --- |
| | **Regular exercise** supports blood circulation, tissue oxygenation, and stress reduction, and relieves menstrual cramps in many women. |
| | Consider **Aromatherapy** section for appropriate remedy. |

# Additional Recommendations

The EZ Care Program consists of basic remedies that are commonly used for menstrual cramps and have been found to work well in most cases. The remedies are most effective when combined, but can be used individually. The options stated below can supplement or replace EZ Care remedies and may be combined when suggested doses are followed.

## Diet

♦ **Avoid overeating,** as this may cause pelvic congestion to worsen.

♦ **Eat high fiber foods**, such as whole grains, legumes, broccoli, raw cabbage, and dark green, leafy vegetables. Avoid constipation; this factor worsens pelvic congestion.

♦ **Reduce salt intake.** High salt intake may contribute to menstrual problems.

♦ **Reduce meat and milk intake.** If required in diet, then select organic varieties. Commercial meats and milk contain hormones that mimic estrogen and can exacerbate menstrual cramping.

## Vitamins

♦ **C** (mineral ascorbates mixed with bioflavonoids) – Dosage: 1,000 to 3,000 mg. daily. Vitamin C plays a role in hormone synthesis, and protects certain B vitamins from oxidation.

♦ **E** (natural d-alpha tocopherol in a base of mixed tocopherols) – Dosage: 800 IU daily with a meal. Vitamin E is essential for normal functioning of reproductive organs. Protects crucial hormones from oxidation.

## Herbs

♦ **Chamomile Flowers** (Matricaria recutitia) – Dosage: 6 oz. warm tea (see Appendix B) three to four times daily or as required. During episodes of acute cramping, take 1 tbsp. every 5 minutes with Mag Phos 6X (see EZ Care Program above).
*Beneficial properties:* A gentle relaxant and antispasmodic that traditionally has been used to relieve menstrual pain.

♦ **Dong Quai** (Angelica sinensis) – Dosage: 1 to 2 capsules three times daily with meals.
*Beneficial properties:* Chinese herbs that may help regulate menstrual function, relieve pelvic congestion, and enhance absorption of vitamin E.

♦ **Red Raspberry Leaf** (Rubus idaeus) – Dosage: 8 oz. tea prepared by infusion (see Appendix B) two to three times daily or as required. If menstrual cramping is chronic, red raspberry leaf tea may be more effective if consumed daily throughout the month.
*Beneficial properties:* May help soothe and tone the uterus.

## Aromatherapy

Mix 3 drops each of essential oils of **Marjoram** (Origanum marjorana) and **Lavender** (Lavendula vera), with 24 drops warm olive oil. Massage gently into area over the uterus. The effects of this gentle, relaxing, antispasmodic blend may be enhanced if massaged in after a warm sitz bath, or if followed with an application of a hot water bottle. Repeat application of this blend two to four times daily or as required. A 5-minute massage of this blend into the area one inch to the right of the lumbar spine also may help.

## Homeopathy

See Appendix E for proper use and handling instruction prior to administering remedies described below.

♦ **Chamomilla 6C** – Spasmodic pain with great nervous sensitivity and irritability. Dosage: Dissolve 5 pellets four times daily or as required, or every 15 minutes during episode of acute cramping.

♦ **Gelsemium 6C** – For menstrual pain accompanied by persistent headache and exhaustion. Dosage: Dissolve 5 pellets four times daily or as required, or every 30 minutes during episode of acute cramping.

♦ **Pulsatilla 6C** – Menstrual pain with scanty flow of black clotted blood. Dosage: Dissolve 5 pellets four times daily or as required, or every 15 minutes during episode of acute cramping.

♦ **Sepia 12C** – Menstrual pain with profuse, early flow, accompanied by emotional distress; especially indicated in spare delicate women with these symptoms. Dosage: Dissolve 5 pellets four times daily or as required, or every 30 minutes during episode of acute cramping.

## Miscellaneous

♦ **Breathing exercise** – Following is a yoga breathing exercise for calming the mind and body: Inhale thorough the nose for a count of 4, hold for a count of 7, exhale through the mouth for a count of 8. Practice two times daily, four to eight sets each time.
*Note:* To enhance concentration and be certain the exercise is performed properly, you might lie down, place a lightweight book on your abdomen, then peacefully observe the book's rise-and-fall-motion as you breathe deeply.

♦ Get plenty of **rest**; over-fatigue can worsen menstrual pain.

♦ **Hot Sitz Bath** (105-115° F.) accompanied by **Hot Foot Soak** (110° F) for up to 10 minutes.

♦ **Natural progesterone cream**. Use product as directed on the container—from the time you ovulate until menstruation begins.
*Note:* Check with a physician before starting use of this or any hormonal product.

# Muscle Spasms and Cramps

Painful contractions of the muscle fibers most commonly occur in the calf or thigh. There are many reasons for these spasms, including vitamin and mineral deficiency, muscle injury, poor circulation, inactivity, dehydration, and hypothyroidism. Certain medications (e.g., diuretics, antipsychotics, and insulin) may cause muscle spasm.

Conventional treatments include assessment of circulation, control of hypertension and cholesterol, proper hydration, replacement of necessary minerals and vitamins, and addressing dietary concerns such as a deficiency in the consumption of fruit. Occasionally, muscle relaxants are prescribed.

| EZ Care Program | |
|---|---|
| Diet | **Drink** 8 glasses of pure, room-temperature water daily. |
| | **Eat** foods that are high in calcium and magnesium, such as yogurt, fish, nuts, broccoli, sesame seeds, bananas, grapes, peaches, plums, pumpkin, potatoes, beets, zucchini, sardines, and dark green vegetables. |
| Vitamins | **C** (mineral ascorbate mixed with bioflavonoids) – Dosage: 1,000 mg., two to three times daily with meals. Vitamin C plays a role in calcium metabolism; deficiency may give rise to muscle pain and spasms. |
| | **E** (natural d-alpha tocopherol in a base of mixed tocopherols) – Dosage: 800 to 1200 IU daily in divided doses with meals. Vitamin E is particularly important if the muscle spasms are partly due to vascular spasm or other forms of circulatory incompetence. |
| Minerals | **Calcium** (elemental calcium from amino acid chelate) – Dosage: 1,000 mg. daily in divided doses with meals and at bedtime. Essential for muscle contraction. Calcium deficiency is the most common cause of leg cramps, especially those occurring at night or during pregnancy. |
| | **Magnesium** (elemental magnesium from amino acid chelate) – Dosage: 1,000 mg. daily in divided doses with meals and at bedtime. Essential for relaxing the skeletal, muscular, and nervous systems. Supplementation of both calcium and magnesium may be required to fully remedy chronic muscle spasms; this combination is often useful for treating "growing pains" in young children. |
| Herbs | **Cayenne Pepper** (Capsicum annuum) – Dosage: 1 to 2 capsules or 1/4 tsp. per meal. *Beneficial properties:* May improve blood circulation, reduce blood vessel spasm, and assist the action of other herbs. |
| Homeopathy | **Mag Phos 6X** – For cramps, stiffness, and numbness caused by prolonged exertion, including writer's cramps. Dosage: Dissolve 5 pellets |

| EZ Care Program | |
|---|---|
| | under the tongue, two to three times daily or as required, or 5 pellets every 15 minutes during actual cramping episode until relief is obtained. |
| Miscellaneous | **Alternating Hot and Cold Foot Soak** (see Appendix D for details) 30 minutes before bed. For greater effect, add 6 drops of the undiluted essential oil blend described above to the basin of hot water. Follow with massaging legs and feet with the diluted essential oil blend described above. May relax muscles and increase circulation to legs. |
| | **Regular exercise** supports blood circulation, tissue oxygenation, and stress reduction. A complete **stretching program** is important for flexibility, and will reduce cramping due to muscle tightness. |

## Additional Recommendations

The EZ Care Program consists of basic remedies that are commonly used for muscle spasms and cramps and have been found to work well in most cases. The remedies are most effective when combined, but can be used individually. The options stated below can supplement or replace EZ Care remedies and may be combined when suggested doses are followed.

### Vitamins

♦ **B Complex -** Dosage 25 to 50 mg daily with a meal.
  *Note:* For highest assimilation, use a multi B complex which contains the vitamins in their coenzyme form and avoid mega-potency B complex products.

### Herbs

♦ **Ginger Root** (Zingiber officinalis) – Dosage: 2 capsules three times a day, or 6-8 oz. dried ginger root tea three times daily (see Appendix B; Jamaican ginger root is preferred). For enhanced effect, add a pinch of cayenne to each serving.
  *Beneficial properties:* May aid circulation.

♦ **Ginkgo Biloba** – Dosage: 2 capsules (80 mg.) 24% standardized extract or 60 drops extract* in 4 oz. water three times daily.
  *Beneficial properties:* May improve general circulation.

♦ **Stinging Nettle** (Urtica dioica) – 1 to 2 capsules or 30 drops extract* in 4 oz. water three times a day for at least one month.
  *Beneficial properties:* Good source of blood-building minerals, including calcium.

### Aromatherapy

Choose 12 drops of one, or six drops of each of the following essential oils: **lavender** (lavendula vera) or **marjoram** (Origanum marjorana. Using equal amounts of the selected essential oils, in an amber glass bottle mix with jojoba, olive, or sweet almond oil in a 1:20 proportion (12 drops essential oil combination per 240 drops jojoba oil). Shake well and stopper. Store in a cool, dark place. Massage into areas of muscle tension or spasm, as required.

## Homeopathy

See Appendix E for proper use and handling instruction prior to administering remedies described below.

- **Arnica 6C** – Cramps in calves caused by fatigue. Dosage: Dissolve 5 pellets every 15 minutes during actual cramping episode until relief is obtained.

- **Calcarea. Carb 6C** – Muscle cramps worse at night in bed, especially when stretching legs. Dosage: Dissolve 5 pellets under the tongue, two to three times daily or as required, or 5 pellets every 15 minutes during actual cramping episode until relief is obtained.

- **Cuprum Metallicum 12C** – Cramps of legs, hands, calves; aggravated by sleep and sexual intercourse; feeling or behaving extremely emotionally closed or "cramped." Dosage: Dissolve 5 pellets under the tongue, two to three times daily or as required.

- **Rhus Tox 12C** – Cramps worse at rest and when first begin moving, better with continued movement; sometimes accompanied by cracking sounds of joints when in motion. Dosage: Dissolve 5 pellets under the tongue, two times daily or as required, or 5 pellets every 15 minutes during actual cramping episode until relief is obtained.

## Miscellaneous

- **Warm Full Bath** - Soak 15 to 30 minutes. While in tub, intermittently massage legs and arms (attempting to move blood back toward heart). Quickly rinse with cool water. Follow with a vigorous towel rub, using a coarse cotton towel. Then massage the body vigorously with the diluted essential oil blend described above. Repeat three times weekly at least three hours after eating dinner.

- * Most herbal extracts contain alcohol. Avoid use if alcohol sensitive or if there is a history of alcohol abuse. *Note:* Alcohol content can be reduced through evaporation by adding extract to very hot water (just below boiling point) and allowing to stand 5 to 7 minutes before drinking.

# Nausea

Nausea may be caused by many different factors, including pregnancy, motion such as car or sea travel, stress, food poisoning, food intolerance, illness, infection, medication, and stimulant use. Treatment for nausea differs according to its etiology. This section is intended to serve as a guide to symptomatic relief. If nausea is ongoing, see a healthcare professional.

Conventional medicines may treat or prevent nausea. Suppositories are commonly used when a person is unable to take oral medication. In addition, great emphasis is placed on replacing fluids and electrolytes. Intravenous agents may be used for patients undergoing chemotherapy or in cases of severe dehydration.

*Pregnancy Note: Pregnant women should always speak to a healthcare practitioner before using any new supplements or therapies.*

| EZ Care Program | |
|---|---|
| Diet | **Eat** low-fat, plain foods, such as dry soda crackers or dry toast. |
| | **Eat** small frequent meals throughout the day. |
| Vitamins | **B6** (pyridoxal 5-phosphate is preferred) – *For morning sickness with pregnancy.* Dosage: 50 – 100 mg. daily with breakfast and dinner. *Notes:* (1) Always use B6 in conjunction with a *complete B complex formula,* because high doses of one B vitamin can lead to imbalance in other B vitamins. (2) Reduce dosage as frequency and intensity of morning sickness diminishes. (3) After delivery, dosage of vitamin B6 should be reduced to no more than 25 mg. daily, because high doses of this vitamin may inhibit the flow of breast milk. |
| Herbs | **Cloves** (Carophyllus aromaticus), **Ginger** (Zingiber officinalis), or **Cinnamon** (Cinnamomum verum) in **Chamomile tea** (Matricaria chamomilla) or **Peppermint tea** – Add a pinch of either powdered cloves, ginger, or cinnamon to 6 oz. warm chamomile or peppermint tea, to allay morning sickness or other forms of nausea. |
| | **Ginger Root** (Zingiber officinalis) – two 500 mg. capsules three times daily, or 6-8 oz. dried ginger root tea three times daily (see Appendix B; Jamaican ginger root is preferred). *Beneficial properties:* Excellent for most cases of nausea. *Notes:* (1) Generally safe and effective for pregnancy; however, always speak to a healthcare practitioner before adding any new herb. (2) To prevent motion sickness, take two 500 mg. capsules 30-60 minutes before trip begins. Additional capsules may be used every four to five hours during travel as needed. |
| | **Peppermint** (Mentha piperita) – 8 oz. warm tea (see Appendix B) 90 minutes after meals. Most beneficial for nausea if taken after the stomach emptied. *Beneficial properties:* May soothe the stomach. |

## Additional Recommendations

The EZ Care Program consists of basic remedies that are commonly used for nausea and motion sickness and have been found to work well in most cases. The remedies are most effective when combined, but can be used individually. The options stated below can supplement or replace EZ Care remedies and may be combined when suggested doses are followed.

## Diet

♦ **Identify personal food sensitivities**. Avoid all common allergenic foods (e.g., dairy, eggs, wheat, corn, sugar, preservatives). Rotate moderately allergic foods on a four-day schedule (see Appendix C).

## Vitamins

♦ **B complex** – Dosage: 25 to 50 mg. daily with a meal.
*Note:* For highest assimilation, use a multi B complex which contains the vitamins in their coenzyme form and avoid mega-potency B complex products.

## Minerals

♦ **Manganese** – Dosage: 5 to 10 mg., (aspartate or citrate) one to three times daily with meals.

♦ **Zinc** – *For morning sickness in pregnant women over 14 years of age*. Dosage: 25 mg. elemental zinc from amino acid chelate with breakfast and dinner. Zinc is a vitamin B6 synergist and also may help prevent post-partum depression. Avoid zinc lozenges, which may cause nausea.

## Herbs

♦ **Goldenseal Root** (Hydrastis canadensis) – *With pregnancy*. Dosage: 1 capsule two times daily after breakfast and dinner.
*Beneficial properties:* May help ameliorate chronic morning sickness.

## Aromatherapy

Blend in a small amber glass dropper bottle 1 part each of the following three essential oils: **Peppermint** + **Ginger** + **Cardamom** (Elletaria cardamomum). During acute episodes of nausea, tap 3 drops of the blend onto a wrist. Then rub the wrists together, and take deep breaths from the wrists until the nausea subsides. Also consider mixing 4 drops of the blend with 12 drops warm sweet almond or jojoba oil; then massage gently into the stomach region, two times daily.

## Homeopathy

See Appendix E for proper use and handling instruction prior to administering remedies described below.

♦ **Cocculus 6C** – *For travel and motion sickness*. Also, dizziness and nausea that are worse after eating or drinking and in fresh air; sense of emptiness in head or stomach, and relief obtained by lying down. Dosage: Dissolve 5 pellets under the tongue, hourly or as required until symptoms subside.

♦ **Ipecac 6C** – *General and pregnancy*. Persistent nausea and vomiting; vomiting preceded by intense nausea that is not relieved by vomiting; often associated with ingesting rich, difficult-to-digest food; may benefit morning sickness. Dosage: Dissolve 5 pellets under the tongue, hourly or as required until symptoms subside.

♦ **Nux Vomica 12C** – *General and pregnancy*. Nausea with much retching; often related to overindulgence in alcohol or food or mental overwork; may be accompanied by sensation as if a stone in stomach; may be specific for morning sickness when nausea is typically accompanied by sour taste in mouth on waking. Dosage: Dissolve 5 pellets under the tongue, hourly or as required until symptoms subside.

♦ **Tabacum 12C** – *For travel and motion sickness*. Dizziness and nausea accompanied by coldness, faintness, sweating, and sinking feeling in stomach. Symptoms worse in stuffy room and better in fresh air, especially if abdomen bared to open air. Dosage: Dissolve 5 pellets under the tongue, hourly or as required until symptoms subside.

### Miscellaneous

♦ **Deep Breathing Exercises** – Calming to the mind and body. Following is a yoga breathing exercise for calming the mind: Inhale through the nose with a deep belly breath for a count of 4, hold for a count of 7, then exhale through the mouth for a count of 8. Practice two times daily, four to eight repetitions each time.
*Note:* To enhance concentration and be certain the exercise is performed properly, you might lie down, place a lightweight book on your abdomen, then peacefully observe the book's rise-and-fall-motion as you breathe deeply.

# Osteoporosis

Osteoporosis is a loss of bone density. It is caused by a loss of calcium and other minerals that are essential to bone formation. Vitamin D deficiency and loss of estrogen production are also responsible for osteoporosis. Affected bones become porous, brittle and are more susceptible to fracture. The condition is usually without symptoms, and can often go undetected. However, severe back pain may occur from vertebral fractures. Osteoporosis is very common among people over age 70, and is seen in post-menopausal women four times more often than men. This is thought to be a result of hormonal changes in women that occur during menopause. Persons affected with osteoporosis are more susceptible to hip fracture after sustaining a fall.

Conventional medicine therapies include over-the-counter analgesics for pain, hormone replacement therapy, and drugs to promote bone rebuilding; as well as mineral supplementation, including calcium, magnesium, and vitamin D. Physician-supervised exercise is part of the standard protocol. Research has proven weight-bearing exercise can improve bone density. Consult with a holistic physician for natural hormone replacement options.

Conventional tests for osteoporosis include the dexa scan, which compares bone density in the spine and hip to indicate degrees of bone loss. The test should be repeated approximately every 18 months. Physicians can measure bone breakdown metabolic studies for a more complete assessment of bone loss. This test can be repeated up to every three months in patients with severe osteoporosis.

| EZ Care Program | |
| --- | --- |
| Diet | **Avoid** caffeine, sugar, sweeteners, alcohol, and soda. The phosphoric acid found in soda increases bone loss. |
| | **Eat a high-water-content diet** consisting predominantly of fresh fruits and vegetables with smaller amounts of whole grains, legumes, nuts, seeds, fowl, and fish. Diets consisting of large amounts of protein—including high protein foods like meat, fowl, fish, and most grains—increase calcium excretion and bone loss. |
| | **Eat calcium- and magnesium-rich foods**, such as sardines, collard greens, sesame seeds, turnip greens, broccoli, almonds, blackstrap molasses, kale, salmon, and apricots. |
| | **Eat generous amounts of soy products**, because they contain diadzein and genistein, that have been shown to help prevent bone loss. Soy has natural estrogenic properties. |
| Vitamins | **B12** (sublingual administration) – Dosage: 2,000 mcg. two times daily. Vitamin B12 deficiency, which is quite common among the elderly, may contribute to osteoporosis. |
| | **C** (mineral ascorbates mixed with bioflavonoids) – Dosage: 1,000 mg., two to three times daily with meals. Plays an essential role in folic acid and calcium metabolism. The need for vitamin C increases with age due to a greater need for collagen regeneration. |
| | **D3** (natural form, derived from fish liver oil) – Dosage: 400 to 1,000 IU daily with meals. Aids in absorption of calcium from the gastrointestinal tract and in assimilation of phosphorus that may be deficient in many of the elderly and post-menopausal women with osteoporosis. |
| Minerals | **Boron** (elemental boron from amino acid chelate) – Dosage: 3 mg. with breakfast. Works with calcium and magnesium to support bone health. |
| | **Calcium** (elemental calcium derived from calcium citrate and hydroxyapatite) – Dosage: 300 mg., three to four times daily with meals and at bedtime. |
| | **Magnesium** (elemental magnesium from amino acid chelate) – Dosage: 300 mg., two to three times daily with meals. Nearly 70% of the body's magnesium is stored in the bones. Magnesium helps promote the absorption and metabolism of both calcium and phosphorus. People with osteoporosis often have low magnesium levels. |

| EZ Care Program | |
|---|---|
| Miscellaneous | **Avoid** all forms of tobacco. |
| | **Betaine Hydrochloride with Pepsin** – One or two 500 mg. capsules at beginning of each meal with 4 oz. warm water. Discontinue use if a burning sensation occurs in the stomach. Do not use with a history of ulcers or gastritis. Absorption of dietary calcium depends on solubility and ionization when mixed with hydrochloric acid secreted in the stomach. Many post-menopausal women and elderly people are deficient in stomach acid. |
| | **Ipriflavone** – Dosage 200 mg. three times daily. Ipriflavone is a synthetic soy derivitave of isoflavone. It has been clinically proven to be effective for osteoporosis in improving bone density. |
| | **Progesterone Cream or Estrogen Cream** (natural products) in 1:1:8 proportion of the three forms of natural estrogen – May help rebuild bone density and prevent further mineral loss without the risk of conventional hormone replacement therapy. Always check with a physician to determine the advisability of using these creams, and to provide guidance regarding proper dosage. |
| | **Weight-bearing Exercises** – May include walking, running, dancing, and weight lifting. Perform daily to maintain bone density. |

# Additional Recommendations

The EZ Care Program consists of basic remedies that are commonly used for osteoporosis and have been found to work well in most cases. The remedies are most effective when combined, but can be used individually. The options stated below can supplement or replace EZ Care remedies and may be combined when suggested doses are followed.

## Vitamins

♦ **B6** (pyridoxal 5-phosphate is preferred form) – Dosage: 25 to 50 mg. daily with breakfast and dinner. Vitamin B6, like folic acid, is required for homocysteine metabolism. Low levels of vitamin B6 are common among the elderly.
*Note:* Always take B6, folic acid, and B12 in conjunction with a complete B complex formula, because high doses of one of the B vitamins may lead to imbalance in the other B vitamins.

♦ **B complex** – Dosage: 50 mg. daily with a meal.
*Note:* For highest assimilation, use a multi B complex which contains the vitamins in their coenzyme form and avoid mega-potency B complex products.

♦ **Folic Acid** – Dosage: 1 to 2 mg., three times daily with meals. Required for metabolism of homocysteine that increases in post-menopausal women. Homocysteine interferes with the maintenance of the collagen content in bones. Collagen is an essential component of the bone matrix.
*Note:* Always take folic acid in conjunction with a complete B complex formula, because high doses of one of the B vitamins may lead to imbalance in other B vitamins.

- **K 1** (phylloquinone) – Dosage: 1 mg. daily with a meal containing raw leafy greens. Required for the retention of calcium in the bones.
  *Medication Note:* If using prescription blood-thinning medications such as warfarin sodium (Coumadin), check with your physician before beginning vitamin K1 supplementation. Vitamin K can reverse the effect of this class of medications.

## Homeopathy

See Appendix E for proper use and handling instruction prior to administering remedies described below.

- **Calc Fluoride 6X** – A safe form of fluoride in a 1:1,000,000 dilution. Fluoride has been shown to increase bone-volume in osteoporosis patients; however, non-homeopathic fluoride supplements may cause significant side-effects. Dosage: Dissolve 5 pellets taken under the tongue, two times daily 60 minutes after meals.

- **Silicea 6X** – Cell salt form of silica, indicated in all disease of bones. Silica may be transmutated in the body into easily assimilated calcium, and may be more effective than calcium supplementation for increasing bone calcium levels in osteoporosis. Dosage: Dissolve 5 pellets taken under the tongue, three times daily 30 minutes before meals.
  *Note:* When using more than one homeopathic cell salt, separate administration of one from another by at least 15 minutes.

# Overweight

Currently 97 million Americans are classified as overweight or obese. Obesity is defined as a body mass index greater than 27. A healthy body mass index is between 18 and 25. To calculate a body-mass index, multiply your weight in pounds x 700 and divide this figure by your height in inches squared. Obesity correlates with the development of cardiovascular disease, diabetes, osteoarthritis, sleep apnea, stroke, hypertension and cancer. Women usually gain approximately 10 pounds during the beginning of menopause.

Perhaps the most complex topic regarding weight loss concerns the question of which diet is best for achieving and maintaining weight loss. Because excessive weight gain has many causes, including stress, emotional problems, poor diet, vitamin or mineral deficiencies, lack of exercise, and hormone imbalances, there is no universal diet that is appropriate for all.

The ideal weight-loss program addresses the actual cause(s) of the problem and is highly individualized. However, effective weight-loss programs have several things in common: they are based on sound nutritional principles, rather than fad dieting. In addition, they offer a holistic approach in which exercise, proper diet, and stress reduction are incorporated into lifestyle changes.

Conventional therapy includes dietary changes, exercise, stress-relieving techniques, and adequate mineral, vitamin, and protein supplementation. Prescription appetite suppressants and fat-blocking agents are also available. Such agents should be used with extreme caution, as some have been shown to cause heart damage and vitamin deficiency.

An evaluation begins with a thorough history, physical, and lab assay. Some hormonal conditions (thyroid, pituitary, adrenal) can cause changes in weight. As weight loss occurs, great changes in electrolytes and other aspects of the metabolism occur.

The following guidelines may prove useful, regardless of which dietary approach to weight loss you employ.

| EZ Care Program | |
|---|---|
| Diet | **Review** entire **Diet** section below. |
| Vitamins | **B complex** – Dosage: 50 mg., two times daily with meals. *Note:* For highest assimilation, look for a multi-B vitamin that contains some of its components in coenzyme form and avoid mega-potency B complex products. May help improve metabolism and the burning of fats while buffering the stress and anxiety that often accompany dieting. |
| | **Chromium** (polynicotinate is preferred form) – Dosage: 200 mcg. two times daily with meals. *Note:* Essential for blood-sugar regulation. Excess blood sugar is converted to fat, while low blood sugar may cause sugar cravings. |
| Herbs | **Chickweed** (Stellaria media) – Dosage: 8 oz. tea prepared by infusion (see Appendix B) using 2 tsp. Chickweed to 8 oz. Pure water four times daily 1 hour before each meal and at bedtime. *Beneficial properties*: Traditionally used with obesity to cleanse the system and break down body fat. *Note:* Consider adding powdered Bladderwrack (see herbs below) into warm Chickweed tea. |
| Miscellaneous | **Eat slowly and chew food well.** Hasty eating and poor chewing encourage overeating and may prevent food from being digested properly. |
| | **Exercise** at least 30 minutes daily. Exercise speeds metabolism and burns excess calories. No weight loss program is complete without a commitment to regular exercise. Consider combining strength training with aerobic exercise as this has proven to produce even greater results than aerobic exercise alone. |
| | **Kelp tablets** – Dosage: 2 to 3 tablets three times daily with meals. One of the most nutrient-rich of all sea vegetables. May support thyroid function and weight loss. |

| EZ Care Program | |
|---|---|
| | **Lecithin granules** – Dosage: 1 tbsp. two times daily with meals. A rich source of choline, a lipotropic B-vitamin that aids in utilizing body fats, thereby supporting weight loss. |
| | **Lemon juice** – Dosage: 1 tbsp. fresh lemon juice in 8 oz. pure water two times daily upon arising and mid-afternoon. A traditional weight-loss remedy that may support liver cleansing and burning of fats. |

# Additional Recommendations

The EZ Care Program consists of basic remedies that are commonly used for weight loss and have been found to work well in most cases. The remedies are most effective when combined, but can used individually. The options stated below can supplement or replace EZ Care remedies and may be combined when suggested doses are followed.

## Diet

♦ **Avoid eating large meals just before going to bed.** The body tends to store more food while asleep, because it is less active then. Also, the body cleanses itself most actively while we sleep, and a large meal might interfere with the cleansing process.

♦ **Avoid eating out too frequently**. Restaurant food is usually much more fattening than home-cooked food; portions are larger, and we tend to eat more and make less healthy choices.

♦ **Avoid high-glycemic foods** (white flour, potatoes, rice, corn, legumes, breads, pasta) during the weight-loss process. These foods can be reintroduced later in moderation (1 to 2 servings, total daily) once ideal body weight has been attained.

♦ **Eat a high-water-content diet** consisting of large quantities of fresh fruits and vegetables and comparatively smaller quantities of whole grains, legumes, seeds, nuts, fish, skinless chicken and turkey. Adequate, but not excessive amounts of protein should be consumed.

♦ Consume a small amount of **mono-unsaturated fats** with each meal. These include nuts, olive oil and avocado.

♦ Eat foods high in **fiber,** such as broccoli, apples, and green, leafy vegetables.

♦ Eat **healthy snacks** at least two times daily between meals. This helps prevent hunger and overconsumption of meals, and as keeps blood sugars balanced.

♦ **Eat smaller, simpler meals; never skip meals**. Smaller, simpler meals are easier to digest, process, and eliminate, rather than accumulate. Also, poorly digested meals contribute to reactive hypoglycemia, because the food is not efficiently converted into blood sugar. Hypoglycemia, in turn, induces hunger and sugar cravings.

- **Eliminate all junk foods**, fast foods, sugar, high-fat foods, refined and denatured foods, highly-seasoned foods, alcohol, caffeine, excess salt, and foods containing artificial sweeteners, preservatives, and colorings.

- **Identify personal food sensitivities**. Avoid all common allergenic foods (e.g., dairy, eggs, wheat, corn, sugar, preservatives). Rotate moderately allergic foods on a four-day schedule (see Appendix C).

- **Increase water** consumption. Drink a minimum of 8 glasses of pure water daily. This helps create a feeling of fullness and also flushes toxins from the body.

- Take a **Fiber Supplement** – Dosage: 1 to 3 tsp. psyllium husk fiber in 8 oz. pure water one or two times daily between meals.
  *Beneficial properties:* Fiber is helpful in weight management because it fills up the stomach, leaving less room for food; it gives a sense of fullness that can help reduce the amount of food eaten; it binds to fat, helping to eliminate it before the body absorbs it.
  *Note:* Carefully read label; some brands require additional water.

## Vitamins

- **Brewer's Yeast** – Dosage: 1 to 2 tbsp. daily with meals. A rich source of B vitamins and amino acids.

- **C** (mixed mineral ascorbates) – Dosage: 1,000 mg., two times daily. Essential for metabolizing vital nutrients, including amino acids, cholesterol, and various vitamins and minerals.

- **Choline** – Dosage: 500 mg., two times daily with meals. A lipotropic B vitamin that aids in utilizing body fats, thereby supporting weight loss.

## Minerals

- **Calcium** (elemental calcium from amino acid chelate) – Dosage: 150 mg., three times daily with meals and at bedtime. Aids utilization of vital nutrients, helps activate certain enzymes involved in metabolism, and helps regulate passage of nutrients in and out of cells. Supplementation may be particularly important if on a high-protein weight-loss diet, because these can produce calcium loss.

- **Magnesium** (elemental magnesium from amino acid chelate) – Dosage: 150 mg., four times daily with meals and at bedtime. Deficiency may cause sugar craving.

- **Potassium** (elemental from potassium citrate or aspartate) – Dosage: 99 mg., two to three times daily with meals and at bedtime. Most beneficial if on a high-protein diet or using diuretics. Regulates water balance and helps with protein and glucose metabolism.

## Herbs

- **Bladderwrack** (Fucus vesiculosis) – Dosage: 1/2 to 1 tsp. powdered bladderwrack stirred into 8 oz. pure warm water two to three times daily between meals. Diuretic and mildly laxative herb that may help support thyroid function as well as counteract constipation, water-retention, and sluggish metabolism.

♦ **Stinging Nettle** (Urtica dioica) – Dosage: 8 oz. of tea prepared by infusion (see Appendix B) using 2 tsp. stinging nettle to 8 oz. pure water two to three times daily between meals. Consider stirring powdered bladderwrack (see above) into warm stinging nettle tea rather than water. Stinging nettle has diuretic and metabolism-supporting properties and traditionally has been used to assist in weight loss.

## Miscellaneous

♦ **Coenzyme Q-10** – Dosage: 50mg., two times daily with meals. A nutrient important to many body energy production systems. Acts as a metabolic stimulant, thus helping to facilitate weight loss.

♦ **Hydroxycitric Acid** (HCA) – Usually found mixed with other substances in tablet or capsule form. Take as directed on package. Plant derivative that decreases conversion of sugar into fat and helps suppress appetite.

♦ **L-5HTP** (hydroxy tryptophan) – Dosage 100 mg. two times daily before meals L-5HTP increases the production of serotonin and aids in appetite suppression.

♦ **L-Carnitine** – Dosage: 1000 - 2000 mg. daily in divided doses with meals. An amino acyl derivitave that enhances fat transport into cells for energy production.

♦ **L-glutamine** – Dosage: 500 mg. two times daily with meals. An amino acid, used by the brain as fuel, which may help reduce cravings for alcohol, sugar, and carbohydrates.

♦ **Pyruvate** – Dosage 1000 mg. twice daily. May increase dose to 4000 – 6000 mg. divided daily. Pyruvate is an intermediate metabolite in the Krebs cycle. The Krebs cycle is the primary series of metabolic events leading to energy production. Pyruvate supplementation may increase metabolism.

♦ **Proteolytic Enzyme Formula** (including protease, bromelain, and papain). May help food digestion and increase fat-burning rate, thus leading to reduced food intake and weight loss. Take as directed on package.
*Note:* Avoid if stomach or duodenal ulcers; proteolytic enzymes may aggravate ulcers and induce bleeding.

♦ Consider **hypnosis** from a qualified practitioner if the above mentioned remedies are ineffective.

♦ Consider **yoga, meditation, flower remedies, aromatherapy, and/or homeopathy** to soothe and strengthen the psycho-spiritual plane of the body. Appetite control is greatly affected by negative emotions. Any weight-loss regimen that considers the need for improved emotional balance and mental discipline has a much greater chance for long-term success.

# Pink Eye (Conjunctivitis)

Pink eye is an inflammation of the mucus membrane that lines the inner surface of the eyelid and the eyeball. The most common cause of conjunctivitis is viral infection. Other causes include bacterial and fungal infections, chemical irritation, and allergies. Symptoms may include bloodshot eyes, itching, swelling, green, yellow or clear discharge, eyelids agglutinated shut in the morning, aversion to bright lights, and increased tearing.

Conventional treatment may include prescription medications such as antibiotic or steroid eyedrops, depending on the cause of the problem. Steroid eyedrops should only be prescribed by an ophthalmologist after a complete corneal exam. If used inappropriately, blindness could occur. Antihistamines, in tablet and eyedrops, may be helpful for allergic conjunctivitis. Application of cool compresses to the eye can also be soothing. Seeing a physician should be considered, in order to rule out any serious conditions, especially if visual changes have occurred or if symptoms have lasted for over one week.

**Pink Eye Note**: Avoid touching your affected eye. This condition can be very contagious, and may be spread from eye to eye, as well as to other people. Be sure to wash hands frequently.

| EZ Care Program | |
|---|---|
| Diet | **Avoid all stressor foods**, such as sugar, white flour, fried foods, caffeine, and coffee, because they weaken the immune system. |
| Vitamins | **A** (natural, from fish liver oil) – Dosage: 10,000 to 25,000 IU daily with meals. Deficiency may cause conjunctivitis symptoms. *Note:* Consult a physician before using higher doses of vitamin A. Avoid use if pregnant. Discontinue use if you experience nausea, dry skin, sore lips, blurred vision, or other signs of vitamin A toxicity. |
| | **C** (mineral ascorbate mixed with bioflavonoids) – Dosage: 1,000 mg., three to four times daily with meals. In addition to being a natural anti-inflammatory agent, vitamin C protects vitamin A and vitamin B2 from oxidation. |
| Herbal Eyewash | **Goldenseal Root** (Hydrastis canadensis) **+ Boric Acid Solution** – Dosage: Add 1 tsp. each of goldenseal root powder and boric acid to 16 oz. boiling water. Shake well and let settle. Let cool, then strain. Bathe the eyes with this solution three times daily. May alternate with marshmallow root/raspberry leaf eyewash described below. |
| Herbs | **Eyebright** (Euphrasia officinalis) – Dosage: 2 capsules three times daily. *Beneficial properties:* Traditionally used for eye irritation. |

| EZ Care Program | |
|---|---|
| Miscellaneous | **Quercitin** – Dosage: 250 mg., three times daily in divided doses between meals until symptoms subside. Then reduce to 1-2 doses daily or as required. One of the most pharmacologically active flavonoids, quercitin inhibits the release of histamine, a substance that gives rise to tissue inflammation. |

# Additional Recommendations

The EZ Care Program consists of basic remedies that are commonly used for "pink eye" and have been found to work well in most cases. The remedies are most effective when combined, but can be used individually. The options stated below can supplement or replace EZ Care remedies and may be combined when suggested doses are followed.

## Diet

♦ **Eat a high-water-content diet** consisting predominantly of fresh fruits and vegetables with smaller amounts of whole grains, legumes, nuts, seeds, fowl, and fish.

## Vitamins

♦ **B2** (riboflavin 5-phosphate is preferred activated form) – Dosage: 25 to 50 mg., two times daily with meals until symptoms subside. Deficiency may cause conjunctivitis symptoms.
*Note:* Always use vitamin B2 in conjunction with a complete B complex formula, because high doses of one of the B vitamins can lead to imbalance in the body's pool of the other B vitamins.

♦ **B6** (pyridoxal 5-phosphate is preferred) – Dosage: 25 to 50 mg., two times daily with meals until symptoms subside. Deficiency may cause conjunctivitis symptoms.
*Note:* Always use vitamin B6 in conjunction with a complete B complex formula, because high doses of one of the B vitamins can lead to imbalance in the body's pool of the other B vitamins.

♦ **B Complex** – Dosage: 25 to 50 mg daily with a meal.
*Notes:* 1) After acute symptoms of conjunctivitis subside, it may be advisable to continue supplementation of a complete B complex formula on a regular basis. 2) For highest assimilation, use a multi B complex that contains the vitamins in their coenzyme form and avoid mega-potency B complex products.

## Herbs

♦ **Echinacea** (Echinacea purpurea) – Dosage: 2 to 4 capsules or 50 drops liquid extract* three times daily for two weeks.
*Beneficial properties:* Traditionally used to fight infections.

♦ **Stinging Nettle** (Urtica dioica) – Dosage: 2 freeze-dried capsules every two to four hours as needed.

*Beneficial properties:* May help to relieve symptoms when conjunctivitis is allergy-related.

## Herbal Eyewashes

♦ **Marshmallow Root** (Althea officinalis) + **Raspberry Leaf** (Rubus idaeus) **tea** – Dosage: Add 2 tbsp. marshmallow root and 1/2 tbsp. raspberry leaves to 24 oz. Pure, cold water. Cover and bring to a boil, then simmer 20 minutes; then lower flame until tea is simmering (below boiling point), then remove lid. Continue to simmer slowly until fluid reduces by 1/3. Let cool. Bathe eyes with cold tea, four to six times daily.

## Homeopathy

See Appendix E for proper use and handling instruction prior to administering remedies described below.

♦ **Belladonna 6C** – Pink, even red, eyes with burning pain; dilated pupils and hypersensitivity to light. Dosage: Dissolve 5 pellets under the tongue, four times daily until symptoms subside, then reduce dosage accordingly.

♦ **Euphrasia 6X or 6C** – Allergic conjunctivitis with eyelid margins that look and feel sore; discharge of pus; constant blinking. Dosage: Dissolve 5 pellets under the tongue, four times daily until symptoms subside, then reduce dosage accordingly.

♦ **Mercurius 6C** – Not at onset of conjunctivitis. Use after symptoms for several days and there is profuse, burning discharge, worse at night and aggravated by heat. Dosage: Dissolve 5 pellets under the tongue, three to four times daily until symptoms subside, then reduce dosage accordingly.

♦ **Pulsatilla 6C or 12C** – Eyes burn and itch at night and water profusely in open air; eyes hypersensitive to light and relieved by cold applications; may be a thick white or yellow discharge upon arising, which glues eyelids together. Dosage: Dissolve 5 pellets under the tongue, three to four times daily until symptoms subside, then reduce dosage accordingly.

## Miscellaneous

♦ **Charcoal Poultice** – Place powdered activated charcoal in a small cotton gauze tea bag (available from many healthfood stores). Dosage: Dip bag into hot or cold water as suits the case (whichever feels best). Place poultice over the eyes and cover with plastic (e.g., cut from a clear plastic produce bag). Keep in place 30-60 minutes, as tolerated. Apply 1 to 2 times daily or as required. This poultice may be alternated with herbal eyewashes (see above).

\*    Most herbal extracts contain alcohol. Avoid use if alcohol sensitive or if there is a history of alcohol abuse. *Note:* Alcohol content can be reduced through evaporation by adding extract to very hot water (just below boiling point) and allowing to stand 5 to 7 minutes before drinking.

# Poison Ivy / Oak / Sumac

This condition is caused when the oily sap found in these particular plants, which contains chemical irritants, rubs off onto exposed skin, producing redness, swelling, blistering, and severe itching. A characteristic lesion of poison ivy, oak or sumac appears similar to numerous long scrapes, as if obtained from a cat or dog. Scratching affected areas can spread the plant oils to other parts of the body, causing additional areas of irritation. If exposure to the plants occurs, immediately cleanse with soap and water, and wash clothes immediately. This will neutralize any of the plant oils and prevent spreading.

Conventional treatments include oatmeal soaks, topical calamine lotion, and oral antihistamines. If there is involvement of large areas, or on the eyes, ears or genitals, immediately seek the attention of a physician, because treatments may entail oral or topical steroids. Antibiotics may be prescribed if the area becomes infected.

Prevention includes gardening with gloves, long sleeves and long pants, and being careful not to touch your face with gloves.

| EZ Care Program | |
|---|---|
| Herbs | **Calendula Cream** – Dosage: apply externally 4 to 6 times daily. |
| | **Goldenseal Root** (Hydrastis canadensis) – Mix Goldenseal Root powder with sufficient pure water to produce a paste. Spread a 1/4-inch layer on a cheesecloth. Fold the cheesecloth over the paste. Position the compress over the affected area. Tape in place and cover with plastic (secure the plastic also) in order to keep the compress moist. |
| Homeopathy | **Rhus Tox 6C** – Use for itching and burning skin eruptions that are made worse by scratching. The rash stings and burns, which contain pus, are worse at night and may be aggravated by the warmth of the bed. Also feels worse when bathing, but extremely hot water and warm applications may be soothing. Dosage: Dissolve 5 pellets every two to three hours until relief is obtained, then reduce dosing frequency, as required. |

| EZ Care Program | |
|---|---|
| Miscellaneous | **Charcoal Wash and Paste** – Dosage: empty 2 to 3 capsules of activated charcoal into a cup of hot water. Allow the charcoal to settle to the bottom. Use the liquid above the sediment at the bottom ("charcoal slurry") to thoroughly wash the exposed area on the skin. Apply a charcoal paste (1 part charcoal plus sufficient water to make a thick paste); smear over the affected area. Change the paste every 10 minutes for 1 hour. Then apply a layer of paste, cover with gauze and plastic, and leave in place 8 hours. |
| | **Oatmeal Poultice** – Blend rolled oats to a fine powder. Mix with water or aloe vera juice to make a paste. Apply in similar fashion to charcoal paste discussed above. |
| | **Wash** the area with **pure lemon juice**. Saturate exposed area with lemon juice. **Apple cider vinegar** used in the same manner may also prove of good service. |

# Additional Recommendations

The EZ Care Program consists of basic remedies that are commonly used for these conditions and have been found to work well in most cases. The remedies are most effective when combined, but can be used individually. The options stated below can supplement or replace EZ Care remedies and may be combined when suggested doses are followed.

## Diet

♦ **Avoid** all sugar.

## Vitamins

♦ **A** (natural, from fish liver oil) – Dosage: 25,000 IU daily with meals for one week. *Note:* Consult a physician before using higher doses of vitamin A. Avoid use if pregnant. Discontinue use if nausea, dry skin, sore lips, blurred vision, or other signs of vitamin A toxicity are experienced.

♦ **C** (mineral ascorbates mixed with bioflavonoids) – Dosage: 500 to 1,000 mg. per hour until bowel tolerance is reached. Bowel tolerance is the point when the dosage exceeds the quantity the body is able to absorb from the gut; the unabsorbed quantity of vitamin C will give rise to gas in the bowels or loose stools. Once bowel tolerance is achieved, reduce dosage to 1,000 mg., four times daily until symptoms have cleared.

## Minerals

♦ **Zinc** (take only if over 14 years of age) 50 mg. elemental zinc from amino acid chelate two to three times daily until the eruptions have cleared.

## Herbs

♦   **Aloe Vera Gel** (cold processed gel from whole leaf aloe is best) – Apply externally 4 to 6 times daily or as required. Also, 1 to 2 oz. aloe vera juice in 6 oz. pure water taken internally three to four times daily may prove of good service.
*Beneficial properties:* May soothe skin and promote the healing of tissue.

♦   **Plantain Leaf** (Plantago major) – Learn to identify this common weed that can be found in many backyards and open fields and is useful for insect bites and stings as well as poison oak and poison ivy. Chop fresh leaves and blend with sufficient water to make a thick paste. Prepare and apply a compress, as with goldenseal root described in the EZ Care Section above.

♦   **White Oak Bark** (Quercus alba) and lime water (available at drug stores). Dosage: Prepare a strong decoction (see Appendix B) of white oak bark, using 1 tbsp. bark to 2 cups pure water. Mix strained decoction with an equal amount of lime water. Saturate a cotton or linen cloth with this solution and apply to affected areas. When dry, resaturate with the solution.

## Aromatherapy

**Thuja** (Thuja occidentalis) – Mix 2 to 3 drops of essential oil of thuja into aloe vera gel and apply to the affected areas, as a follow-up to goldenseal root or plantain poultices.

## Homeopathy

See Appendix E for proper use and handling instruction prior to administering remedies described below.

♦   **Sulphur 6C** – Burning and itching aggravated by warm bathing and warmth of bed; scratching provides temporary relief but worsens burning sensation; frantic scratching ultimately may lead to bleeding. Dosage: Dissolve 5 pellets every two to three hours until relief is obtained, then reduce dosing frequency or as required.

## Miscellaneous

♦   **Warm Hydrogen Peroxide Baths** – Dissolve 1 to 2 cups of peroxide in bath water. Peroxide also may be dabbed directly on lesions to ascertain relief.

♦   **Banana Peel Rub** – Temporary relief from itching can be obtained in some cases by rubbing the affected areas with the inside of a banana peel.

# Premenstrual Syndrome (PMS)

PMS is characterized by a constellation of symptoms that may include mood swings, acne, cravings, forgetfulness, insomnia, fatigue, bloating, breast tenderness, palpitation, irritability, backache, headache, anxiety, and depression. It usually begins seven to fourteen days before menstruation, and often continues through the first few days of the menstrual cycle. While the exact cause is unknown, hormonal, psychological, and nutritional factors all influence the condition.

Conventional medicine often treats this condition with pain relievers, such as acetaminophen and nonsteroidal anti-inflammatory drugs (NSAIDs) like ibuprofen. Warm compresses and baths, along with a regular exercise program, are recommended. Hormonal treatments such as the oral contraceptive pill, are commonly prescribed to reduce hormone fluctuations.

| EZ Care Program ||
| --- | --- |
| Diet | **Avoid** all caffeine containing products, including coffee, chocolate, black tea, orange pekoe tea, soda, etc. Avoid alcohol during the premenstrual phase. |
| | **Avoid** all foods containing estrogens, including nonorganic meats, poultry, eggs, and dairy products. Strong, chemical estrogen mimics, known as xenoestrogens should be avoided. These compounds, found in plastic beverage and storage containers, can aggravate PMS and increase the risk of breast cancer. <br> *Note:* Meat, poultry, and eggs organically produced and certified hormone-free may be acceptable if desired. |
| | **Avoid dairy foods** – Even hormone-free dairy foods may worsen PMS by evoking allergic responses, increasing congestion, and impairing the absorption of magnesium from the gut. |
| | **Avoid excess intake of salt**, because this may aggravate premenstrual edema. |
| Vitamins | **B6** (pyridoxal 5-phosphate is preferred form) – Dosage: 25 to 50 mg., two times daily with morning and evening meals. Especially important during the 10 days preceding menstruation to help prevent premenstrual swelling and soreness. B6 is a natural diuretic (water pill). <br> *Note:* Always use B6 in conjunction with a complete B complex formula, because high doses of one of the B vitamins may lead to imbalance in the body's pool of the other B vitamins. |

| | **EZ Care Program** | | |
|---|---|
| | **E** (natural d-alpha tocopherol in a base of mixed tocopherols) – Dosage: 800 to 1200 IU daily with a meal. Reduces breast tenderness. |
| Minerals | **Calcium** (elemental calcium from amino acid chelate) – Dosage: 800 mg. daily in divided doses with meals and at bedtime. May help prevent premenstrual edema and menstrual cramping, especially if taken during the 10 days prior to onset of menstruation. |
| | **Magnesium** (elemental magnesium from amino acid chelate) – Dosage: 800 mg. daily in divided doses with meals. Essential for relaxing the muscular and nervous systems.<br>May help reduce nervous sensitivity, depression, breast tenderness, and uterine pain associated with PMS. |
| | **Zinc** (elemental zinc from amino acid chelate) – Dosage: 25 mg taken separately from calcium and magnesium; may compete with magnesium for absorption from the gut.<br>May help reduce depression, mood-swings, headaches, dizziness, and craving for sweets. |
| Herbs | **Chaste Tree Berries** (Vitex agnus castus) – Dosage: two 1,000 mg. capsules or 1 tsp. liquid extract* upon arising for at least 90 days.<br>*Beneficial properties:* May encourage hormonal harmonization in women. |
| | **Evening Primrose Oil** (Oenothera biennis) – Dosage: 1300 mg., two times daily with meals for at least 6 to 8 weeks. Thereafter, 500 mg., two times daily during the ten days proceeding each period. Contains gamma-linoleic acid (GLA), a natural anti-inflammatory.<br>*Beneficial properties:* May help balance hormones and reduce breast swelling and tenderness.<br>*Note:* Black currant or borage oil, also rich sources of GLA, may be used as alternatives to evening primrose oil. |
| Miscellaneous | **Avoid** all forms of **tobacco.** |
| | **Exercise daily**, incorporating 30 minutes of aerobic exercise. Promotes detoxification, increased circulation, and overall well being.<br>*Note:* Consult a healthcare practitioner before starting any new exercise program. |
| | **Natural Progesterone Skin Cream** (3% progesterone, not wild yam cream) – Apply topically 1 to 2 times daily for the two-weeks beginning with ovulation until the first day of menstrual flow. Then discontinue use until time of ovulation of the next cycle. |
| | **Review Homeopathy** and **Aromatherapy** sections for appropriate remedies. |

## Additional Recommendations

The EZ Care Program consists of basic remedies that are commonly used for premenstrual syndrome and have been found to work well in most cases. The remedies are most effective when combined, but can be used individually. The options stated below can supplement or replace EZ Care remedies and may be combined when suggested doses are followed.

## Diet:

♦ **Drink** 6 to 8 glasses of pure **water** daily.

♦ **Eat a high-water-content diet** consisting of large quantities of fresh fruits and vegetables with comparatively smaller quantities of whole grains, legumes, seeds, nuts, fish, skinless chicken and turkey.

♦ **Fiber Supplement** – Dosage: 1 to 3 tsp. psyllium husk fiber in 8 oz. pure water one to two times daily between meals.
*Note:* Carefully read label; some brands require additional water.

## Vitamins

♦ **A** (natural, from fish liver oil) – Dosage: 10,000 to 25,000 IU daily with meals during second half of menstrual cycle.
*Note:* Consult a physician before using higher doses of vitamin A. Avoid use if pregnant or attempting pregnancy. Discontinue use if you experience nausea, dry skin, sore lips, blurred vision, or other signs of vitamin A toxicity.

♦ **B3** (niacin)'– Dosage: 100 mg., two times daily with meals. May help reduce headache, dizziness, and craving for sweets.
*Notes:* (1) Niacin, which initiates the release of histamine from mast cells, may cause an uncomfortable flushing sensation that generally lasts as much as 30 minutes. If this occurs, change to a flush-free form of niacin (niacin with inositol). (2) Always use B3 in conjunction with a complete B complex formula, because high doses of one of the B vitamins may lead to imbalance in the body's pool of the other B vitamins.

♦ **B Complex** – Dosage: 50 to 100 mg daily with a meal.
*Note:* For highest assimilation, use a multi B complex which contains the vitamins in their coenzyme form and avoid mega-potency B complex products.

♦ **C** (mixed mineral ascorbate) – Dosage: 1,000 mg., twice daily with breakfast and dinner. Protects some of the B vitamins, vitamin A, and vitamin E from oxidation. Also helps control allergic reaction and aids in formation of red blood cells.

## Herbs

♦ **Dandelion Root** (Taraxacum officinalis) – Dosage: two 500 mg. capsules two to three times daily with meals.
*Beneficial properties:* Liver tonic that may help the body metabolize hormones. For water retention, consider a tea prepared by infusion (see Appendix B): 1 part **Dandelion Root** to 1 part **Cleavers herb** (Galium aparine). Take 6-8 oz. of this tea two to three times daily during the premenstrual phase.

♦ **Dong Quai** (Angelica sinensis) – Dosage: two 500 mg. capsules two times daily with meals.
*Beneficial properties:* A Chinese herb that may help balance hormones.

♦ **False Unicorn Root** (Helonias dioica) – Dosage: two 1,000 mg. capsules or 60 drops liquid extract* two times daily between meals for 60-90 days. For synergistic action, take with chaste tree berries capsules or liquid extract.
*Beneficial properties:* Regenerative tonic for ovaries and uterus, which may encourage hormonal harmonization in women.

♦ **Milk Thistle Seed Extract** (silybum marianum) – Dosage: 250 mg. daily of standardized extract or 30-60 drops liquid extract* in 4 oz. water three times daily with meals.
*Beneficial properties:* May help protect the liver, which is the body's major detoxification organ, from toxins. The liver is responsible for the breakdown and elimination of excess estrogens. Hyperestroginism is commonly a contributing factor to PMS.

♦ **Motherwort** (Leonurus cardiaca) + **Passion Flower tea** (Passiflora incarnata) with **Oat Seed Extract** (Avena sativa) (see Appendix B). Proportion: 1 part **motherwort** to 1 part **passionflower**. Pour into a cup. While still hot, add 35 drops liquid extract of oat seed. Let stand 7 minutes before drinking. If a quantity of tea + extract is saved for later use, warm-up gently using low heat before serving. Dosage: 8 oz. of this tea two to three times daily or as required.
*Beneficial properties:* Calming blend that may help relieve premenstrual agitation, anxiety, and insomnia.

## Aromatherapy

**Neroli** (Citrus aurantium var. amara) + **Chamomile** (Matricaria chamomilla) + **Rose** (Rosa damascena) – Add 2 drops each of these essential oils into a warm (but not hot) full bath. Soak up to 30 minutes. After gently drying, massage a blend consisting of 2 drops each of these essential oils mixed with 1-1/2 tsp. sweet almond or jojoba oil into the chest, throat, abdomen, hands, and feet. May help alleviate premenstrual depression and irritability.

## Homeopathy

See Appendix E for proper use and handling instruction prior to administering remedies described below.

♦ **Belladonna 12C** – Severe premenstrual uterine pain and discomfort with sudden, violent, spasmodic contractions that are worse with sudden movement, jarring, or pressure; may be accompanied by flushes of facial heat and diverse burning sensations. Dosage: Dissolve 5 pellets under the tongue, two times daily or as required.

♦ **Platina 12C** – Burning pain or discomfort, especially of left abdominal or ovarian region, with early painful and heavy periods; may have increased libido and tendency to be critical, suspicious and jealous of others. Dosage: Dissolve 5 pellets under the tongue, two times daily or as required.

♦ **Pulsatilla 12C** – Changeable moods, tearfulness, anxiety, and hysteria; nausea with lightheadedness and fainting; cycle irregular, with absence of, or short, menstrual periods. Dosage: Dissolve 5 pellets under the tongue, two times daily or as required.

♦ **Sepia 15C** – Exhaustion, irritability, low back pain, abdominal cramping, loss of libido, anger, intolerance, indifference, depression, and moodiness. Dosage: Dissolve 5 pellets under the tongue, one to two times daily or as required.

### Miscellaneous

♦ **Deep Breathing Exercises** – Calms the mind and body. Following is a yoga breathing exercise for calming the mind: Inhale through the nose with a deep belly breath for a count of 4, hold for a count of 7, exhale through the mouth for a count of 8. Practice two times daily, four to eight repetitions each.
*Note:* To enhance concentration and be certain the exercise is performed properly, you might lie down, place a lightweight book on your abdomen, then peacefully observe the book's rise-and-fall motion as you breathe deeply.

\* Most herbal extracts contain alcohol. Avoid use if alcohol sensitive or if there is a history of alcohol abuse. *Note:* Alcohol content can be reduced through evaporation by adding extract to very hot water (just below boiling point) and allowing to stand 5 to 7 minutes before drinking.

# Prostate Enlargement (BPH)

This condition occurs when the prostate gland enlarges, causing obstruction of the proper flow of urine. This may result in frequent urination, decreased force of urination, difficulty starting and stopping urination, dribbling, and a sensation of incomplete emptying. This is the leading cause of urinary obstruction in men ages 45 to 70. A physician should be consulted by men who have these symptoms, to properly diagnose the cause and rule out any potentially serious condition, such as prostate cancer.

Conventional medicine may choose not to treat cases with mild symptoms, or may use several prescription medicines to help shrink the prostate, or alleviate urinary difficulties. Antibiotics also may be used when there is an associated bacterial infection that has caused inflammation of the prostate. More advanced cases are treated with a surgical procedure called transurethral resection of the prostate (TURP). Other surgical procedures include transurethral needle ablation of the prostate (TUNA), and microwave prostate obliteration. Of these choices, TUNA may be the safest and most effective treatment for prostate hypertrophy.

| EZ Care Program | |
|---|---|
| Diet | **Avoid** all caffeine containing products, including coffee, chocolate, black tea, orange pekoe tea, and soda. Avoid **alcohol**, refined sugar, excessive salt, and strong spices, all of which may cause irritation and decrease blood flow to the prostate gland. |
| | **Drink 8 glasses of pure, room-temperature water** daily. Important to control tissue inflammation and help facilitate the voiding of urine. However, avoid most fluid intake after 6 PM, to decrease the need to void at night. |
| | **Eat a high-water-content diet** consisting of large quantities of fresh fruits and vegetables and soy protein. Men who consume a large soy protein diet have lower incidences of prostate cancer and less prostatism. |
| | **Eat** generous amounts of raw **pumpkin seeds**, because they contain zinc and essential fatty acids that are beneficial for prostate health. Dosage: Pumpkin seed oil capsules 1,000 mg., two times for three months may prove helpful. |
| | **Eat** 2 to 3 tbsp. **lecithin granules** (help the body process cholesterol) daily with meals. Elevated cholesterol levels may lead to harmful accumulation of cholesterol metabolites in the prostate gland. |
| | **Flaxseed Oil** – Dosage: 1 to 2 tsp. daily. Rich source of omega-3 essential fatty acids, a deficiency of which may be a factor in BPH. |
| Vitamins | **B6** (pyridoxal 5-phosphate is preferred) – Dosage: 50 to 100 mg., two times daily with morning and evening meals. An important zinc synergist and essential for proper fatty acid metabolism. *Note:* Always use B6 in conjunction with a complete B complex formula, because high doses of one of the B vitamins may lead to imbalance in the body's pool of the other B vitamins. |
| | **Lycopene** – Dosage 5 mg., two to three times daily with meals. A natural carotenoid (tomatoes are an excellent source) that may support prostate health. Clinically proven to reduce the incidence of prostate carcinoma. |
| Minerals | **Zinc** – Dosage: 25 mg. elemental zinc from amino acid chelate two to three times daily with meals. May help reduce prostate enlargement. |
| Herbs | **Pygeum africanum** – Dosage: 40 mg. standardized extract two times daily with saw palmetto extract. *Beneficial properties:* May exert a positive influence on testosterone metabolism. Works as a synergist with saw palmetto in treating BPH. |
| | **Saw Palmetto** (Serenoa repens) – Dosage: 160 mg. standardized extract two to four times daily in divided doses between meals. *Beneficial properties:* Supports proper prostate and urinary function. |
| Miscellaneous | **Avoid** use of all forms of **tobacco.** |
| | **Combination** of these amino acids: **L-glutamic acid + L-alanine + L-glycine**. Dosage: two 500 mg. capsules three times daily for two weeks. Then 1 capsule three times daily thereafter or as required. May help relieve many symptoms of BPH. |

| | **EZ Care Program** |
|---|---|
| | **Soy capsules** - Dosage 1000 mg. twice daily. Soy isoflavones promote healthy hormone metabolism and inhibit prostate enlargement. In population studies, high soy consumption is associated with lower incidences of prostate hypertrophy, prostate cancer, and cardiovasuclar disease. |

# Additional Recommendations

The EZ Care Program consists of basic remedies that are commonly used for BPH and have been found to work well in most cases. The remedies are most effective when combined, but can be used individually. The options stated below can supplement or replace EZ Care remedies and may be combined when suggested doses are followed.

## Diet:

♦ **This salad may prove beneficial for supporting a healthy prostate gland:** Slice 1 large tomato or 2 medium-size ones into a bowl. Add 1/3 cucumber plus 1-2 tbsp. chopped parsley. Then mix 1 tbsp. unfiltered apple cider vinegar, 2 tbsp. olive oil and a dash of ginger powder; pour over the vegetables. Serve 1 to 2 times daily with meals.

## Vitamins

♦ **B complex** – Dosage 25 to 50 mg daily with a meal.
*Note:* For highest assimilation, use a multi B complex which contains the vitamins in their coenzyme form and avoid mega-potency B complex products.

♦ **C** (mineral ascorbates mixed with bioflavonoids) – Dosage: 1,000 mg., two times daily with breakfast and dinner. Important factor in prostaglandin synthesis, amino acid, and hormone metabolism; and protects the B-vitamins and vitamin E from oxidation.

♦ **E** (natural d-alpha tocopherol in a base of mixed tocopherols) – Dosage: 600 to 800 IU daily with a meal. Vitamin E is specific for reproductive organs. Required for normal fatty acid metabolism.

## Minerals

♦ **Selenium** – Dosage: 200 mcg. daily from l-selenomethionine.
*Note:* Selenium and vitamin E are synergistic; thus, they enhance each other's activity in the body.

## Herbs

♦ **Burdock Root** (Arctium lappa) – Dosage: two 1,000 mg. capsules two times daily upon arising and mid-afternoon with 1 to 2 cups pure water or raw vegetable juice.
*Beneficial properties:* Traditionally used in treating prostate enlargement.

## Homeopathy

See Appendix E for proper use and handling instruction prior to administering remedies described below.

- **Populus 3X** – Enlarged prostate, with scalding urine passed spasmodically with pain and difficulty; pain behind pubic bone after urination. Dosage: Dissolve 5 pellets under the tongue, two to four times daily or as required.

- **Sabal Serrul 3X** – Chronic or acute enlargement, with difficulty passing urine, burning sensation while urinating, chronic bladder infections, and a constant desire to urinate at night. Dosage: Dissolve 5 pellets under the tongue, two to four times daily or as required.

## Hydrotherapy

- **Hot Sitz Bath (105° F to 115° F)** – Sitz baths can be hot, cold, or an alternation of both as the condition requires. Complete procedure in Appendix D. The hot sitz bath is the most common. For BPH, sit in the tub (with feet in water) for 4 to 12 minutes. Relaxes and dilates the urinary passageway. Follow with a cool sponging of the pelvic region. Avoid hot sitz baths if there is acute inflammation or infection of the prostate. Sitz baths can be used 1 to 2 times daily or several times weekly or as required.

- **Cold Sitz Bath (55°F-75°F)** for 1 to 6 minutes is generally used in BPH to tone the organs of the pelvic region after the enlargement has subsided. To enhance reaction to the cold stimulation, precede the cold sitz bath with a 2-4 minute *warm* sitz bath. To help prevent chilling, the water level of the cold sitz bath should be one inch less than that of the hot bath; and the feet should be in a basin of hot water. During the cold sitz bath, briskly rub the hips and lower abdominal region with a dry wash cloth to support circulatory reaction to the cold water. Sitz baths can be used 1 to 2 times daily or several times weekly or as required.
  *Note: If seriously ill or debilitated, avoid cold sitz baths unless under the guidance of a physician.*

## Miscellaneous

- **Exercise** at least 30 minutes daily. May benefit blood circulation to prostate.

- **Fish Oil Capsules** – Dosage: 1000 mg., two to three times daily with meals. A rich source of omega-3 EPA and DHA fatty acids that may inhibit production of inflammatory compounds leading to prostate enlargement.

- **Di-indolymethane** (DIMM) – Dosage: 60 mg., two times daily with meals. A phyto-chemical extracted from cruciferous vegetables, which promotes healthy metabolism. Excess estrogens can be metabolized into testosterone, causing prostate enlargement.

# Psoriasis

Psoriasis is a skin disorder characterized by patches of raised, reddish plaques covered with silvery scale. It usually affects the scalp, knees and elbows, but can spread over large areas. This condition tends to be persistent and recurrent, and is one of the most common skin diseases. The cause is unknown.

Conventional treatments include topical moisturizing creams, vitamin D analogs, cortisone creams, and oral cortisone tablets. A procedure combining exposure to ultra violet light with the drug psoralen known as PUVA may be effective for more severe cases. Powerful vitamin A derivatives may be used in some cases. For severe cases, anti-cancer drugs may be used to inhibit the immune system.

Alternative medicine physicians may also screen and treat for candida overgrowth, mineral deficiency, fatty acid imbalances, food allergies, and heavy metal toxicity. All can contribute to the condition.

| EZ Care Program | |
|---|---|
| Diet | **Avoid** citrus juices. |
| | **Avoid** or reduce dairy products, fried foods, sugar, citrus, white flour, caffeine, and alcohol. |
| | **Drink 8** glasses of pure, room-temperature **water** daily. Important for the control of tissue inflammation. |
| | **Eat a high-water-content diet** consisting of large quantities of fresh fruits and vegetables with comparatively smaller quantities of whole grains, legumes, seeds, nuts, fish, skinless chicken and turkey. |
| | **Identify personal food sensitivities**. Avoid all common allergenic foods (e.g., citrus, dairy, eggs, wheat, corn, preservatives, sugar). Rotate moderately allergic foods on a four-day schedule (see Appendix C). |
| | **Eat fish**, such as mackerel, herring, trout, and salmon, because they contain anti-inflammatory omega-3 fatty acids. |
| | **Flaxseed Oil** (cold-pressed) – Dosage: 1 to 2 tbsp. daily with meals. Rich source of alpha-linoleneic acid, which may benefit the treatment of psoriasis. Flaxseed oil can also be taken in capsule form of 1000 – 1250 mg. twice daily. *Note:* Keep refrigerated at all times. Add 1 capsule of vitamin E extract to bottle to prevent rancidity. |
| | **Fish Oil** (Max EPA) – Dosage: 4,000 to 10,000 mg. divided daily with meals. A rich source of omega-3 fatty acids clinically proven to reduce symptoms of psoriasis. Inhibits inflammatory compounds necessary for formation of skin irritation. |

| EZ Care Program | |
| --- | --- |
| Vitamins | **A** (emulsified) – Dosage: 50,000 to 100,000 IU daily for 30 days. Then reduce to 25,000 IU daily for 90 days. Repeat this cycle as required. *Note:* Because vitamin A is fat-soluble and stored in the body, it has the potential for toxicity. Always check with a physician before beginning supplementation with this level of vitamin A. Avoid use if pregnant. Discontinue use if you experience nausea, dry skin, sore lips, blurred vision, or other signs of vitamin A excess. May inhibit the endogenous synthesis of certain toxic substances that have been linked to psoriasis. |
| | **D** (from fish liver oil) – Dosage: 400 IU two to three times daily with meals. *Note:* Vitamin D is fat-soluble and stores in the body, giving it the potential for toxicity. Always check with a physician before beginning supplementation with this level of vitamin D. |
| | **E** (natural d-alpha tocopherol in a base of mixed tocopherols) – Dosage: 1,200 IU daily in divided doses with meals. Helps maintain the biological integrity of vitamin A and helps protects the skin from free radical damage due to the oxidation of polyunsaturated fats. |
| Minerals | **Zinc** (take only if over 14 years of age) – Dosage: 25 mg. elemental zinc from amino acid chelate two to three times daily with meals. Necessary for absorbing alpha-linoleneic acid, a deficiency of which increases the risk for developing psoriasis. |
| Herbs | **Burdock Root** (Arcium lappa) – Dosage: 2 capsules with 8 oz. pure water two to three times daily between meals. *Beneficial properties:* May help bowel detoxification and be beneficial as a blood purifier. |
| | Prepare an infusion (see Appendix B) using equal parts of: **Red Clover** (Trifolium praetense) + **Echinacea** (Echinacea purpurea) + **Sarsaparilla Root** (Smilax officinalis) + **Yellow Dock Root** (Rumex crispus). Dosage: drink 6 oz. three to four times daily between meals. *Beneficial properties:* May exert potent blood-cleansing and skin-purifying actions. |
| Miscellaneous | Expose skin to **direct sunlight** or ultraviolet light up to 30 minutes daily, being careful not to overdo and suffer sunburn. Sunbathing is best practiced before ten a.m. or after three p.m. to avoid the most intensive period of ultraviolet (UV) ray exposure. |
| | **Reduce** lifestyle **stress** and implement a relaxation program. Harmonizing practices (e.g., biofeedback, meditation, yoga, Tai Chi exercise) may prove beneficial. |
| | **Review** the **Homeopathy** section and **ocean bathing** for appropriate remedies. |

## Additional Recommendations

The EZ Care Program consists of basic remedies that are commonly used for psoriasis and have been found to work well in most cases. The remedies are most effective when combined, but can be used individually. The options stated below can supplement or replace EZ Care remedies and may be combined when suggested doses are followed.

### Vitamins

♦ **B12** – Dosage: 2,000 mcg. daily for 30 days, then every other day for two months. Sublingual forms are preferred for maximal absorption. May prove beneficial in psoriasis treatment.
*Note:* Always use a complete B complex formula in addition to vitamin B12, because high doses of one of the B vitamins may lead to imbalance in the body's pool of the other B vitamins.

♦ **B complex** – 25 to 50 mg. daily with a meal.
*Note:* For highest assimilation, use a multi B complex which contains the vitamins in their coenzyme form and avoid mega-potency B complex products.

♦ **Biotin** – Dosage 1000 mg. twice daily. Biotin is a vitamin in the B family important for the integrity of skin, hair, and nails.

♦ **C** (mineral ascorbate mixed with bioflavonoids) – Dosage: 2,000 to 3,000 mg. daily in divided doses with meals. Required for forming and maintaining collagen, an important component of skin.

♦ **Folic Acid** – Dosage: 800 mcg. one to two times daily with meals. Commonly given with vitamin B12, because they are intimately related regarding red blood cell production. Green, leafy vegetables are an excellent source of folic acid. It is not coincidental that the words *folic* and *foliage* derive from the same word root. Psoriasis patients may be deficient in folic acid.
*Note:* Always use a complete B complex formula (preferably in coenzyme form) in addition to folic acid, because high doses of one of the B vitamins may lead to imbalance in the body's pool of the other B vitamins.

### Minerals

♦ **Selenium** – Dosage: 200 mcg. daily from l-selenomethionine. Parallels the antioxidant and free radical-scavenging action of vitamin E and, thus, may enhance its action.

### Herbs

♦ **Dandelion Root** (Taraxacum officinalis) – Dosage: 1 capsule or 30 drops extract* in 4 oz. water before each meal up to three times daily.
*Beneficial properties:* A liver cleanser and blood purifier that may benefit skin conditions.

♦ **Milk Thistle Seed Extract** (silybum marianum) – Dosage: 250 mg. daily of standardized extract or 30-60 drops liquid extract* in 4 oz. water three times daily with meals.
*Beneficial properties:* May help support the liver's detoxification function and inhibit inflammation. Abnormal liver detoxification function may be a contributing factor to psoriasis.

♦ **Sarsaparilla (**Smilax officinalis) – Dosage: 1 capsule three times daily for at least three months.

*Beneficial properties:* May help condition by promoting excretion of toxins from the lymph and circulatory systems and neutralization of microbial substances in the bloodstream.

## Aromatherapy

**Essential Oil of Lavender** (Lavendula vera) – Mix 4 drops in 1 tsp. aloe vera gel. Apply topically as required.

## Homeopathy

See Appendix E for proper use and handling instruction prior to administering remedies described below.

♦ **Graphites 6C** – Psoriasis behind ears, on palms or back of hands, characterized by thick skin with cracks that may ooze a thick, yellow, honey-like fluid. Dosage: Dissolve 5 pellets under the tongue, two to three times daily or as required.

♦ **Kali Arsenicum 12C** – Patches of psoriasis on back, arms, and elbows; burning, itching scales that, when they detach, leave red skin; withered skin in the crooks of elbows and knees; condition becomes worse when undressing and with exposure to cold substances and conditions. Dosage: Dissolve 5 pellets under the tongue, two to three times daily or as required.

♦ **Petroleum 12C** – Fissured psoriasis lesions on hands that are worse when exposed to cold substances and conditions and in winter; fissures often deep and bloody; may scratch the skin until raw, and a cold sensation of the skin after scratching. Dosage: Dissolve 5 pellets under the tongue, two to three times daily or as required.

♦ **Sulphur 1M** – Consider administering as a general remedy when first beginning homeopathic therapy for psoriasis. Dosage: Dissolve 5 pellets under the tongue, once only. No other homeopathic remedy is given for at least 15 days afterward. Then proceed with one of the specific remedies listed in this section, selected in accordance with associated characteristic symptoms.

## Miscellaneous

♦ **Apple Cider Vinegar Massage** – Add 1/2 cup unfiltered apple cider vinegar to a small basin of 2 to 3 cups warm water. Dip both hands into the mixture and thoroughly massage entire skin surface. Wet the skin with the mixture several times. Massage the skin with bare hands until completely dry. Do not rinse afterward; allow the apple cider vinegar to thoroughly penetrate the skin layers. Perform one to three times weekly or as desired.

♦ **Applications of therapeutic mud**, particularly from the Dead Sea. May be very beneficial for psoriasis. Apply to dry skin and allow to dry until a clay texture has formed. Rinse thoroughly and apply calendula oil (Calendula officinalis).

♦ **Fumaric Acid** – Dosage: 250 mg. daily. Fumaric acid can reduce symptoms of psoriasis but should only be used with physician supervision. Side effects include nausea, diarrhea, headaches, and liver and kidney toxicity.

♦ **Lecithin granules** – Dosage: 4 tbsp. daily with meals for two months, than reduce to 2 tbsp. daily. A rich source of phospholipids that plays an important role in fat transport. Disturbance of fat metabolism may be an important factor in psoriasis.

♦ **Ocean Bathing or Salt Baths** – Regular immersion in mineral-rich sea water has proven to be of benefit for many psoriasis sufferers. When regular sea-bathing is not feasible, the salt bath is an option. Add 2 to 3 lb. unscented Dead Sea salt (first choice, available in many healthfood stores) or unrefined sea salt to a half-full bath of cool water (85° F to 90° F). If frail, begin with 2 lb. salt, gradually increasing quantity in subsequent baths in accordance with improved tolerance. Using a thermometer, adjust water temperature until it is in the range indicated. A cooler temperature may cause chilliness; hotter temperature may cause depletion or aggravate a case of psoriasis that worsens with warmth. Bathe for 10 to 30 minutes. The first baths should be of shorter duration; increase bath time in accordance with expanding tolerance. While in tub, rub briskly with the salty water. Then rub body with a coarse cotton towel until skin is warm and glowing. Perform one to three times weekly according to tolerance.
*Note:* If frail or have a heart condition or other serious health problem, consult a physician regarding the advisability of these tub baths in your case.

♦ **Proteolytic Enzyme Formula** (including protease, bromelain, and papain). May help with digestion. Take as directed on package.
*Note:* Avoid if stomach or duodenal ulcers; proteolytic enzymes may aggravate ulcers and induce bleeding.

\* Most herbal extracts contain alcohol. Avoid use if alcohol sensitive or if there is a history of alcohol abuse. *Note:* Alcohol content can be reduced through evaporation by adding extract to very hot water (just below boiling point) and allowing to stand 5 to 7 minutes before drinking.

# Rash

A rash can be defined as a skin eruption, generally typified by reddening and itching. It may be a local skin reaction, or an outward sign of internal problems. When a rash develops, it is important to discover the cause rather than treat the rash symptomatically. Any new food or medication can cause a rash. Speak with your health care practitioner to determine the causes of any unknown rash.

Conventional treatments vary, but may include emollients for dry, scaly rashes, and drying agents for weeping rashes. Medications that cause a rash should be stopped under a physician's supervision.

| EZ Care Program | |
|---|---|
| Diet | **Drink 8** glasses of pure, room-temperature **water** daily. Important for flushing toxins from the tissues. |
| Vitamins | **C** (mineral ascorbate with bioflavonoids) – Dosage: 1,000 mg., three to five times daily. May be very helpful as an anti-inflammatory and detoxificant. |
| Herbs | **Burdock Root** (Arcium lappa) and **Echinacea Root** (Echinacea purpurea) – Dosage: 2 capsules of each three to four times daily with meals and at bedtime, or use in combination in tea form. Prepare tea by decoction (see Appendix B) using 3 parts burdock root to 2 parts echinacea root. Drink 6 oz. four to five times daily between meals. *Beneficial properties:* Burdock Root may be beneficial as a blood purifier. Echinacea supports immune system function. |
| | **Calendula Cream** (Calendula officinalis) – Apply externally 4 to 6 times daily. *Beneficial Properties:* May promote soothing and healing of skin tissue and prevent infections. In some cases, may help avoid need for topical cortisone. Especially noted in treating diaper rash. *Note:* Avoid use of calendula lotions that contain alcohol; alcohol may exacerbate irritation and dryness. |
| | **Red Clover Blossom** (Trifolium praetense) and **Chickweed** (Stellaria media) **tea** – Prepare a strong infusion (see Appendix B) using 3 parts red clover to 2 parts chickweed. Drink freely between meals. Red clover is a blood purifier; chickweed soothes and heals inflamed tissue. |
| Miscellaneous | **Oatmeal Bath** – Cook 2 cups rolled oats in 4 cups water. Place oatmeal gruel into a cheesecloth bag (i.e., fold cheesecloth around the gruel and secure with a string or rubber band). Place the bag into bathtub while filling with warm water. Soak in tub for 15 to 30 minutes. After bath, pat dry without rinsing to allow demulcent substances from the oatmeal to remain on skin. Repeat 1 to 2 times daily as needed. Soothes itchy rashes and diaper rash. |
| | **Review Homeopathy** section for appropriate remedies. |

# Additional Recommendations

The EZ Care Program consists of basic remedies that are commonly used for rashes and have been found to work well in most cases. The remedies are most effective when combined, but can be used individually. The options stated below can supplement or replace EZ Care remedies and may be combined when suggested doses are followed.

## Diet

♦ **Consider a two-to-seven day juice fast** (i.e., intake restricted to fresh fruit, vegetable juices, and pure water) **or complete fast** (i.e., intake restricted to pure water only). Most suitable length and type of fast varies with each person.
*Note*: If you have a serious health problem, or are taking prescription medication, always consult with a physician before undertaking a fast. Fasting provides the body with a respite from needing to react to substances that may be causing a rash, and allows the body to focus on the process of detoxification. If fasting is not feasible, consider a diet

consisting exclusively of raw fruits, vegetables, and fresh juices for a period of 4 to 7 days.

♦ **Eat a high-water-content diet** consisting of large quantities of fresh fruits and vegetables and comparatively smaller quantities of whole grains, legumes, seeds, nuts, fish, skinless chicken and turkey.

♦ **Flaxseed Oil** – Dosage: 1 to 2 tbsp. daily. Contains omega-3 fatty acids that may help control inflammatory reactions.

♦ **Identify personal food sensitivities** for chronic rashes. Avoid all common allergenic foods (e.g., dairy, eggs, wheat, corn, sugar, preservatives). Rotate moderately allergic foods on a four-day schedule (see Appendix C).

## Vitamins

♦ **A** (natural, from fish liver oil) – Dosage: 25,000 IU one to three times daily with meals for seven to ten days. Then reduce to a maintenance level of 10,000 to 25,000 IU daily. Helps maintain, smooth, disease-free skin.
*Note:* Consult a physician before using higher doses of vitamin A. Avoid use if pregnant. Discontinue use if you experience symptoms of overload, such as dry skin, nausea, sore lips, and headache.

♦ **B complex** – Dosage: 25 to 50 mg. daily with meals.
*Note:* For highest assimilation, use a B complex that contains the vitamins in their coenzyme form and avoid mega-potency B complex products. B complex vitamins are essential for the health of the skin, liver detoxification, and cortisone secretion by the adrenal glands. Also crucial for normal functioning of nervous system; chronic rashes are often related in part to emotional stress.

♦ **E** (natural d-alpha tocopherol in a base of mixed tocopherols) – Dosage: 800 IU daily with meals. Vitamin E prevents oxidation of adrenal hormones and vitamin A; and promotes proper functioning of essential fatty acids.

## Minerals

♦ **Selenium** – Dosage: 200 mcg. daily from l-selenomethionine. An antioxidant that delays oxidation of essential fatty acids, preserves elasticity of skin tissue, and stimulates formation of antibodies.
*Note:* Selenium and vitamin E are synergistic; thus, they enhance each other's activity in the body.

♦ **Zinc** –Dosage: 25 mg., two to three times daily with meals until rash clears, then reduce intake to once daily or as required. Plays an important role in collagen formation, wound healing, and functioning of the skin's normal oil gland function. Zinc is a vitamin A synergist.

## Herbs

♦ Mix equal parts of **Goldenseal Root** (Hydrastis canadensis) + **Echinacea Root** + **Yellow Dock Root** (Rumex crispus) + **Witch Hazel Bark** (Hamamelis virginiana) – Prepare a strong infusion (see Appendix B) using 1 heaping tbsp. of the mixture to 16 oz. pure water. Steep for 1 hour; strain, discard herbs, and add 1 tbsp. boric acid to the recovered liquid. Use this preparation to wash the affected area, or saturate a white cotton cloth and apply as a compress four to five times daily or as required.
*Beneficial properties:* May exert a local soothing and healing action.

## Aromatherapy

Mix 3 drops of **Calendula** essential oil with 1/2 tsp. **Aloe Vera Gel** and apply topically several times daily or as required.

## Homeopathy

See Appendix E for proper use and handling instruction prior to administering remedies described below.

♦ **Apis 12C** – Rash with sudden appearance of pink or pale swelling that may progress to purplish color accompanied by severe itching, burning, stinging sensation, and soreness; better with cold applications. Dosage: Dissolve 5 pellets under the tongue, one to three times daily or as required.

♦ **Rhus Tox 12C** – Small fluid-filled eruptions grouped together in clumps with surrounding inflammation; itching relieved by warm applications. Dosage: Dissolve 5 pellets under the tongue, one to three times daily or as required.

♦ **Urtica Urens 3C** – Prickly heat rash with sweatiness, burning, swelling, and severe itching; condition worse with cold applications, and with bathing and washing in general. Dosage: Dissolve 5 pellets under the tongue, two to four times daily or as required.

## Miscellaneous

♦ **Clay Poultice** – *For dry, scaly rash:* mix 1 tbsp. clay with 2 tbsp. olive oil plus 1 tbsp. pure water. For either, use a spatula or wooden spoon to spread the clay paste 1/4 inch to one inch thick on a piece of undyed cotton or linen cloth (cut to the dimensions of the rash). Place the clay side down on the rash. Secure and leave in place two hours. Apply one to three times daily or as required.

♦ **Lactobacillus Probiotic** (friendly intestinal bacteria that aids digestion, nutrient assimilation, and toxin elimination) (L. acidophilus with bifidus and fructo-oligosaccharides) – Follow directions on label.
*Note:* Particularly indicated when antibiotics have been used.

♦ **Psyllium Powder** – Dosage: 1 to 2 tsp. in 8 oz. pure water (followed by another 8 oz. pure water) one to two times daily upon arising and before bedtime. Psyllium facilitates full, easy bowel movements. Sluggish bowel function and accumulation of intestinal toxins are often an important contributory factor to various skin conditions.

# Sinusitis

Sinusitis is an inflammation of one or more of the facial sinus cavities, generally caused by infection. It may be classified as acute, which is a temporary infection that often follows a cold or flu, or chronic, which is a recurring condition often caused by environmental irritants and allergies like dust, pollen, smoke, or an unresolved case of acute sinusitis. Symptoms include chills or fever, pressure over the eyes or in the cheekbones, swelling of the eyelids, tenderness over the affected sinus, congestion, yellowish green discharge, headache or dizziness, and tooth pain.

Allergies play a significant role in both types of sinusitis. Immediate exposure to an allergen causes mucus membrane swelling, leading to the build-up of sinus pressure and increasing the risk of infection. Chronic allergy exposure causes permanent changes in the anatomy of the palate and nasal septum, resulting in improper sinus drainage and airway obstruction.

Conventional treatments include inhalation of steam, warm facial compresses, over-the-counter decongestants, steroid nasal sprays, antibiotics, or surgery for severe cases. Seek the advice of a holistic physician to obtain advanced allergy testing and evaluation for yeast overgrowth.

| EZ Care Program | |
|---|---|
| Diet | **Drink 8** glasses of pure, room-temperature **water** daily. Important for controlling tissue inflammation |
| | **Avoid milk** and all milk products, because they increase mucus formation. Consider dairy alternatives like soy or nut milks and cheeses. |
| Vitamins | **C** (mixed mineral ascorbates) – Dosage: 1,000 mg., three to four times daily with meals. May resolve sinus infection. Decreases the body's response to allergies. Boosts the immune system. |
| | **Bioflavonoids** (full potency) – Dosage: 500 mg., three to four times daily with vitamin C. Essential for proper absorption of vitamin C, and for resisting infection |
| Herbs | **Garlic** (Allium sativa) – Add raw garlic liberally and 1 tbsp. unfiltered apple cider vinegar to salads 2 times daily. *Beneficial properties:* May help resolve infection and catarrhal discharge. |

| | EZ Care Program |
|---|---|
| | **Echinacea** (Echinacea purpurea) – Dosage: 50 drops liquid extract* or 2 capsules dried flowers every two to three hours for acute sinusitis. For added benefit, combine with goldenseal. *Beneficial properties:* An immune stimulant used to fight viral infections. |
| Miscellaneous | **Horseradish** (Amoracia lapathifolia) – Eat 1/2 tsp. fresh, grated horseradish two times daily, morning and afternoon. Do not eat or drink anything for at least 15 minutes after each dose. **Lemon juice** and horseradish work as synergists in treating sinus infections; express juice from 1 lemon (if organic, juice the peel also) and mix with 4 oz. grated horseradish + 12 oz. **pure water**. Mix in blender. **Note:** Juice lemon peel only when using an organically-grown lemon whose peel is chemical-free. Otherwise, juice only the lemon pulp. Serve 8 oz. of either juice combination 2 times daily between meals. In chronic cases, it may be necessary to continue this treatment for several months. May help sinuses to drain. |
| | **Nasal irrigation** to flush out the sinuses. Dissolve 1/4 tsp. Kosher salt in 1 cup warm water. Snort solution from a cupped hand, directly from the cup prepared in, or by tilting head back and squirting gently with a rubber bulb syringe. Irrigate one nostril at a time, holding the other closed with other hand. Perform several times daily for acute condition, gently blowing nose after each time. *Note:* May be performed daily as a preventive measure. |
| | Review **Homeopathy** and **Aromatherapy** sections for appropriate remedies. |

# Additional Recommendations

The EZ Care Program consists of basic remedies that are commonly used for sinusitis and have been found to work well in most cases. The remedies are most effective when combined, but can be used individually. The options stated below can supplement or replace EZ Care remedies and may be combined when suggested doses are followed.

## Diet

♦ **Eat a high-water-content diet** consisting of large quantities of fresh fruits and vegetables and comparatively smaller quantities of whole grains, legumes, seeds, nuts, fish, skinless chicken and turkey.

♦ For chronic sinusitis, **identify personal food sensitivities**. Avoid all common allergenic foods (e.g., dairy, eggs, wheat, corn, preservatives, sugar). Rotate moderately allergic foods on a four-day schedule (see Appendix C). This procedure is crucial to identify foods responsible for sinus congestion.

## Vitamins

♦ **A** (natural, from fish liver oil) – Dosage: 25,000 IU one to three times daily with meals for seven to ten days. Then, reduce to a maintenance level of 10,000 to 25,000 IU daily. Helps maintain healthy mucous membrane of the nose and throat.

*Note:* Consult a physician before using higher doses of vitamin A. Avoid use if pregnant. Discontinue use if symptoms of toxicity, such as dry skin, nausea, sore lips, or headache.

♦ **Beta-Carotene** – Dosage: 50,000 IU two times daily for up to two weeks. Then, in chronic cases, reduce to a maintenance dose of 50,000 IU daily. Non-toxic, precursor of vitamin A derived from vegetable sources.

## Minerals

♦ **Zinc** (take only if over 14 years of age) – Dosage: 25 mg. elemental zinc from amino acid chelate two to three times daily taken with meals. After two weeks, reduce to a maintenance dose of 25 mg. daily. May inhibit the growth of infectious microorganisms and stimulate the immune system.
*Note:* Zinc and vitamin A are synergistic and work well together in this context.

## Herbs

♦ **Bayberry Bark** (Myrica cerifera) – Prepare a decoction of bayberry root bark (see Appendix B) using 1 tsp. bayberry bark to 1 cup pure water. Simmer 30 minutes. Let cool and strain. Sniff strained decoction into the nose, alternating between nostrils. Continue until each side is thoroughly treated.
*Beneficial properties:* Excellent when sinus mucosa has lost tone and is discharging profusely. May help both clean and heal the sinuses.

♦ **Goldenseal** (Hydrastis canadensis) – Dosage: 1 to 2 capsules or 30-50 drops liquid extract* every four hours for acute infections.
*Beneficial properties:* Traditionally used to treat acute bacterial sinus infection.

♦ **Grapeseed Extract or Pine Bark Extract** (Pycnogenol) – Dosage: 50 mg., three times daily.
*Beneficial properties:* A powerful antioxidant that may benefit allergy-related sinusitis.

♦ **Peppermint** (Mentha piperita) – Dosage: 8 oz. warm tea prepared by infusion (See Appendix B) three to four times daily between meals.
*Beneficial properties:* May help open the sinus passages.

♦ **Stinging Nettle** (Urtica dioica) for allergy-related sinusitis – Dosage: 1 to 2 capsules or 30 drops liquid extract* in 4 oz. water every two hours until relieved.
*Beneficial properties:* May relieve allergy-related sinusitis.

## Aromatherapy

**Aromatherapy Head Vapor (steam inhalation) followed by Cold Water Sniffling** (see Appendix D for head vapor instructions) – Dosage: 1 to 3 times daily to open and drain sinus passages, enhance oxygenation, and destroy pathogenic bacteria. Bring 1 qt. pure water to a boil in a glass or stainless steel pot (avoid aluminum). Remove from heat. When water has cooled below boiling point, add the following essential oil combination:

*To relieve blockage, pain & counteract infection:* 3 drops **Eucayptus** (Eucalyptus globulus) + 3 drops **Pine** (Pinus sylvestris) + 2 drops **Tea Tree** (Melaleuca alternifolia).

Follow with **Cold Water Sniffling,** as follows: Fill a basin with pure, cold water. Scoop up water with cupped hands. Sniff water up into both nostrils. Perform 15 to 20 deep sniffs.

## Homeopathy

See Appendix E for proper use and handling instruction prior to administering remedies described below.

♦ **Calcarea Carb 12C** – Sinus headache from forehead to nose; nose dry during day and drains constantly at night; yellow discharge clogs nose and may smell like manure, rotten eggs, or gunpowder; wings of nose thickened and ulcerated. Dosage: Dissolve 5 pellets under the tongue, two to three times daily.

♦ **Hepar Sulph 12C** – Boring, aching pain at root of nose and above eyes, with thick yellow or green discharge; scalp very sensitive to touch; cold air, motion, stooping, and riding in a car worsen the condition, while warmth helps it. Dosage: Dissolve 5 pellets under the tongue, three to four times daily.

♦ **Silicea 30C** – Chronic stuffed nose; head feels as if will burst; pain over the right eye; mental exertion makes it worse; pain relieved by tight wrapping of head and heat application; Dosage: Dissolve 5 pellets under the tongue, three to four times daily to help promote drainage.

## Miscellaneous

♦ **Avoid all smoke**, including second-hand smoke, damp, and other conditions. Nose drops may induce a rebound effect in which stuffiness is actually worse after the drug effect wears off. Swimming and diving may wash the nasal infection into the sinuses. Flying, which exposes the sinuses to sudden changes in pressure may worsen the condition.

♦ **Address constipation** with a high-fiber diet, psyllium seed powder, adequate water intake, and exercise. Constipation is often an important factor in sinusitis.

♦ **Use hot and cold facial compresses**. May relieve congestion and stimulate the immune system in the sinus area. Alternate one minute of a hot (to tolerance) compress with thirty seconds of a cold (ice cold preferably) compress. Alternate these two compresses 5 to 7 times. Perform this therapy as needed for pain relief as often as every half-hour.

♦ **Hot foot bath** (*see* Appendix D for details) – Soak feet in hot water for 20 to 30 minutes. Conclude treatment with a brief (5 to 10 seconds) pouring of cold water over the feet. Then rest in bed until the perspiring stops. This treatment may help break up head congestion and open nasal passages. Perform one to two times daily or as required.

♦ **N-Acetylcysteine** – Dosage: 500 mg., three times daily. An amino acid that may help loosen and liquefy mucus in the sinuses, enabling them to drain.

\* Most herbal extracts contain alcohol. Avoid use if alcohol sensitive or if there is a history of alcohol abuse. *Note:* Alcohol content can be reduced through evaporation by adding extract to very hot water (just below boiling point) and allowing to stand 5 to 7 minutes before drinking.

# Sore Throat

Sore throat is pain in the back of the mouth, commonly due to bacterial or viral infection, low humidity environment, or a post-nasal drip caused by allergies. Areas typically affected are the tonsils, larynx, and pharynx. There may be throat pain, difficult or painful swallowing, headache, fever, and chills. Streptococcal infections are highly contagious, and can lead to greater health problems, such as rheumatic heart disease, if left untreated. If you have been exposed to someone with a streptococcal throat infection, or fever, headache, swollen glands, and skin rash accompany your sore throat, you should be under the supervision of a physician.

Conventional treatments include over-the-counter pain medications and antibiotics to treat the infection.

| EZ Care Program | |
|---|---|
| Diet | **Avoid** milk, dairy, alcohol, coffee, caffeine, and sugars, because they weaken the immune system. |
| | **Drink pure water freely upon arising and between meals** to soothe inflamed throat tissues and flush toxic substances from the body. |
| | **Eat small light meals** and consider a soft-food diet to decrease food irritation. |
| Vitamins | **A** (natural, from fish liver oil) – Dosage: 25,000 to 50,000 IU daily with meals for one week. Essential for maintenance of mucous membranes, including those of the throat. *Note:* Consult a physician before using higher doses of vitamin A. Avoid use if pregnant. Discontinue use if you experience nausea, dry skin, sore lips, blurred vision, or other signs of vitamin A toxicity. |
| | **C** (mineral ascorbates mixed with bioflavonoids) – Dosage: 1,000 - 2,000 mg., four times daily or to bowel tolerance, the point at which tissue saturation with vitamin C is reached and the body will not absorb vitamin C from the gut. Stimulates immune function and aids in prevention or treatment of infection. |

| | EZ Care Program |
|---|---|
| Minerals | **Zinc** (take only if over 14 years of age) – Dosage: zinc lozenges containing 23 mg. elemental zinc dissolved in mouth every two hours during waking hours. Limit intake at this high dosage to no more than 7 to 10 days. Zinc plays an important role in immune function and greater amounts are required during acute or chronic infection. Also, zinc and vitamin A are synergistic and work well together in this context. *Note:* May cause nausea. If this occurs, discontinue. |
| Herbs | **Goldenseal** (Hydrastis canadensis ) – Gargle, then swallow, 40 to 50 drops liquid extract* in 4 oz. warm water every three hours until throat symptoms subside. *Beneficial properties:* Traditionally used to cleanse mucous membranes. An antibacterial that may have specificity for streptococcal infection. |

# Additional Recommendations

The EZ Care Program consists of basic remedies that are commonly used for sore throats and have been found to work well in most cases. The remedies are most effective when combined, but can be used individually. The options stated below can supplement or replace EZ Care remedies and may be combined when suggested doses are followed.

## Diet

♦ **Consider a two-to-three day juice fast** (intake restricted to fresh, unsweetened fruit and vegetable juices and pure water only)
**Note**: If fasting is not feasible, consider (if well-tolerated) adherence to a diet consisting exclusively of raw fruits, steamed vegetables, and fresh juices for a period of two to three days. *Avoid with serious health problems, or usage of prescription medication. Always consult your physician before undertaking a fast.*

♦ **Include** mineral-rich vegetable broth, herbal tea, and raw vegetable juices for their nutritional value and easy swallowing. **Eat small, light meals** to ensure ready absorption of vital nutrients.

## Vitamins

♦ **Beta-Carotene** – Dosage: 50,000 to 75,000 IU three times daily with meals. Converts to vitamin A in the body and does not have the toxic potential of pre-formed vitamin A.

## Herbs

♦ **Cayenne (Capsicum annuum) + Apple Cider Vinegar Gargle** – Mix 1 tsp. Cayenne powder + 8 oz. Sage (salvia officinalis) tea prepared by infusion (*see* Appendix B*)* + 2 tbsp. unfiltered apple cider vinegar + 2 tbsp. sea salt + 2 tbsp. raw honey. Steep sage infusion mixed with cayenne for 15 minutes, then mix in the remaining ingredients. Dosage: gargle with a mouthful of the blend 4 to 8 times daily. After spitting out the gargle, take orally and swallow 1 to 2 tbsp. of the same blend.
*Beneficial properties:* May help stimulate local circulatory and immunological activity.

♦ **Echinacea** (Echinacea purpurea) – Dosage: 2 to 4 capsules or 50 drops liquid extract* every two hours until throat symptoms subside. *Echinacea has a noteworthy affinity with garlic,* so these two can be used to greater effect when taken in combination.
*Beneficial properties:* Traditionally used to stimulate the immune system and help fight infection.

♦ **Garlic capsules** (Allium sativum) – Dosage: 1 to 2 capsules per meal of standardized allicin garlic or aged garlic extract. Fresh, raw garlic (a whole, living food) is preferable, but capsules should be considered if raw garlic is used inconsistently. Raw garlic should be served with steamed vegetables. Additionally, stir 1 tsp. garlic juice (by using a garlic press) into servings of broth and raw vegetable juice. *Garlic has a noteworthy affinity with echinacea,* so these two can be used in combination for greater effect.
*Beneficial properties:* Powerful antiviral and antibacterial.
*Note:* Raw parsley taken with raw garlic helps prevent "garlic breath" and enhances garlic's blood-cleansing effects.

♦ **Ginger Root** (Zingiber officinalis) – Dosage: 2 capsules three times daily or 6-8 oz. dried ginger root tea three times daily (see Appendix B; Jamaican ginger root is preferred). For enhanced effect, add a pinch of cayenne to each serving.
*Beneficial properties:* May help relieve sore throat through stimulation of local blood circulation.

♦ **Myrrh** (Commiphora myrrha) – Dosage: 30 to 50 drops liquid extract* three times daily in unsweetened pineapple juice or diluted lemon juice. Also, add 25 drops liquid extract to pineapple juice or lemon juice gargle. Consider adding a similar amount liquid extract to dilute the lemon juice; spray into the mouth and down the throat several times daily.
*Beneficial properties:* May exert a powerful antiseptic action on the mucous membranes, help relieve inflamed throat, and stimulate immune system.
*Note:* Combines well with echinacea and goldenseal.

♦ **Slippery Elm** (Ulmus fulva) – slippery elm lozenges; use according to directions on label.
*Beneficial properties:* May provide soothing relief to inflamed throat.

## Homeopathy

See Appendix E for proper use and handling instruction prior to administering remedies described below.

♦ **Aconite 6C** – First stage of sore throat, perhaps accompanied by fever; comes on suddenly and intensely after exposure to cold air or dry, cold wind; throat very red, burning ,dry, and swollen. Dosage: Dissolve 5 pellets under the tongue, every two to four hours or as required.

♦ **Belladonna 6C** – A leading remedy for acute tonsillitis. Throat very dry, with intense burning; tonsils and tongue bright red; tickling of larynx; face red and hot, but hands and feet cold; restless and agitated, great difficulty swallowing due to pain, yet a constant desire to swallow and crave lemon juice. Dosage: Dissolve 5 pellets under the tongue, every one to four hours or as required.

♦ **Lachesis 12C** – Sore throat worse on left side; left throat gland more swollen and sensation of a fishbone caught in, or lump in, throat; pain worse with empty swallowing or drinking warm liquids, but eased by swallowing food; throat hypersensitive to touch; pain goes to ear when swallowing. Dosage: Dissolve 5 pellets under the tongue, every three to four hours or as required.

♦ **Mercurius Sol 12C** – Pain or choking sensation when swallowing, yet must swallow because of increased saliva; a thick, yellow coating on tongue, and foul breath; a great thirst and sensation of dryness despite excessive salivation; throat may be ulcerated and worse on right side. Dosage: Dissolve 5 pellets under the tongue, every three to four hours, in alternation with Ferrum Phos or as required.

## Miscellaneous

♦ **Heating compress** – Place a cold, damp cloth (wring it out) on the throat and wrap the entire neck with a dry towel. Leave on the throat one hour (towel should feel warm). May help soothe the throat and stimulate the immune system.

♦ **Gargle** with **Kosher salt water**. Dosage: 1/2 tsp. salt in a glass of warm water. May help fight throat infections. Repeat this gargle every three hours.

♦ **Charcoal tablets or liquid** – Take 4 charcoal tabs three times daily. Allow to dissolve in the mouth and drain down the throat. Option: empty 2 capsules charcoal in 4 oz. warm water; gargle with and swallow this mixture two to three times daily. May help remove bacteria and disease by-products, both locally and systemically.

\* Most herbal extracts contain alcohol. Avoid use if alcohol sensitive or if there is a history of alcohol abuse. *Note:* Alcohol content can be reduced through evaporation by adding extract to very hot water (just below boiling point) and allowing to stand 5 to 7 minutes before drinking.

# Sprains and Strains

Sprains and strains are tears in the muscles, tendons, or ligaments. They are commonly caused from trauma, twisting or pulling injuries, overuse, or excessive activity. Sprains and strains are graded by the degree of injury. Grade 1 tears are mild and heal quickly, while grade 4 tears are complete, often requiring surgery. Symptoms include pain, swelling, bruising, loss of movement, and weakness. Spasm of nearby muscles may occur. A physician should evaluate any serious injury.

Conventional treatments include rest, ice, elevation and compression, over-the-counter pain medications, muscle relaxants, physical therapy, and surgery for severe cases. Although widely prescribed, non-steroidal anti-inflammatory drugs (NSAIDs) should be avoided. While these drugs may offer pain relief, they interfere with natural healing processes and may lead to incomplete healing.

Chronic strains and sprains can be treated with **Prolotherapy**, a reconstructive techinque that utilizes the body's natural healing processes to repair damaged tissue. Only a properly trained physician should perform prolotherapy. See Appendix F for more information.

| EZ Care Program | |
| --- | --- |
| Vitamins | **C** (mineral ascorbate) – Dosage: 1,000 mg., four to six times daily with meals. Vitamin C is crucial for collagen formation. Collagen is the material involved in repair of ligaments and tendons. |
| Herbs | **Curcumin** (extracted from Tumeric) – Dosage: 300 mg., two to three times daily between meals.<br>*Beneficial properties:* Traditionally used to relieve inflammation and joint, tendon, and muscle pain. |
| | **Bromelain** – Dosage: two 5,000 mcu (measure of bromelain activity) capsules three times daily between meals. Enzyme derived from pineapple, which may help reduce inflammation and speed healing. |
| Miscellaneous | **Apply ice** to injured area **immediately** to reduce inflammation and pain. Keep ice pack in place for 5 minutes. Remove for 1 to 2 minutes. Then repeat. Continue as required. For the first 24 hours, use only cold applications. |
| | **Arnica Oil or Gel** – Use externally by rubbing a small amount into the affected area three to four times daily. May reduce swelling and pain and speed healing.<br>*Important note: Toxic when taken internally. Avoid mouth, eyes, and any open cuts.* May help reduce swelling and speed healing. For best results, use immediately after injury. |
| | **Massage** damaged tissue to reduce pain and increase circulation in the area. |
| | **Rest** the injured area to allow it to heal. Use crutches if necessary. |
| | **Support bandages**, such as elastic wrap bandages, can be used to protect the damaged tissue. Wrap the injured joint with a figure-of-eight bandage. For instance, with an *injured ankle:* Start above the ankle and wrap under the foot. Then cross back-and-forth over the top of the foot, continuing back-and-forth in a figure-eight pattern.<br>*Caution:* Do not wrap elastic bandages too tightly. This will compromise the circulation. |
| | **Warm compresses** should be applied after the first 24 hours of injury. Warmth stimulates blood flow, allowing for a more efficient delivery of nutrients to the damaged area. |

# Additional Recommendations

The EZ Care Program consists of basic remedies that are commonly used for sprains and strains and have been found to work well in most cases. The remedies are most effective when combined, but can be used individually. The options stated below can supplement or replace EZ Care remedies and may be combined when suggested doses are followed.

## Diet

◆ **Eat** generous amounts of **pineapple** for its high bromelain content. Bromelain is an enzyme that may help reduce swelling.

## Vitamins

◆ **A** (natural, from fish liver oil) – Dosage: 10,000 to 25,000 IU daily with meals.
*Beneficial properties:* May help with formation and repair of connective tissue.
*Note:* Consult a physician before using higher doses of vitamin A. Avoid use if pregnant. Discontinue use if you experience nausea, dry skin, sore lips, blurred vision, or other signs of vitamin A toxicity.

◆ **Bioflavonoids** (full potency) – Dosage: 500 mg., two to three times daily with vitamin C. May help limit ruptures in capillaries and connective tissues. Provides synergy in utilization of vitamin C.

## Minerals

◆ **Zinc** (take only if over 14 years of age) – Dosage: 50 mg. elemental zinc from amino acid chelate one to three times daily with meals. Through its influence on immune function and collagen formation, zinc may help speed wound healing.
*Note:* Zinc and vitamin A are synergistic and work well together in this context.

## Herbs

◆ **Grapeseed Extract** is very beneficial for its healing properties – Dosage: 100 mg., three times daily for one month.

## Aromatherapy

Add 3 drops of **Blue Chamomile** (Matricaria chamomilla) or **Lavender** (Lavendula vera) essential oil to a mixture of 1-1/2 tbsp. olive oil plus 3/4 tbsp. finely grated garlic. Store in a sealed jar in a cool, dark spot. *Lightly* massage this essential oil compound into the injured tissue, several times daily.

## Homeopathy

See Appendix E for proper use and handling instruction prior to administering remedies described below.

- **Arnica 6C** – Dosage: Dissolve 5 pellets every 10 minutes for the first 3 hours of treatment, then every hour for 4 hours. Then decrease to two to four times daily (in accordance with severity of injury), for the next two days.
- **Bryonia 6C** – Joint painful and distended with fluid, aggravated by least amount of motion and worse with continued motion. Dosage: Dissolve 5 pellets under the tongue, three to four times daily.

- **Rhus Tox 6C** – Primary homeopathic medicine for sprains and muscle strains from overexertion. Joints hot, swollen, stiff, and painful; worse with initial motion but loosens up with continued motion; pain relieved by warmth, gentle rubbing, and change of position. Dosage: Dissolve 5 pellets under the tongue, three to four times daily.

- **Ruta Graveolens 12C** – Pain feels closer to the bone (e.g., shin or wrist) and hot to the touch; may be associated with a wrenching or tearing of a tendon, with hard swelling where it inserts into the bone; an aching pain that becomes worse with movement of the injured part. Dosage: Dissolve 5 pellets under the tongue, three to four times daily. Sometimes alternated with arnica.

### Miscellaneous

- **Clay Poultice** – Place affected part under a stream of cold water for 20 to 30 minutes. Then make a paste by mixing the clay (see Appendix B) and water and spread a thick layer on a cotton or linen bandage. Apply to injured part and leave in place three to four hours or overnight.

- **Proteolytic Enzyme Formula** (including protease, bromelain, and papain) – Dosage: 3 or more capsules three times daily between meals. Can decrease inflammation and speed healing of tissues if taken between meals.
  *Note: Avoid if stomach or duodenal ulcers; proteolytic enzymes may aggravate ulcers and induce bleeding.*

- **Salt Water** – Cold, wet compresses using 1 tbsp. sea salt per 8 oz. cold water may prove of good service during the first 24 hours after injury. Place wet compress on injured part and apply ice pack as described in EZ Care section above.

# TMJ Syndrome

The Temporomandibular Joint (TMJ) is the area at where the jaw hinges on the bones of the skull. This joint can become damaged, which causes pain, muscle spasms, difficulty opening the jaw, cracking and popping when opening and closing the mouth, headaches, neck pain, and ear pain. Possible causes include gum chewing, an improper bite, cervical spine misalignment, grinding of the teeth, dental procedures, and trauma.

Conventional treatments include avoidance of teeth grinding and gum chewing, over-the-counter pain relievers, tranquilizers or muscle relaxants, dental corrections, custom mouthpieces while sleeping, and relaxation therapies.

*Special Note:* **Prolotherapy**, a reconstructive injection therapy, can be highly successful in relieving symptoms of TMJ pain. Prolotherapy injections stimulate tissue regrowth, allowing for normal joint function. Contact a physician skilled in prolotherapy for treatment. See Appendix F for more information.

| EZ Care Program | |
|---|---|
| Vitamins | **B complex** – Dosage: 50 mg., one to two times daily with meals. Helps the body cope with stress. <br> *Note:* For highest assimilation, use a B complex which contains the vitamins in their coenzyme form and avoid mega-potency B complex products. |
| | **B5** (pantothenic acid) – An anti-stress factor that may help reduce grinding of teeth. Dosage: 250 mg., two times daily with breakfast and at bedtime; take bedtime dose with vitamin C. <br> *Note:* Always use B5 in conjunction with a complete B complex formula, because high doses of one B vitamin may lead to imbalance in the body's pool of the other B vitamins. |
| | **C** (mineral ascorbates mixed with bioflavonoids) – Dosage: 1,000 mg., three to four times daily with meals, and at bedtime with pantothenic acid; these two vitamins taken together may support the adrenal glands. Helps repair damaged joint tissue. |
| Minerals | **Magnesium** (elemental magnesium from amino acid chelate) – Dosage: 1,000 mg. daily at bedtime. Essential for relaxing the muscles and nervous system. |
| Miscellaneous | **Consider** regular chiropractic care, massage, therapeutic bodywork, and cranial manipulation, such as craniosacral therapy or etiopathy, performed by a qualified healthcare professional. |
| | Consider a **dental** consultation with a qualified dentist. |
| | **Methyl sulfonyl methane** (MSM) – Dosage: 1000 mg. twice daily. Provides a source of natural sulfur, which aids in the structure of ligaments and tendons. MSM also has analgesic properties, and can boost the immune system, aid in liver detoxification, and relieve allergies. Most effective in oral forms; less effective in creams. |
| | **Reduce** lifestyle **stress** and implement a relaxation program. Harmonizing practices (e.g., biofeedback, meditation, yoga, and Tai Chi exercise) may prove beneficial. |

# Additional Recommendations

The EZ Care Program consists of basic remedies that are commonly used for TMJ syndrome and have been found to work well in most cases. The remedies are most effective when combined, but can be used individually. The options stated below can supplement or replace EZ Care remedies and may be combined when suggested doses are followed.

## Diet

♦ **Identify personal food sensitivities**. Avoid all common allergenic foods (e.g., dairy, eggs, wheat, corn, sugar, preservatives). Rotate moderately allergic foods on a four-day schedule (see Appendix A).

♦ **Avoid** foods that require **extensive chewing**, and **cut food** into small pieces. During acute phases, consume soft fruits, steamed vegetables, and stews.

## Minerals

♦ **Calcium** (elemental calcium from amino acid chelate) – Dosage: 1,000 mg. daily at bedtime. Essential for relaxing the nervous system. Considered a "lullaby" mineral. In combination with pantothenic acid, may help reduce grinding of teeth.

## Herbs

♦ **Chamomile Flowers** (Matricaria recutita) – Dosage: 2 to 3 capsules three times daily with meals or 4 to 8 oz. tea three times daily between meals (*see* Appendix B).
*Beneficial properties:* Antispasmodic and soothing to nerves (*see* Appendix B).

♦ **Valerian Root** (valeriana officinalis) – Dosage: 2 capsules or 30-60 drops liquid extract* in 4 oz. water two to three times daily.
*Beneficial properties:* Sedative and soothing to nerves. Traditionally used as antispasmodic and muscle relaxant.

♦ **Antispasmodic Extract** – Dosage: 25 to 40 drops liquid extract* in 4 oz. warm water one to four times daily or as required. Grind the following herbs in blender or coffee grinder and add to a quart mason jar: 3 tbsp. **Lobelia Seed** (Lobelia inflata) + 2 tbsp. **Scullcap** (Scutellaria lateriflora) + 2 tbsp. **Skunk Cabbage Root** (Symplocarpus foetida) + 3 tbsp. **Gum Myrrh** (Commiphora myrrha) + 3 tbsp. **Black Cohosh Root** (Cimicifuga racemosa) + 1 tbsp. **Cayenne Powder** (Capsicum annum). Pour 80 proof vodka over the mix (alcohol level about two inches above level of herbs). Seal jar tightly and store in a warm, dark spot. Shake well daily. After two to three weeks, strain off the liquid and squeeze or press out as much fluid as possible from the herb mass. Store the finished fluid extract in amber glass dropper bottles. May help reduce spasmodic contraction in the jaw muscles.

## Aromatherapy

Add 20 drops each of the following essential oils to a 1 oz. dropper bottle filled with olive or emu oil: **Blue Chamomile** (Matricaria chamomilla) + **Marjoram** (Origanum marjorana). Shake well. *Use as follows:* Several times weekly take a warm bath or shower to effect general relaxation of the musculature. Consider taking the **Antispasmodic Extract** mentioned above just prior to hydrotherapy. Immediately after hydrotherapy, deeply knead a small amount of this oil blend into the muscles of the neck and shoulders; gently massage the blend into the facial muscles around the TMJ (temporomandibular) joint.

## Homeopathy

See Appendix E for proper use and handling instruction prior to administering remedies described below.

♦ **Causticum 12C** – TMJ spasms, especially on right side; sincere, idealistic, intense person, unable to tolerate the suffering of others; spasms worse when opening mouth; local paralysis of flexor muscles; worsens with cold, but helped with sips of cold water; better in cloudy or rainy weather; crave smoked foods; generally feel aggravated about four p.m. Dosage: Dissolve 5 pellets one to two times daily or as required.

♦ **Rhus Tox 12C** – Restless, timid, apprehensive at night, superstitious, depressed, morose; cannot find rest in any position; TMJ worse when jaw muscles inactive; better with continued motion; worse when cold and damp and in morning upon arising; helped by warmth. Dosage: Dissolve 5 pellets one to two times daily or as required.

## Miscellaneous

♦ **Deep Breathing Exercises** – Calms the mind and body. Following is a yoga breathing exercise to calm the mind: Inhale through the nose with a deep belly breath for a count of 4, hold for a count of 7, exhale through the mouth for a count of 8. Practice two times daily, four to eight repetitions each time.

♦ **Reduce** lifestyle **stress** and implement a relaxation program. Harmonizing practices (e.g., biofeedback, meditation, yoga, Tai Chi exercise) may prove beneficial.

* Most herbal extracts contain alcohol. Avoid use if alcohol sensitive or if there is a history of alcohol abuse. *Note:* Alcohol content can be reduced through evaporation by adding extract to very hot water (just below boiling point) and allowing to stand 5 to 7 minutes before drinking.

# Ulcers (Peptic)

Ulcers occur when there is damage to the lining of the stomach. Once thought to be as a result of stress, the bacteria Helicobacter pylori (H. pylori) causes ninety percent of cases. Additional causes include stress, poor digestion, and overuse of aspirin and nonsteroidal anti-inflammatory agents like ibuprofen and naproxen.

Symptoms usually consist of abdominal pain occurring 30 minutes after eating, although it can be at other times, and can be accompanied by regurgitation and burning in the throat and esophagus. Some ulcers may not produce symptoms of pain, but may cause a serious bleeding condition.

*Note: Ulcers should be cared for under the supervision of your physician, as bleeding ulcers can be life threatening.*

Conventional treatments include histamine blockers, proton pump inhibitors and antibiotics. Invasive procedures such as endoscopy may be warranted for diagnosis or to rule out bleeding or infection.

| EZ Care Program | |
|---|---|
| Diet | **Avoid** all **sour fruits**. Bananas and papaya may be well tolerated. |
| | **Avoid bedtime feeding**, because this will cause a rise in acid secretion in the middle of the night when the body is least able to the cope with the acid load. |
| | **Avoid salt and strong spices**, such as white and black pepper, mustard, chili, and vinegar, because these increase gastric secretions that may irritate the stomach lining. |
| | **Avoid milk** and all milk products, because they increase stomach acid secretion. Consider nondairy alternatives like soy or nut milks and cheeses. |
| | **Carefully review** other diet remedies, because they are also very important for ulcer treatment. |
| | **Chew food thoroughly.** Urogastrone, a polypeptide in saliva, protects the stomach lining from the erosive effects of acidity. |
| | **Drink** 8 to 10 glasses of pure water daily. |
| | **Eliminate** coffee (regular and decaffeinated), black tea, chocolate, soda, alcohol, processed sugar, and refined flour (white bread acts similarly to tobacco in ulcer development), because they may irritate the stomach. |
| | **Identify personal food sensitivities**. Avoid all common allergenic foods (e.g., dairy, eggs, wheat, corn, preservatives, sugar). Rotate moderately allergic foods on a four-day schedule (see Appendix C). |
| Vitamins | **A** (water-soluble, emulsified, natural, from fish liver oil) – Dosage: 25,000 IU one to two times daily with meals. Helps maintain the gastrointestinal mucosa and may help prevent the development of stress ulcers. *Note:* Consult a physician before using higher doses of vitamin A. Avoid use if pregnant. Discontinue use if you experience nausea, dry skin, sore lips, blurred vision, or other signs of vitamin A toxicity. |
| | **E** (water-soluble, emulsified, natural d-alpha tocopherol in base of mixed tocopherols) – Dosage: 400 IU two to three 3 times daily with meals. A natural anti-inflammatory that may protect against stress ulceration. |

| EZ Care Program | |
| --- | --- |
| Herbs | **Golden seal Root** (hydrastis canadensis) and **Gum Myrrh** (commiphora myrrha) – Prepare tea by decoction (see Appendix B) consisting of 1 tsp. goldenseal root plus 1 tsp. myrrh plus 16 oz. water. Simmer 20 minutes, then let cool. Serve 4 oz. four times daily, 30 minutes before meals and at bedtime. Traditional herbal combination for cleansing and healing ulcerated surfaces. |
| Raw Juices | **Drink** any of the following freshly made juices two to four times daily: green cabbage, red or yellow potato or papaya juice. |
| Miscellaneous | **Avoid antacids**, because some of these products may irritate the gastric mucosa, causing a reactive increase in stomach acid production that may cause a wide array of side effects. |
| | **Avoid aspirin**, because it may induce gastrointestinal bleeding. |
| | **Avoid** all forms of **tobacco**, because this may irritate the stomach. |
| | **L-Glutamine** – Dosage: 500 mg., three times daily one hour before meals. An amino acid that helps stimulate production of mucin, thus helping regenerate gastric mucosa. Cabbage juice is a rich source. |
| | **Sialic Acid** – Dosage: 500 mg, three times daily with meals. A substance extracted from mucin, the chief constituent of protective mucous. |

## Additional Recommendations

The EZ Care Program consists of basic remedies that are commonly used for peptic ulcers and have been found to work well in most cases. The remedies are most effective when combined, but can be used individually. The options stated below can supplement or replace EZ Care remedies and may be combined when suggested doses are followed.

### Diet

♦ **Eliminate all fried foods.** Heated vegetable oils can be a contributing factor to developing ulcers.

♦ **Fiber Supplement** – Dosage: 1 to 3 tsp. Psyllium Husk fiber in 8 oz. pure water one to two times daily between meals. Constipation greatly worsens ulcer symptoms and must be avoided.
*Note:* Carefully read label; some brands require additional water.

♦ **The following foods may be beneficial:**

*Raw (uncooked) green cabbage* – Serve finely minced. Contains an anti-ulcer factor referred to as vitamin U.
*Note*: Avoid raw vegetables for the first few weeks of treatment, then experiment with small servings.

*Green leaf lettuce* – May contain vitamin U.
*Note*: Avoid raw vegetables for the first few weeks of treatment, then experiment with small servings.

*Steamed yellow or red potatoes* – Contain ulcer healing factors and assists in acid-neutralization.

*Millet* – Soothes gastrointestinal tract. One of the few grains generally well tolerated by many ulcer patients.

*Almonds* – Soak overnight and serve in the form of almond milk. *To prepare:* Blend for 1 minute 5 tbsp. soaked almonds with 7 oz. pure water plus 1 tsp. flaxseed. Almonds decrease gastric acid production, bind excess acid in the stomach, and provide high-quality protein.
*Note*: Pure, store-bought almond milk is acceptable.

*Ripe, black oil-cured olives* – Black olives soothe the stomach and provide valuable fatty acids and protein. Avoid olives preserved in vinegar or brine. Soak oil-cured olives in pure water for 10 minutes, then rinse to remove excess salt. Serve 4 to 6 olives per meal.

*Other foods that may be well tolerated:* Papaya, baked squash, bananas, yams, and avocados.

## Vitamins

♦ **B6** (coenzymated form, pyridoxal 5-phosphate) – Dosage: 25 mg., one to two times daily with meals. May be deficient in some patients with peptic ulcers and may help heal stress ulcers.

♦ **B complex** – Dosage: 50 mg. daily with meal. Essential for proper functioning of the nervous system and helps the body cope with stress.
*Note:* For highest assimilation, use a B complex which contains the vitamins in their coenzyme form and avoid mega-potency B complex products.

♦ **C** (non-acidic, mixed calcium and magnesium ascorbate powder) – Dosage: 1,000 mg. dissolved in warm water three times daily with meals. Vitamin C deficiency may contribute to developing peptic ulcers and their subsequent hemorrhaging.

## Minerals

♦ **Copper** (from amino acid chelate) – Dosage: 3 mg. elemental copper daily when indicated. Take separately from zinc.
*Notes:* High doses of zinc may cause a copper deficiency over time. Since copper is potentially toxic and may be present in water or soil, consult a physician to determine if a deficiency exists before supplementing with copper.

♦ **Zinc** (take only if over 14 years of age) – Dosage: 25 mg. elemental zinc from amino acid chelate one to three times daily with meals. May increase mucin production and inhibit degenerative change in the stomach mucosa, thus protecting the stomach lining.
*Note:* Zinc and vitamin A are synergistic in this context.

### Herbs

♦ **Alfalfa tablets** (medicago sativa) – Dosage: 1 to 2 tablets every two to four hours or as required. A restorative tonic that has been used long in treating peptic ulcers.
*Beneficial properties*: May improve assimilation of food.

♦ **Aloe Vera Juice** – Dosage: 1 to 2 oz. organic, cold-pressed, whole-leaf aloe vera juice in 7 oz. water three to four times daily between meals and at bedtime.
*Beneficial properties*: May inhibit gastric acid secretion and help heal ulcers.

♦ **Chamomile tea** (matricaria chamomilla) – Prepare a very strong infusion (*see* Appendix B) using 6 to 10 tbsp. Chamomile to 3 cups water. Drink 8 oz. three times daily between meals.
*Beneficial properties:* Considered by herbalists as a specific for gastric spasm, inflammation, and ulceration.

♦ **Irish Moss** (chondrus crispus) **Jelly** – Add 1 tbsp. powdered Irish moss to 16 oz. raw almond milk. Bring to a boil, lower to a simmer, and stir until Irish moss dissolves. Remove from heat and let cool. Stir in 1 tsp. raw honey. Serve 8 oz., warm, two times daily.
*Beneficial properties:* Soothing, nourishing, restoring, mucilaginous and highly nutritious. The jelly may serve as a strengthening meal when digestive powers are reduced and coarser foods are not well tolerated by the inflamed gastric mucosa.

♦ **Licorice Root** (Glycyrrhiza uralensis or glabra) – Dosage: 1 to 2 capsules or 40-50 drops liquid extract* between meals. Also consider DGL (deglycyrhizinated licorice) which is a side-effect free licorice extract; dosage: 500 mg., four times daily between meals.
*Beneficial properties:* May stimulate the defense mechanisms, including production of mucous, that prevent ulcer formation. Soothing and healing to the stomach lining.
*Notes:* If you have high blood pressure, consult a physician before using this herb, because it may increase blood pressure via increased water retention. Chinese licorice root (uralensis) is less problematic in this regard than the western variety (glabra).

♦ **Slippery Elm** (Ulmus fulva) + **Marshmallow Root** (althea officinalis) **Gruel** – *To prepare:* Make a paste from 3/4 tsp. each of slippery elm powder and marshmallow root powder mixed with 1 tsp. raw honey. Bring 8 oz. raw almond milk to a boil (see instructions above in Diet section for raw almond milk preparation) and stir in the slippery elm/honey paste. Immediately remove from heat and stir for 5 to 10 seconds. Let cool and serve.
*Beneficial properties:* May simultaneously provide strengthening nutrition and soothe inflamed mucosa.

### Homeopathy

See Appendix E for proper use and handling instruction prior to administering remedies described below.

♦ **Arsenicum Album 12C** – Ulceration of stomach with extreme burning pain; burning in stomach with desire to frequently drink small sips of water; desire fat and sour, especially lemon. Dosage: Dissolve 5 pellets under the tongue, one to two times daily or as required.

♦ **Lycopodium 12C** – Feel bloated after a few mouthfuls of food, and heartburn with sour or bitter belching; stomach pains helped by rubbing abdomen and lying on side; loud rumbling in abdomen; indigestion after eating onions; pain after eating fruit; crave sweets. Dosage: Dissolve 5 pellets under the tongue, one to two times daily or as required.

♦ **Phosphorus 12C** – Bleeding ulcer, with vomiting of bright red blood, or vomit that looks like coffee grounds; burning pain with nausea; symptoms relieved by cold drinks but return as soon as liquids become warmed in stomach; ravenous appetite, even getting up in middle of night to eat, and crave foods like chocolate, ice cream, cold foods, salt, spice, rice, milk, alcohol (especially wine); aversion to sweets and tremendous thirst for cold drinks. Dosage: Dissolve 5 pellets under the tongue, one to two times daily or as required.

♦ **Pulsatilla 12C** – Peptic ulcer and suffer indigestion from fats, yet crave foods like butter, cream, whipped-cream, pork, peanut butter, and cheese; bloating and abdominal distention present, and lack thirst; symptoms improve in open air. Dosage: Dissolve 5 pellets under the tongue, one to two times daily or as required.

## Miscellaneous

♦ **Lactobacillus Probiotic Product** (friendly intestinal bacteria that aid digestion, nutrient assimilation, and toxin elimination) (L. acidophilus with bifidobacteria) – Use according to directions on label.

♦ **Reduce** lifestyle **stress** and implement a relaxation program. Harmonizing practices (e.g., biofeedback, meditation, yoga, Tai Chi exercise) may prove beneficial.

\* Most herbal extracts contain alcohol. Avoid use if alcohol sensitive or if there is a history of alcohol abuse. *Note:* Alcohol content can be reduced through evaporation by adding extract to very hot water (just below boiling point) and allowing to stand 5 to 7 minutes before drinking.

# Urinary Tract Infection

Urinary tract infections (cystitis) are infections of the bladder and/or urethra that are often caused by the bacteria E. Coli. This bacterium is a normal inhabitant of the bowel flora, and can migrate to the urethra after sexual intercourse. Therefore, urination before and after sexual contact is highly recommended to prevent urinary tract infections. Symptoms may include burning with urination, a constant burning in the general area, an urgency to urinate, frequency in urination, urinating in small amounts, and fatigue. The urine also may be cloudy, bloody, and/or have a strong odor. Back pain, fevers, nausea and shaking chills may be a sign that the infection has spread to the kidneys. This condition, known as pyleonephritis, should be treated by a physician.

Conventional treatments include antibiotics and increased fluid intake. Older individuals with symptoms of cystitis may require vaginal estrogen suppositories to decrease inflammation and reduce the chance of an infection.

| EZ Care Program | |
|---|---|
| Diet | **Drink** 4 to 8 glasses unsweetened **cranberry juice** daily. May help kidney and urinary tract inflammations. If not feasible, take a 500 mg. capsule of cranberry concentrate three to four times daily. |
| | **Drink** 8 to 10 glasses pure **water** daily to flush the infection. Drinking with meals interferes with digestion by diluting digestive juices. Thorough chewing promotes saliva production to properly moisten food in the mouth. Small amounts of water may be sipped with meals or as required. |
| | **Eat a high-water-content diet** as described in Diet section below. |
| Herbs | **Echinacea** (Echinacea purpurea) + **Goldenseal** (Hydrastis canadensis) – Dosage: 1,000 to 2,000 mg capsules of each herb every two hours for the first eight hours of acute infection, then reduce dosage accordingly. *Beneficial properties:* Natural antibiotic combination that may help resolve infection. |
| | **Uva Ursi** (Arctostaphylos Uva-ursi) – Dosage: 10 drops of tincture or 2 capsules, three times daily. *Beneficial properties:* An aniseptic for the urinary tract. |
| Miscellaneous | Review **Homeopathy**, **Aromatherapy,** and **Sitz Baths.** |

## Additional Recommendations

The EZ Care Program consists of basic remedies that are commonly used for urinary tract infection and have been found to work well in most cases. The remedies are most effective when combined, but can be used individually. The options stated below can supplement or replace EZ Care remedies and may be combined when suggested doses are followed.

### Diet

♦ **Eat a high-water-content diet** consisting of large quantities of fresh fruits and vegetables and comparatively smaller quantities of whole grains, legumes, seeds, nuts, fish, skinless chicken and turkey. Because the waste products of protein metabolism are eliminated via the urinary tract, with acute infection or stubborn chronic infection, it is important to temporarily restrict food intake to raw fruits and vegetables (include generous amounts of parsley) and raw vegetable juices. Consider a two-to-three day melon fast, including watermelon, honeydew, and papaya. Watermelon is especially soothing; cut it into bite-size pieces and eat 1 piece every 15 minutes throughout the day. After infection clears, gradually reintroduce protein foods.

- **Identify personal food sensitivities** for chronic infections. Avoid all common allergenic foods (e.g., dairy, eggs, wheat, corn, sugar, preservatives) as well as coffee. Rotate moderately allergic foods on a four-day schedule (see Appendix C).

- **Avoid** all sugar and citrus fruits (except cranberries and cherries), because these may irritate the urinary tract during an infection.

## Vitamins

- **A** (from fish liver oil) – Dosage: 25,000 IU two to three times daily with meals for several days until acute symptoms diminish, then reduce dosage to once daily as required. Essential for maintaining integrity and secretions of urinary tract mucous membranes.
  *Note:* Consult a physician before using higher doses of vitamin A. Avoid use if pregnant. Discontinue use if you experience nausea, dry skin, sore lips, blurred vision, or other signs of vitamin A toxicity.

- **C** (mineral ascorbates mixed with bioflavonoids) – Dosage: 1,000 mg., four to six times daily with meals. May ward off or clear infection.

## Minerals

- **Zinc** (take only if over 14 years of age) – Dosage: 25 mg. elemental zinc from amino acid two to three times daily with meals. Zinc levels may be suppressed during acute and chronic infections.

## Herbs

- **Chamomile** (Matricaria recutita) – Prepare an infusion (See Appendix B) using 1 heaping tsp. chamomile to 8 oz. pure water. Take 6 oz., three to four times daily between meals, alternating with one of the herbal combinations described in the EZ Care Program above.
  *Beneficial properties*: May reduce spasm of the urinary tract and counteract inflammation of its mucous membrane lining.

## Aromatherapy

Use equal parts of essential oils **Bergamot** (Citrus bergamia) + **Sandalwood** (Santalum album) in the following application:

**Hot Compress** – Prepare a hot compress using 1 qt. pure water (kept warm on stove) and 4 to 5 drops of the 2 essential oils. Place 2 washcloths in the water. Apply one of the washcloths to the lower abdomen immediately above the pubic bone and cover with a thick, dry towel. When the wet cloth cools, replace with the hot, wet cloth. Place the cool cloth back in the pot of hot water. Alternate in this manner or as required. Continue this compress for about 30 minutes.
*After completing compress,* mix 2 drops each of the 3 essential oils in 1 tsp. warm olive oil; massage into lower abdomen and inner thighs. May help relieve cystitis by reducing bladder congestion and spasm.

### Homeopathy

See Appendix E for proper use and handling instruction prior to administering remedies described below.

- **Aconite 6C** – Use at onset of symptoms of bladder infection, especially if brought on by exposure to cold; indicated in first 48 hours if bladder infection accompanied by high fever, hot painful urination, restlessness, and anxiety or fear. Dosage: Dissolve 5 pellets under the tongue, two to three times daily or as required.

- **Belladonna 6C** – Bladder irritation with great urgency due to burning urethral spasm and irritation; worse with slightest pressure, touch, or movement. Dosage: Dissolve 5 pellets under the tongue, two to three times daily or as required.

- **Berberis 6X** – Bladder infection with pain from motion or jarring; burning, stitching pain while urinating; aching in bladder when not urinating. Dosage: Dissolve 5 pellets under the tongue, three to four times daily or as required.

- **Cantharis 12C** – Sudden, frequent urge to urinate, yet passing only a little urine; painful drop-by-drop burning before, during, and after urination; violent spasms of searing, lancing pain when passing urine. Dosage: 2 pellets under the tongue, three times daily until condition improves. If burning relieved by heat and urine reddish or cloudy, Dosage: Dissolve 5 pellets two to three times daily or as required.

- **Pulsatilla 6C** – Use at onset of bladder infection after becoming chilled during hot weather; frequent urge to urinate, with pain before and during passing of urine; commonly indicated for chronic bladder infection and moody, weepy, thirstless, and intolerant of heat. Dosage: Dissolve 5 pellets under the tongue, two to three times daily or as required.

### Miscellaneous

- **Lactobacillus Probiotic Product** (friendly intestinal bacteria that aids digestion, nutrient assimilation, and toxin elimination) (L. acidophilus, with bifidobacterium powder or capsules) – Use according to directions on label.

- **Standardized Extract of Oil of Oregano** – Dosage: one 50 mg. capsule three to four times daily with meals and at bedtime. May help bacterial and fungal infections of the urinary tract.

- **Warm Shallow Sitz Bath** – Fill tub with very warm water (105°-110°F) high enough to cover the anus. Sit in tub 15 minutes. Repeat several times daily. May enhance circulation in the urinary tract and help heal irritated tissue.

# Vaginal Yeast Infection

Yeast infections occur when there is an overgrowth of yeast in the vagina. Symptoms include itching, burning, offensive odors, vulvar irritation and redness, fissuring and swelling, pain during intercourse or urination, and white curdish discharge. Possible causes include destruction of the body's natural bacterial balance as a result of antibiotic and steroid use, pregnancy, birth control pills, overconsumption of sugar and simple carbohydrates, and low immunity. Diabetics also have an increased incidence of yeast infections.

Conventional treatments include using anti-fungal over-the-counter and prescription creams, suppositories, and pills. Alternative medicine physicians may treat patients with chronic yeast infections with several months of antifungal medication to rid the yeast from the gastrointestinal system. Specialized testing is available to measure candida antibodies and to confirm yeast overgrowth.

| EZ Care Program | |
|---|---|
| Diet | **Eliminate** sugar and foods that contain processed sugar (all forms), alcohol, white flour, fruit juices, dried fruits, breads and baked goods, cheese, and mushrooms, because they encourage yeast growth. |
| | Limit intake of **high carbohydrate foods,** including potatoes, yams, and grains to once daily. |
| Vitamins | **B complex** (yeast free) – Dosage: 25 to 50 mg. daily with meals. *Note:* For highest assimilation, use a B complex which contains the vitamins in their coenzyme form and avoid mega-potency B complex products. B vitamins are necessary for carbohydrate metabolism, hormonal regulation, and normal immune function. Biotin, a B vitamin, may have particular value in treating candida infection. |
| | **C** (mineral ascorbates mixed with bioflavonoids) – Dosage: 1,000 mg., three to four times daily with meals. May inhibit bacterial proliferation. Vitamin C supports immune function and connective tissue integrity, thus helping to control the spread of infection in the vagina. |
| Minerals | **Magnesium** (elemental magnesium from amino acid chelate) – Dosage: 150 mg., four times daily with meals and at bedtime. Deficiency may cause craving for sugar and alcohol. Supplementation may help some symptoms of candida overgrowth, including anxiety, fatigue, and depression. |
| Miscellaneous | **Apple Cider Vinegar Douche** – Dosage: 1 to 2 times daily or as required. Prepare douche solution using 2 tbsp. unfiltered apple cider vinegar in 1 qt. warm water. May help restore normal acidity of vagina. Candida organisms prefer a less acidic environment. May also be used for trichomoniasis. |
| | **Avoid** pantyhose, girdles, tight-fitting pants and jeans, and panties made of synthetic materials. Wear cotton underwear to decrease moisture build-up. Warm, moist, poorly drained environments are ideal breeding grounds for yeast. |
| | **Avoid sexual relations** during active infection. |
| | **Avoid** using feminine hygiene sprays, synthetic detergents, tampons, and colored toilet tissue, because they contain irritating chemicals. |

| EZ Care Program |
|---|
| **Lactobacillus Probiotic Product** (friendly intestinal bacteria that aid digestion, nutrient assimilation, and toxin elimination) (L. acidophilus with bifidobacteria and fructo-oligosaccharides powder or capsules) – For oral use, take as directed on container. Keep refrigerated. In addition, insert 1 capsule one to two times daily directly into vagina and cover with a pad. May help restore healthy vaginal ecology by competing with overgrown yeast. |
| **Boric Acid** – Dosage: Insert 1 capsule of about 600 mg. boric acid into vagina and cover with a pad, morning and evening, *for no more than to two weeks*. Discontinue if treatment causes local irritation or symptoms in other parts of the body due to absorbing Boric Acid into the blood. May change the pH balance, making it uncomfortable for yeast to live. <br> *Note:* Perform treatment several hours before or after any other form of douche. |
| **Standardized Extract of Oil of Oregano Capsules** – Dosage: 50 mg., four times daily with meals and at bedtime. <br> *Beneficial properties:* May help resolve bacterial or fungal infections. |
| **Tea Tree Oil** (Melaleuca alternifolia) – soak small tampon with tea tree oil and insert into vagina twice daily. Tea tree oil is a natural anti-fungal agent and can reduce the duration of yeast infections. |
| **Review Homeopathy** section for appropriate remedy. |

# Additional Recommendations

The EZ Care Program consists of basic remedies that are commonly used for vaginal yeast infections and have been found to work well in most cases. The remedies are most effective when combined, but can be used individually. The options stated below can supplement or replace EZ Care remedies and may be combined when suggested doses are followed.

## Diet

♦ **Drink** 6 to 8 glasses of pure water daily.

♦ **Eat a high-water-content diet** consisting of large quantities of fresh fruits and vegetables and comparatively smaller quantities of whole grains, legumes, seeds, nuts, fish, skinless chicken and turkey.

♦ **Identify personal food sensitivities**. Avoid all common allergenic foods (e.g., dairy, eggs, wheat, corn, sugar, preservatives). Rotate moderately allergic foods on a four-day schedule (see Appendix C).

♦ **Psyllium Seed and Husk Powder** – Dosage: 2 tsp. in 8 oz. warm water, followed with another 8 oz. warm water , once daily either upon arising or before bedtime. Fiber helps bind toxins in the bowel and alleviate or prevent constipation, which is a top priority for treating yeast infections, because a toxic, waste-choked bowel is an ideal breeding ground for all types of pathogenic microbes, including yeast.

### Vitamins

- **A** (natural, from fish liver oil) – Dosage: 25,000 IU daily with meals. Required for normal growth and integrity of the vaginal mucosa and resistance to infection.
  *Note:* Consult a physician before using higher doses of vitamin A. Avoid use if pregnant. Discontinue use if you experience nausea, dry skin, sore lips, blurred vision, or other signs of vitamin A toxicity.

- **Beta-Carotene** – Dosage: 150,000 to 200,000 IU in divided doses with meals. A non-toxic source and precursor of vitamin A, which safely supports the immune system's functions.

- **E** (natural d-alpha tocopherol in a base of mixed tocopherols) – Dosage: 800 to 1200 IU daily with a meal. Vitamin E helps regulate vitamin A and hormone metabolism, supports immune function, and may reduce vaginal inflammation and itching.

### Minerals

- **Chromium** (polynicotinate is preferred form) – Dosage: 200 mcg. two times daily with meals. Essential for blood-sugar regulation. High blood-sugar peaks contribute to yeast overgrowth.

- **Selenium** – Dosage: 200 mcg. daily from l-selenomethionine. Supports immune function and tissue integrity, and its antioxidant actions parallel those of vitamin E.

- **Zinc** (take only if over 14 years of age) – Dosage: 25 to 75 mg. elemental zinc from amino acid chelate in divided doses with meals. Required for utilization of vitamin A and normal immune function.

### Herbs

- **Chickweed Douche** (Stellaria media) – Prepare an infusion (see Appendix B) using 3 tbsp. Chickweed to 1 qt. water. Steep 30 minutes, then strain. Use as a douche one to two times daily or as required.
  *Beneficial properties*: May soothe and help heal irritated and inflamed vaginal mucosa.

- **Garlic** (Allium sativum) – Dosage: 1 to 2 capsules per meal of standardized allicin garlic or aged garlic extract. Fresh, raw garlic (a whole, living food) is preferable and should be generously added to salads twice daily, but capsules should be considered if use of raw garlic is problematic. Also can be used as a vaginal suppository: Peel, but don't nick, a garlic clove. Wrap in gauze with a clean string attached to it, forming a tampon-like suppository. Insert 1 to 2 of these suppositories daily or as required.
  *Beneficial properties*: Powerfully antifungal and antibacterial.
  *Note:* Raw parsley taken with raw garlic helps prevent "garlic breath" and enhances garlic's blood-cleansing effects.

- **Goldenseal** (Hydrastis canadensis) – Dosage: 1 to 2 capsules or 30-50 drops liquid extract* two to four times daily or as required. May also prove of good service as a douche in combination with **Myrrh** (Commiphora myrrha): Prepare by decoction (see

Appendix B) using 1 tbsp. each of goldenseal and myrrh in 3 cups pure water. Simmer 30 minutes. Let cool and strain. Administer 1 to 2 times daily or as required.

*Beneficial properties*: Goldenseal contains the antibacterial alkaloid berberine and may soothe inflamed vaginal mucosa. The combination of goldenseal and myrrh has been used traditionally to treat infections of the skin and mucous membranes.

♦ **Pau d'Arco tea** (Tabebuia impetiginosa) – Prepare a decoction (see Appendix B) using 1 tbsp. pau d'arco to 2 cups pure water. Simmer 30 minutes. Let cool and strain. Drink 4 to 6 oz. three to four times daily between meals.

*Beneficial properties*: Pau d'arco is a South American tree long used to treat yeast infections, allergies, and other immunological disorders.

## Aromatherapy

**Vaginal douche with diluted essential oils** – Administer 1, or a combination of 2, of the following fungicidal essential oils in a vaginal douche: **Lavender** (Lavendula vera), or **Tea Tree** (Melaleuca alternifolia). Prepare the douche by dissolving 20-40 drops of one essential oil, *or* 10-20 drops each of two oils for a combination (number of drops varies with individual tolerance; do not use more than a total of 40 drops), in 1 tsp. vodka. Add the oil/vodka solution to 16 oz. boiled, pure water after it has cooled, and shake vigorously.

## Homeopathy

See Appendix E for proper use and handling instruction prior to administering remedies described below.

♦ **Graphites 12C** – Thin, watery, burning discharge; may be accompanied by excessive sexual drive or aversion to sex; itching of vagina before menses, or vaginitis during menopause. Dosage: Dissolve 5 pellets under the tongue, once daily to twice weekly or as required

♦ **Nitric Acid 6C** – Thick and cloudy, burning discharge, with a sore, raw feeling accompanied by cracking and burning of local skin area. Dosage: Dissolve 5 pellets under the tongue, one to two times daily or as required.

♦ **Pulsatilla 6C** – Yellowish-green, or clear or white watery discharge; worse during first part of menstrual cycle; often feel chilly yet aversion to warmth. Dosage: Dissolve 5 pellets under the tongue, one to two times daily or as required.

♦ **Sepia 12C** – Offensive, yellowish discharge, with dragging sensation in lower abdomen and uterine discomfort; vulva may be hot and itchy, or become sore just before menstrual period; constipation, irritability, exhaustion. Dosage: Dissolve 5 pellets under the tongue, once daily to twice weekly or as required.

♦ **Sulphur 6C** – Chronic vaginitis, with offensive discharge accompanied by diarrhea and local eczema; symptoms worse in morning, or may be a sinking sensation in stomach mid-morning. Dosage: Dissolve 5 pellets under the tongue, one to two times daily or as required.

**Miscellaneous**

♦ **Warm Sitz Bath** – Dosage: 1 to 3 times daily or as required (see Appendix D for instructions). Water temperature 105° -110°F. May help reduce infection and local irritation.

# Varicose Veins

Varicose veins are caused when the superficial veins become dilated, and are easily visible at the skin surface. Variosities are caused by an incompetent valve structure. This condition is most common in the legs, but can occur in the anus. Varicose veins result from a variety of factors, including nutritional deficiencies, pregnancy, obesity, prolonged sitting or standing, lack of exercise, heredity, and increased abdominal pressure. Varicose veins can cause aching and pain, which may be worse during menstruation. Complications can include skin ulceration, bleeding or development of blood clots, known as phlebitis.

Conventional treatments include preventive measures as described below. Also recommended are compression support stockings, analgesics for pain, and diuretics to relieve swelling. Sclerotherapy, an injection technique similar to prolotherapy, can be used to obliterate the varicose vein. In a severe case, a surgical procedure called "vein stripping" may be used to tie off or remove the effected veins.

| EZ Care Program | |
|---|---|
| Diet | **Fiber Supplement** – Dosage: 1 to 3 tsp. Psyllium Husk fiber in 8 oz. pure water one to two times daily between meals. *Note:* Carefully read label; some brands require additional water. Constipation may cause or worsen varicose veins. |
| Vitamins | **C** (mineral ascorbates mixed with bioflavonoids) – Dosage: 1,000 mg., three to four times daily with meals. May strengthen integrity of blood vessels and support their elasticity. |
| Minerals | **Calcium** (elemental calcium from calcium citrate or amino acid chelate) – Dosage: 1,000 mg. daily in divided doses with meals. Crucial for normal blood clotting and cardiovascular tone. |
| Herbs | **Horse Chestnut** (Aesulus hippocastanum) – Dosage: 1 capsule or 30 drops extract* in 4 oz. water three times daily. *Beneficial properties:* May improve blood vessel tone and ability to contract. |

| | EZ Care Program |
|---|---|
| | **White Oak Bark** (Quercus alba) **Wash and Compress** – Prepare a strong decoction (see Appendix B) using 1 tsp. of herb per 1 cup pure water. Bathe affected areas two to three times daily with the decoction; allow it to dry on skin. Also apply a compress in a similar fashion as the bayberry root bark/witch hazel bark compress described below.<br>*Beneficial properties:* White oak bark is a powerful astringent that may help shrink and tone varicose veins.<br>*Note:* May be substituted by the bayberry/witch hazel remedy described below. |
| Homeopathy | **Calc Fluor. 6X** – The chief cell salt remedy for varicose veins and ulceration of varicose veins. Specific for laxity of elastic fibers in veins. Dosage: Dissolve 5 pellets under the tongue, two to four times daily or as required. |
| Miscellaneous | **Avoid** wearing **tight clothing** like girdles, tight jeans, panties, or stockings with tight elastic bands, because these may further restrict venous drainage of the legs. |
| | **Regular exercise** – Dosage: 30 minutes aerobic exercise daily may help tone blood vessels and increase circulation. Take a 15 minute walk three to four times daily. |
| | **Rutin** – Dosage: 500 mg., two to three times daily with meals. A bioflavonoid that may increase the integrity of the vein's wall, thus helping to relieve the symptoms of varicose veins. |

# Additional Recommendations

The EZ Care Program consists of basic remedies that are commonly used for varicose veins and have been found to work well in most cases. The remedies are most effective when combined, but can be used individually. The options stated below can supplement or replace EZ Care remedies and may be combined when suggested doses are followed.

## Diet

♦ **Drink** 6 to 8 glasses of pure **water** daily.

♦ **Eat a high-water-content diet** consisting of large quantities of fresh fruits and vegetables and comparatively smaller quantities of whole grains (especially buckwheat and millet), legumes, seeds, nuts, fish, skinless chicken and turkey.

♦ **Eat cherries, blueberries**, and **blackberries** for their high levels of proanthocyanidins and anthocyanidins, which may benefit blood vessel health.

♦ **Eat generous amounts of raw garlic and onions**, which are considered to be potent cleansers and strengtheners of the circulatory system, and may help prevent or break down clots in varicose veins.

## Vitamins

♦ **B complex** – Dosage: 25-50 mg. two times daily with meals.

*Note:* For highest assimilation, use a B complex which contains the vitamins in their coenzyme form and avoid mega-potency B complex products.

♦ **E** (natural d-alpha tocopherol in a base of mixed tocopherols) – Dosage: 800 IU daily with a meal. May increase elasticity of blood vessels and prevent blood clots.

## Minerals

♦ **Magnesium** (elemental magnesium from amino acid chelate) – Dosage: 500 to 1,000 mg. daily in divided doses with meals and at bedtime. Promotes absorption of other minerals, including calcium. Helps the body utilize vitamins C, E, and B complex. May help speed the healing of affected veins.

## Herbs

♦ **Bayberry Root Bark** (Myrica cerifera) + **Witch Hazel Bark** (Hamamelis virginiana) **Compress** –Prepare a strong decoction (see Appendix B) using 1 tsp. of each herb per 1 cup pure water. Each evening before bedtime, dip a wide gauze bandage or folded cotton kitchen towel in the decoction and wrap around the affected area. Cover with a dry flannel or cotton towel. Cover all with plastic (e.g., plastic supermarket bag). *Be careful not to wrap too tightly; will impair circulation.* Keep the bandaged area warm. Remove the compress in the morning upon arising. Continue this procedure nightly for several weeks or as required.
*Beneficial properties*: Witch hazel bark may improve circulation and soothe and reduce inflammation of swollen veins. Bayberry root bark tightens and tones blood vessels.

♦ **Bilberry** (Vaccinium myrtillus) – Dosage: 80 to 160 mg., three times daily for a minimum of three months.
*Beneficial properties*: May increase integrity of the venous wall and venous tone.

♦ **Cayenne** (Capsicum annuum) – Dosage: 1,000 to 2,000 mg., two to three times daily with meals. May nourish the structural tissues of the veins, restore their elasticity, and normalize blood pressure.
*Beneficial properties:* Equalizes circulation.

♦ **Ginkgo Biloba** – Dosage: 1 to 2 capsules (40-80 mg.) of 24% standardized extract or 30-60 drops extract* in 4 oz. water three times daily.
*Beneficial properties*: May improve general circulation and blood flow to the heart.

♦ **Grapeseed Extract** – Dosage: 50 to 100 mg., two to three times daily with meals.
*Beneficial properties*: Contains anthocyanidins that may strengthen veins and reduce swelling.

## Aromatherapy

*Prepare an **ointment** using the following ingredients and proportions:* 5 drops **Cypress** (Cupressus semipervirens) per 1 tsp. **Aloe Vera Gel,** two to three times daily. With fingertips, *very gently* massage the ointment into the varicose veins and the region immediately *above it. Do not massage the area below the varicose veins, because this will increase the congestion.* For synergistic effect, perform this essential oil massage immediately after the herbal compresses described above. Also, add these essential oils into a bath (see procedure below under Miscellaneous).

## Homeopathy

See Appendix E for proper use and handling instruction prior to administering remedies described below.

♦ **Hamamelis 6C** – Homeopathic form of Witch Hazel. Use for varicose veins with stinging and pricking pain and feeling of fullness in leg. Dosage: Dissolve 5 pellets under the tongue, two to three times daily or as required. Also, consider applying Hamamelis lotion several times daily to affected area.

♦ **Millefolium 6C** – Varicose veins accompanied by spongy and enlarged capillaries that break easily when congested; also for varicose veins during pregnancy, especially if they ulcerate and bleed. Dosage: Dissolve 5 pellets under the tongue, two times daily or as required.

## Miscellaneous

♦ **Avoid Prolonged Standing**. If unavoidable, take frequent breaks to walk or elevate feet. Support stockings may be helpful in this situation.

♦ **Avoid** sitting with crossed legs, squatting, or sitting on heels.

♦ **Coenzyme Q-10** - Dosage: 50 mg., two times daily. May help oxygenate tissues, including the vascular system

♦ **Consider raising foot of bed** 4 to 6 inches to assist venous blood flow from the lower extremities to the heart.

♦ **Take several rest periods** during the day and elevate legs to allow gravity to assist venous drainage.

* Most herbal extracts contain alcohol. Avoid use if alcohol sensitive or if there is a history of alcohol abuse. *Note:* Alcohol content can be reduced through evaporation by adding extract to very hot water (just below boiling point) and allowing to stand 5 to 7 minutes before drinking.

# Warts

Warts are small, benign growths in the skin, usually caused by a virus. They are most commonly found on the hands, fingers, forearms, knees, face, feet and genital area but may appear on any part of the body. Genital warts may cause serious complications and should be seen by your health care practitioner.

Conventional treatments include the use of over- the-counter wart medications and prescription topical salicylic acid (these should not be used on the face or genitals), removal by freezing, laser surgery, and electrical wart ablation. Alternative medicine physicians can also treat warts with dilute injections of candida extract. This treatment has a reported 70% success rate.

| EZ Care Program | |
|---|---|
| Vitamins | **A** (natural, from fish liver oil) –Dosage: 10,000 to 25,000 IU per day, taken with meals. Vitamin A is essential for the maintenance of the epithelium and in the prevention against infectious diseases. <br> *Note:* Consult a physician before using higher doses of vitamin A. Avoid use if pregnant. Discontinue use if you experience nausea, dry skin, sore lips, blurred vision, or other signs of vitamin A toxicity. |
| | **E** (natural d-alpha tocopherol in a base of mixed tocopherols) –Dosage: 800 IU daily taken with a meal. Apply externally by squeezing the contents of a vitamin E capsule on a band-aid and placing over the wart. Repeat this procedure daily for 2 to 3 weeks. Vitamin E is a potent antioxidant that helps protect the tissues of the skin and is commonly used to treat skin lesions. <br> *Note:* Vitamin E should not be applied to any open skin lesions. |
| Herbs | **Garlic** –(Allium sativum) Dosage: 1 to 2 capsules per meal of standardized allicin garlic or aged garlic extract. Fresh, raw garlic, a whole, living food is preferable, but capsules should be considered if use of raw garlic is inconsistent. Externally, rub warts with a slice of fresh garlic several times daily. Garlic has potent antiviral properties and has long been used in folk medicine for the treatment of warts. <br> *Beneficial properties*: Powerful antiviral. <br> Garlic Note**:** Raw parsley taken with raw garlic will help prevent "garlic breath" and enhance garlic's blood cleansing effects**.** |
| Aromatherapy | Mix 2 drops of essential oil of **Thuja** (Thuja occidentalis) with ¼ teaspoon aloe vera gel and apply topically several times daily. Alternatively**,** apply 1 undiluted drop upon the center of the wart and cover with a band-aid. Repeat daily for several weeks. This oil is commonly used in aromatherapy in the treatment of warts**.** |

| EZ Care Program | |
|---|---|
| Homeopathy | **Thuja 6C-** Commonly used homeopathic remedy for crops of flat black warts that are seedy, sometimes oozing moisture and bleeding easily. Dosage: Dissolve 5 pellets under tongue 2 to 3 times daily as required. |
| Miscellaneous | **Imagery** Close your eyes while in a quiet, comfortable place and take 4 deep belly breaths to relax. Then picture yourself at the beach. Make sure that your images are very clear, so that you can feel the sun and sand and smell the salt water. See yourself going into the ocean and rinsing your wart with the salt water. Feel the salt begin to dissolve the wart all the way down to the root. Now see yourself lying on a blanket in the sand while the sun dries out what is left of the wart, until it just flakes away. Do this twice daily for three to four weeks. The whole process should only take three to five minutes.<br>*Note*: You can visualize other environments or locations, such as mountains or a stream, if you prefer. Create your own healing image that is very real and clear in your mind. |

## Additional Recommendations

The EZ Care Program consists of basic remedies that are commonly used for warts and have been found to work well in most cases. The remedies are most effective when combined, but can be used individually. The options stated below can supplement or replace EZ Care remedies and may be combined when suggested doses are followed.

### Diet

♦ **Eat a high-water-content diet** consisting of large quantities of fresh fruits and vegetables and comparatively smaller quantities of whole grains, legumes, seeds, nuts, fish, skinless chicken and turkey.

### Vitamins

♦ **C** (mineral ascorbates mixed with bioflavonoids) – Dosage: 1,000 mg., three to four times daily with meals. May enhance immune function and protect against viral infection.

### Minerals

♦ **Zinc** (take only if over 14 years of age) – Dosage: 50 mg. elemental zinc from amino acid chelate with meals. Plays an important role in immune function and wound healing. Is often useful in treating a variety of skin problems.
*Note:* Zinc and vitamin A are synergists and work well together in this context.

### Herbs

♦ **Dandelion** (Taraxacum offinalis) – Squeeze the milky sap from a stalk of fresh dandelion onto the warts several times daily. Traditional herbal remedy for warts.
*Beneficial properties*: May help break down warts

- **Lomatium** (Lomatium dissectum) – Dosage: 30 drops liquid extract* three times daily for four weeks.
  *Beneficial properties*: Helps stimulate the immune system to fight viral infections.

- **Echinacea** (Echinacea purpurea) – Dosage: 2 to 4 capsules or 50 drops liquid extract* three times daily for two weeks.
  *Beneficial Properties*: Traditionally used to fight infections.

## Homeopathy

See Appendix E for proper use and handling instruction prior to administering remedies described below.

- **Calc Carb 6C** – Large numbers of small, hard warts that itch and sting and may be inflamed or ulcerated. Dosage: Dissolve 5 pellets under the tongue, two to three times daily or as required.

- **Causticum 6C** – Clusters of many small warts that are soft at the base and hard at the top, appearing on arms and hands, eyelids and face. Dosage: Dissolve 5 pellets under the tongue, two to three times daily or as required.

- **Sulphur 6C** – Hard warts with throbbing pain. Dosage: Dissolve 5 pellets under the tongue, two to three times daily or as required.

## Miscellaneous

- **Banana** – Tape the inner surface of a fresh banana peel over the warts. Change once daily. May be particularly effective for plantar warts.

- **Castor Oil** – Soak a piece of gauze with castor oil and place over the warts. Secure in place for 30 minutes two times during the day, and keep a third application in place overnight. Continue treatment for several weeks to several months.

- **Figs** – Squeeze the milky juice from fresh, barely ripe figs and apply directly to warts several times daily. Traditional folk remedy.

- **Onion** – Mix 2 parts onion juice to 1 part unfiltered apple cider vinegar. Rub into warts several times daily. Traditional herbal remedy.

- **Papaya** – Apply the juice of green papaya to warts, several times daily. Contains powerful proteolytic enzymes that may assist in degrading warts.

- **Pineapple** – Apply a piece of crushed, fresh pineapple pulp over the warts and tape in place. Change two times daily. Contains powerful proteolytic enzymes that may assist in degrading warts.

- **Salt Water Soak** – Soak wart in a salt water solution 30 minutes, two to three times daily. Continue treatment several weeks. *To prepare solution*: 1-1/2 tsp. sea salt to 8 oz. pure water.

♦   **Sunlight** – Direct sunlight exposure may be helpful in treating warts.

*   Most herbal extracts contain alcohol. Avoid use if alcohol sensitive or if there is a history of alcohol abuse. *Note:* Alcohol content can be reduced through evaporation by adding extract to very hot water (just below boiling point) and allowing to stand 5 to 7 minutes before drinking.

# Appendix A: Vitamins and Minerals

## *Vitamins*

*Note:* Although RDA requirements are listed, the dosages supplied by the RDA are not recommended to achieve optimal health. The requirements are derived to provide the minimal amount of a nutrient to prevent deficiency.

### *Fat Soluble Vitamins*

| | |
|---|---|
| Vitamin A<br>Retinol | ◆ **Functions:** growth, vision, reproduction, healthy skin and hair, resistance to infection<br>◆ **Recommended Daily Allowance** (RDA): 1000 IU<br>◆ **Sources:** yellow, orange and red fruits and vegetables, green, leafy vegetables, milk, butter, eggs, liver<br>◆ **Complimentary nutrients:** niacin, C, D, E, pantothenic acid, zinc<br>◆ **Symptoms of deficiency:** night blindness, itching, dry skin, lost sense of taste<br>◆ **Increases need:** alcohol, coffee, cortisone, mineral oil, nitrates |
| Vitamin D<br>Cholecalciferol<br>Ergocalciferol | ◆ **Functions:** bones, teeth, optimum calcium-phosphorus absorption<br>◆ **Recommended Daily Allowance** (RDA): 10 IU<br>◆ **Sources:** sunlight, fortified milk, cod liver oil, herring, tuna, salmon, eggs, and dark green, leafy vegetables<br>◆ **Complimentary nutrients:** vitamin A, vitamin C, calcium, phosphorus<br>◆ **Symptoms of deficiency:** Soft bones and teeth, spontaneous fractures, bone curvature<br>◆ **Increases need:** mineral oil |
| Vitamin E<br>d-alpha tocopherol | ◆ **Functions:** antioxidant, protects cell membrane and tissues, maintains circulatory system<br>◆ **Recommended Daily Allowance** (RDA): 30 IU<br>◆ **Sources:** vegetable oil, grains, wheat germ, green, leafy vegetables, nuts, eggs<br>◆ **Complimentary nutrients:** selenium, vitamin C, B12, manganese<br>◆ **Symptoms of deficiency:** poor muscular and circulatory performance, reproductive disorders<br>◆ **Increases need:** air pollution, mineral oil, birth control pills |
| Vitamin K | ◆ **Functions:** blood clotting (coagulation)<br>◆ **Recommended Daily Allowance** (RDA): 45 mcg.<br>◆ **Sources:** green, leafy vegetables, molasses, yogurt, alfalfa, liver, asparagus, soy lecithin, egg yolk, cauliflower<br>◆ **Symptoms of deficiency:** diarrhea, increased tendency to bruise, prolonged bleeding<br>◆ **Increases need:** aspirin, antibiotics, mineral oil, rancid fat, X-ray therapy |

## Water Soluble Vitamins

| Vitamin B1 Thiamin | ♦ **Functions:** heart and cardiovascular system, growth, nervous system, energy production, digestion<br>♦ **Recommended Daily Allowance** (RDA): 1.5 mg.<br>♦ **Sources:** whole grains, brown rice, oats, fish, lean meat, liver, poultry, milk, brewer's yeast, nuts, seeds<br>♦ **Complimentary nutrients:** B-complex, B12, vitamin C<br>♦ **Symptoms of deficiency:** fatigue, poor appetite, pins and needles in legs, depression<br>♦ **Increases need:** depleted by physical and mental stress, alcohol, coffee, excessive sugar, tobacco |
|---|---|
| Vitamin B2 Riboflavin | ♦ **Functions:** growth and energy production, healthy skin, tissue repair, antibody and red-blood cell formation<br>♦ **Recommended Daily Allowance** (RDA): 1.7 mg.<br>♦ **Sources:** whole grain cereals, yeast, dairy, eggs, green, leafy vegetables, lean meat, soy beans<br>♦ **Complimentary nutrients:** vitamin A, niacin, B-complex, B1<br>♦ **Symptoms of deficiency:** cracks at corners of mouth, sore tongue, light sensitivity to eyes<br>♦ **Increases need:** depleted by physical and mental stress, alcohol, coffee, sugar, tobacco |
| Vitamin B3 Niacin or Niacinamide | ♦ **Functions:** healthy skin, nervous system, cell metabolism, converts food to energy, development of sex hormones<br>♦ **Recommended Daily Allowance** (RDA): 18 mg.<br>♦ **Sources:** whole grain products, liver, eggs, legumes, broccoli, figs, avocados, poultry, fish, yeast, lean meat<br>♦ **Complimentary nutrients:** B-complex, B1, B2, B6, tryptophan<br>♦ **Symptoms of deficiency:** weakness, skin rash, memory loss, irritability, insomnia<br>♦ **Increases need:** depleted by physical and mental stress, alcohol, coffee, sugar, antibiotics |
| Vitamin B5 Pantothenic Acid | ♦ **Functions:** immune system, cell growth; helps convert proteins, carbohydrates, and fats into energy<br>♦ **Recommended Daily Allowance** (RDA): 7.0 mg.<br>♦ **Sources:** beef, eggs, brewer's yeast, vegetables, liver, legumes, mushrooms, nuts, saltwater fish<br>♦ **Complimentary nutrients:** B-complex, folic acid, biotin<br>♦ **Symptoms of deficiency:** weakness, depression, hair loss, low blood pressure, decreased resistance to infection<br>♦ **Increases need:** depleted by physical and mental stress, alcohol, coffee |
| Vitamin B6 Pyridoxine | ♦ **Functions:** healthy red-blood cells, gums, teeth, blood vessels, nervous system, B12 absorption, production of stomach acid<br>♦ **Recommended Daily Allowance** (RDA): 2.0 mg.<br>♦ **Sources:** whole grains, wheat germ, yeast, meat, bananas, vegetables, egg yolk, nuts, seeds, cantaloupe, peas, oats<br>♦ |

| | |
|---|---|
| | • **Complimentary nutrients:** B-complex, vitamin C, biotin, pantothenic acid, niacin, magnesium<br>• **Symptoms of deficiency:** fatigue, anemia, nerve dysfunction, irritability, fluid retention<br>• **Increases need:** depleted by physical and mental stress, alcohol, coffee, tobacco, birth control pills |
| Vitamin B12<br>Cyanocobalamin | • **Functions:** development of red-blood cells, growth, nervous system maintenance<br>• **Recommended Daily Allowance** (RDA): 3.0 mcg.<br>• **Sources:** brewer's yeast, eggs, fish, lean meat, liver, dairy, kelp<br>• **Complimentary nutrients:** B-complex, folic acid, A, B1, B6, niacin, biotin, pantothenic acid<br>• **Symptoms of deficiency:** anemia, poor memory, weakness, fatigue, red and sore tongue, nerve degeneration<br>• **Increases need:** alcohol, coffee, tobacco, calcium deficiency |
| Biotin | • **Functions:** skin, circulatory system; metabolism of carbohydrates, proteins, and fats<br>• **Recommended Daily Allowance** (RDA): 200 mcg.<br>• **Sources:** nuts, egg yolk, soybeans, legumes, green, leafy vegetables, milk, organ meats<br>• **Complimentary nutrients:** vitamin A, B2, B6, niacin<br>• **Symptoms of deficiency:** hair loss, depression, non-specific skin rash, memory loss<br>• **Increases need:** alcohol, coffee, raw egg white, antibiotics |
| Choline | • **Functions:** nerve transmission, regulates liver and gallbladder, metabolizes fat and cholesterol, cell-membrane structure<br>• **Recommended Daily Allowance** (RDA): not established<br>• **Sources:** yeast, green, leafy vegetables, eggs, fish, lecithin, wheat germ, organ meats, soybeans, legumes, cauliflower<br>• **Complimentary nutrients:** vitamin A, B-complex, inositol, folic acid<br>• **Symptoms of deficiency:** growth problems, impaired liver and kidney functions<br>• **Increases need:** alcohol, coffee, sugar |
| Folic Acid<br>Folacin<br>Or<br>Folate | • **Functions:** red blood-cell production, development of nervous system, tissue cells, normal growth, healthy intestinal tract<br>• **Recommended Daily Allowance** (RDA): 200 mcg.<br>• **Sources:** brewer's yeast, green, leafy vegetables, whole grains, salmon, tuna, lentils, dairy, legumes, brown rice, meats<br>• **Complimentary nutrients:** B-complex, vitamin C, B6, B12, niacin<br>• **Symptoms of deficiency:** anemia, poor memory, intestinal problems, pale tongue, infertility<br>• **Increases need:** depleted by physical and mental stress, alcohol, oral contraceptives, tobacco |

| Inositol | • **Functions:** fat and cholesterol metabolism, nerve function.<br>• **Recommended Daily Allowance (RDA):** not established<br>• **Sources:** molasses, brewer's yeast, lecithin, fruits, meat, milk, nuts, lima beans, cabbage.<br>• **Complimentary nutrients:** B-complex, choline, B12<br>• **Symptoms of deficiency:** hair loss, eczema, constipation, depression, eye abnormalities, high cholesterol, anxiety<br>• **Increases need:** alcohol, coffee |
|---|---|
| PABA<br>Para-<br>Aminobenzoic<br>Acid | • **Functions:** blood cell formation, pigmentation of skin, formation of folic acid<br>• **Recommended Daily Allowance (RDA):** not established<br>• **Sources:** molasses, whole grains, eggs, liver, milk, rice, brewer's yeast, wheat germ, bran<br>• **Complimentary nutrients:** B-complex, folic acid, vitamin C<br>• **Symptoms of deficiency:** constipation, fatigue, eczema, depression, headaches, irritability<br>• **Increases need:** alcohol, coffee, sulfa drugs |
| Vitamin C<br>Ascorbic Acid | • **Functions:** antioxidant, wound healing, supports immune system; maintenance of healthy gums, skin, blood, and bones; iron absorption, connective tissue formation<br>• **Recommended Daily Allowance (RDA):** 60 mg.<br>• **Sources:** citrus fruits, green peppers, broccoli, melons, berries, cabbage, Brussels sprouts, green, leafy vegetables, tomatoes, potatoes<br>• **Complimentary nutrients:** vitamin A, B6, pantothenic acid, zinc<br>• **Symptoms of deficiency:** bruise easily, slow wound healing, teeth/gum problems, aching joints<br>• **Increases need:** depleted by physical and mental stress, antibiotics, aspirin, stress, cortisone |

*Minerals*

| | |
|---|---|
| Boron | ♦ **Functions:** healthy bones; metabolism of calcium, magnesium, and phosphorus<br>♦ **Recommended Daily Allowance (RDA):** not established<br>♦ **Sources:** apples, grapes, green, leafy vegetables, honey, nuts, grains, carrots, whole grains, legumes<br>♦ **Symptoms of deficiency:** bone loss |
| Calcium | ♦ **Functions:** bone and teeth formation and maintenance, muscle contraction, nerve transmission<br>♦ **Recommended Daily Allowance (RDA):** 1000-1,500 mg.<br>♦ **Sources:** dairy products, sardines, almonds and other nuts, green, leafy vegetables, figs, sesame seeds, kelp, tofu<br>♦ **Complimentary nutrients:** vitamin A, vitamin C, vitamin D, phosphorus<br>♦ **Symptoms of deficiency:** heart palpitations, muscle cramps, teeth/bone weakening, osteoporosis<br>♦ **Increases need:** excess saturated fat in diet |
| Chromium | ♦ **Functions:** balances blood sugar, carbohydrate metabolism, and energy<br>♦ **Recommended Daily Allowance (RDA):** 50-200 mcg.<br>♦ **Sources:** brewer's yeast, whole grains, brown rice, corn and corn oil, legumes, clams, chicken, mushrooms<br>♦ **Symptoms of deficiency:** poor glucose tolerance, weight gain, low blood sugar levels<br>♦ **Increases need:** excess iron |
| Copper | ♦ **Functions:** enzyme function, hemoglobin production, connective tissue formation<br>♦ **Recommended Daily Allowance (RDA):** 2-3 mg.<br>♦ **Sources:** nuts, seeds, organ meats, raisins, poultry, avocado, bran, oysters<br>♦ **Complimentary nutrients:** cobalt, iron, zinc (helps balance)<br>♦ **Symptoms of deficiency:** anemia, fatigue, weakness, bone fragility<br>♦ **Increases need:** Fructose, exhaust fumes, cadmium |
| Iodine | ♦ **Functions:** thyroid hormone production, metabolism regulation<br>♦ **Recommended Daily Allowance (RDA):** 150 mcg.<br>♦ **Sources:** onions, seafood, kelp, iodized salt<br>♦ **Symptoms of deficiency:** enlarged thyroid gland in neck, low thyroid function<br>♦ **Increases need:** certain raw vegetables may interfere with absorption, including spinach, cauliflower, Brussels sprouts, kale and turnips |

| Iron | • **Functions:** production of red-blood cells to carry oxygen to tissues; enzyme functions |
| | • **Recommended Daily Allowance** (RDA): 10-18 mg. |
| | • **Sources:** whole grain cereals, organ meats, beef, egg yolks, black strap molasses, nuts, green, leafy vegetables, parsley |
| | • **Complimentary nutrients:** B6, vitamin C, B12, folic acid |
| | • **Symptoms of deficiency:** fatigue, weakness from anemia, brittle fingernails, hair loss, heart problems, decreased growth |
| | • **Increases need:** excess saturated fat in diet, excess protein |
| Magnesium | • **Functions:** enzyme activity, healthy heart arteries, protein production, nerve function |
| | • **Recommended Daily Allowance** (RDA): 300-400 mg. |
| | • **Sources:** whole grains, wheat germ, corn, peas, figs, carrots, bananas, seafood, green vegetables |
| | • **Complimentary nutrients:** B6, vitamin C, calcium, phosphorus |
| | • **Symptoms of deficiency:** high blood pressure, growth failure, leg cramps, nervousness, confusion |
| | • **Increases need:** excessive iron |
| Manganese | • **Functions:** enzyme activity in reproduction, growth, and fat metabolism |
| | • **Recommended Daily Allowance** (RDA): 2.5-5.0 mg. |
| | • **Sources:** whole grains, eggs, nuts, blueberries, peas, beets, avocados, blackberries, green, leafy vegetables |
| | • **Symptoms of deficiency:** poor growth |
| | • **Increases need:** alcohol, coffee, cortisone, diuretics, excessive processed sugar |
| Phosphorus | • **Functions:** bone and teeth formation, muscle contraction, energy production, kidney function, nerve and muscle activity |
| | • **Recommended Daily Allowance** (RDA): 600-1250 mg. |
| | • **Sources:** legumes, nuts, eggs, fish, meat, poultry, whole grains, dairy |
| | • **Complimentary nutrients:** calcium, iron, magnesium, manganese, vitamins A, D |
| | • **Symptoms of deficiency:** digestive problems, continuous thirst, dry skin, general weakness |
| Potassium | • **Functions:** pH balance of blood, kidney and adrenal function; nerve and muscle function |
| | • **Recommended Daily Allowance** (RDA): 99 mg. |
| | • **Sources:** dates, raisins, figs, apples, oranges, carrots, fish, legumes, whole grains, peaches, sunflower seeds |
| | • **Complimentary nutrients:** sodium |
| | • **Symptoms of deficiency:** irregular heartbeat, muscular weakness, build-up of lactic acid |
| | • **Increases need:** mercury, cadmium |

| Selenium | • **Functions:** antioxidant, protects cell membrane and internal structures, chelates, heavy metals<br>• **Recommended Daily Allowance** (RDA): 50-70 mcg.<br>• **Sources:** whole grains, seafood, eggs, organ meat, brown rice, brewer's yeast, tomatoes, broccoli<br>• **Complimentary nutrients:** vitamin E<br>• **Symptoms of deficiency:** anemia, breakdown of cartilage and muscle, heart muscle enlargement, irregular beat<br>• **Increases need:** coffee, excess zinc or copper |
|---|---|
| Sodium | • **Functions:** proper water regulation; muscle, nerve, and stomach function<br>• **Recommended Daily Allowance** (RDA): 1.1 – 3.3 mg. daily<br>• **Sources:** most foods (sea salt preferred form)<br>• **Complimentary nutrients:** must be balanced with potassium<br>• **Symptoms of deficiency:** abdominal cramps, confusion, dehydration, fatigue, dizziness, low blood pressure<br>• **Increases need:** diuretics |
| Zinc | • **Functions:** immune system, wound healing, reproductive organ development, male hormone production<br>• **Recommended Daily Allowance** (RDA): 15 mg.<br>• **Sources:** pumpkin seeds, oysters, eggs, green, leafy vegetables, fish, dairy products, yeast, whole grains, liver, sunflower seeds<br>• **Complimentary nutrients:** calcium, phosphorus, vitamins A, C, D; increases absorption<br>• **Symptoms of deficiency:** depression, poor sense of smell and taste, poor growth and wound healing |

# Appendix B: Herbs

## *Herbs*

Herbs are derived from plants that have natural healing properties. Their versatility allows them to be used internally, externally and as aromatics. They can be prepared as liquids, pills, pastes, powders, teas and oils. In this section, we will describe these different preparations and their uses.

When choosing an herb, it is important to purchase herbs that are fresh and potent. Herbs can be obtained in standardized and non-standardized extracts, and whole herb forms. Standardized herbs guarantee that a certain amount of the useful component is contained in each dosage. This process is very useful for certain herbs; however, in standardizing the herb, other parts, which may be beneficial as well, are discarded. Whole herbs, on the other hand, use the entire content of the herb. Various remedies throughout the book inform you as to when it is appropriate to use standardized forms. When the individual remedy does not call for standardization, the whole herb form should be used if available. Below is a description of herbal preparations.

## Internal Uses

### *Liquid extracts*

Liquid extracts, also known as tinctures, are concentrated forms of herbal medicine. They are prepared by soaking the herb in diluted alcohol to extract the herb's beneficial properties. In this extract form, the herbs are extremely potent and are usually taken mixed in herbal tea or pure water. Caution should be taken when combing several tinctures, as this can cause high levels of alcohol to be ingested. Most tinctures have a shelf life of several years.

Those wishing to avoid alcohol should not take tinctures, even if the alcohol content is reduced. The alcohol content can be lowered by adding the extract to very hot water (just below the boiling point) which has been poured into a cup and allowing it to stand for at least 5 to 7 minutes. As alcohol has a lower boiling temperature than water, this procedure causes alcohol to evaporate while leaving behind the pure herbal extract.

## *Glycerites*

Glycerites are alcohol free, syrupy liquid extracts. They are prepared by using glycerine instead of alcohol. Although they have a sweet taste, they generally do not affect blood sugar levels. Glycerites are most often diluted in herbal tea or pure water, because they can irritate the mouth if taken full strength, and are very drying. They are not as potent as alcohol extracts, but they are often recommended for use with children and adults wishing to avoid alcohol. One problem is that only a limited number of herbs produce effective glycerites, thus there is a smaller selection available.

## *Pills*

Pills come in both tablet and capsule form. They are generally made from either dried herbs, or powdered liquid tinctures, combined with a filler. The advantage of taking pills is that they are convenient, are alcohol free, and you do not taste the herb when swallowing. This can be a disadvantage with some herbs, such as bitters, for which the taste makes them more effective. Pills have a shorter shelf life than tinctures, and are less potent. Vegetarians should be careful to avoid gelatin capsules that are made from meat derivatives. To assure freshness, break open a capsule and make sure the smell, color, and taste are similar to that of the original herb.

## *Teas*

Teas are one of the least expensive ways to take herbs. They are prepared as either infusions, or decoctions.

**Infusion: (Hot)** Although tea bags are the most common form of infusion, loose herbs can often create a fresher and more powerful tea. Hot infusions are prepared by placing one tablespoon of herb in a non-aluminum cooking pot (preferably glass), and pouring two cups of pure boiling water over the herbs. Cover and let steep for 15 to 30 minutes. Strain and drink while still warm. Infusions are used for the soft part of herbs, which contain volatile oils. If these delicate oils are boiled, they can be destroyed. That is why hot water is poured over the herbs as opposed to a decoction which is placed in the boiling water.

**Decoctions:** Decoctions are used to make a tea out of hard or woody objects such as roots, bark, nuts, and seeds. They are prepared by breaking up herbs into small pieces, and adding one cup of pure water to two teaspoons of dried herb, or four teaspoons of fresh herbs. Bring the water to a boil and then reduce the heat to gently simmer the herbs for 20 to 35 minutes. After boiling, allow to stand and cool prior to straining.

# External Applications

## *Compress*

A compress is an easy way to use herbs externally. To prepare a compress, take a clean cloth (white cotton or linen is preferred) and soak it in warm, strong herbal tea. Loosely wring out so that cloth is wet but not dripping, and place the warm cloth over the affected area. Cover the wet cloth with a dry cloth, and cover both with plastic or waxed paper. A hot water bottle can be placed on top to keep compress warm.

## *Poultice*

Poultices are made from fresh or dry plants which have been cut, mashed or blended, and then mixed with a sufficient amount of water to form a thick, spreadable (not too watery) paste. This paste can be applied directly to the affected area, or placed between one or two thin layers of gauze, and then applied. The poultice should be kept moist with a plastic bag or appropriate vegetable leaf, and covered with a towel to keep warm. A hot water bottle can then be placed on the towel to prolong heating.

**Clay Poultice:** Bentonite clay or French green clay are most commonly used. To prepare, mix dry clay with water or other recommended liquid, to make a paste. Spread a 1/2-inch layer of clay on a cotton or linen cloth. Place the poultice clay side down over the affected area. If the affected area is covered with hair (i.e., pubic area), place gauze over the hair prior to application of the poultice, then cover the area with a cabbage leaf to help keep the area moist. The longer the clay is moist, the more effective it is. Secure the poultice in place. Keep it on for 1 to 2 hours during the day or overnight.

## *Herb Caution*

Although herbs are natural substances, they have medicinal properties, and should be used with caution. Never take herbs or any other supplements if you are pregnant, nursing, being treated for any other illness, or taking any other medications without consulting a medical doctor. If you experience any side affects, discontinue use and notify your medical doctor. Parents should not give any herbs to children without prior consultation with their pediatrician.

Never discontinue any prescribed medication without consulting your medical doctor.

| Traditional Usage | |
|---|---|
| **Aloe**<br>*Aloe barbadenis* | ◆ Burns, sunburn, dry skin and skin irritations, bug bites, rashes from poisonous plants.<br>◆ Digestive irritation, constipation |
| **American ginseng**<br>*Panax quinquefolium*<br>Panax Ginseng | ◆ Mental or physical stress<br>◆ Stressed adrenal glands<br>◆ Fatigue, lethargy, low stamina<br>◆ Poor physical or mental performance |
| **Angelica**<br>*Angelica sinensis*<br>Tang-quei<br>Dong quai | ◆ Premenstrual syndrome, menopause, painful or irregular menses<br>◆ Colic, gas, indigestion, hepatitis, heartburn<br>◆ Inflammation<br>◆ Estrogen deficiency<br>◆ *Note: Do not use if you have diabetes.* |
| **Arnica**<br>*Arnica Montana*<br>Leopard's bane | ◆ Externally*:* bruises, strain, sprain<br>◆ *Note: Do not use on broken skin*<br>◆ Internally*:* as a homeopathic remedy for bruises, strain, sprain<br>◆ *Note: Use Internally only as a homeopathic remedy.* |
| **Astragalus**<br>*Astragalus membranosus* | ◆ Weak metabolism or digestion<br>◆ Weak immune system<br>◆ Chronic or recurring infection<br>◆ Excessive water weight |
| **Bearberry**<br>*Arctostaphylos uva-ursi*<br>Uva Ursi | ◆ Bloating from excessive water retention<br>◆ Bladder infection<br>◆ Kidney infection<br>◆ Kidney stones |
| **Bilberry**<br>*Vaccinium myrtillus*<br>Huckleberry | ◆ Vision ailment, such as cataract, macular degeneration, diabetic retinopathy, or night blindness |
| **Black cohosh**<br>*Cimicifuga racemosa* | ◆ Delayed and painful menstruation<br>◆ Menopause symptoms<br>◆ Muscle spasms<br>◆ Depression<br>◆ Bronchial coughing |
| **Blue cohosh**<br>*Caulophyllum thalictroides* | ◆ Painful periods with cramping<br>◆ Stomach cramping<br>◆ Arthritis cramping<br>◆ *Note: Do not use if pregnant, have high blood pressure or heart disease. Do not eat the seeds of this plant.* |

## Traditional Usage

| | |
|---|---|
| **Black currant**<br>*Ribies nigrum*<br>Quinsy berry | ♦ Skin condition<br>♦ Inflammatory disorder<br>♦ Bleeding gums<br>♦ Auto-immune disorder, including systemic lupus erythematosis<br>♦ Hair or nail problem<br>♦ Premenstrual syndrome |
| **Burdock root**<br>*Arctium lappa* | ♦ Blood needs purifying<br>♦ Fever, inflammation, hepatitis, swollen glands<br>♦ Toxic liver or congested bile flow<br>♦ Psoriasis, acne, or other skin condition |
| **Butcher's broom**<br>*Ruscus aculeatus* | ♦ Hemorrhoids, varicose veins<br>♦ Poor circulation in hands or feet<br>♦ Inflammation<br>♦ Overdilated veins |
| **Calendula**<br>*Calendula officinalis* | ♦ Skin irritation, eczema, acne, rash (including diaper rash)<br>♦ Chapped skin or lips<br>♦ Wounds, cuts, abrasions, burns |
| **Cascara sagrada**<br>*Rhammnus Punshiana* | ♦ Constipation<br>♦ Poor digestion |
| **Cat's claw**<br>*Uncaria tomentosa*<br>Una de gato | ♦ Inflammation<br>♦ Weak immune, intestinal, or cardiovascular system<br>♦ Chronic infections<br>♦ Parasites<br>♦ Arthritis, gastritis, tumors, dysentery, female hormonal imbalance, ulcers<br>♦ *Note: Do not take if chemically immuno-suppressed or have received an organ transplant.* |
| **Cayenne**<br>*Capsicum annuum*<br>Chili pepper | ♦ Arthritis and muscle aches<br>♦ Chills<br>♦ High cholesterol<br>♦ Poor circulation; heart conditions<br>♦ Poor digestion<br>♦ Bleeding external cuts<br>♦ Pain and inflammation |
| **Chamomile**<br>*Matricaria recuttia*<br>German or blue chamomile | ♦ Inflammation or spasms in digestive tract<br>♦ Upset stomach, heartburn, colic, indigestion, acid reflux<br>♦ Nervousness<br>♦ Ulcers<br>♦ Menstrual cramps<br>♦ Insomnia (mild sedative properties) |

## Traditional Usage

| | |
|---|---|
| **Chasteberry**<br>*Vitex agnus castus*<br>Vitex | ◆ Irregular menses<br>◆ Hormonal imbalance<br>◆ Cystic ovaries<br>◆ Premenstrual syndrome<br>◆ Menopausal symptoms |
| **Cineraria**<br>*Cineraria maritima*<br>Dusty miller | ◆ Cataracts |
| **Cinnamon Bark**<br>*Cinnamomum verum* | ◆ Poor circulation<br>◆ Colds, flu, chills<br>◆ Poor digestion<br>◆ Loss of appetite |
| **Coltsfoot**<br>*Tussilago farfara*<br>Coughwort | ◆ Inflammation or bronchial irritation<br>◆ Emphysema<br>◆ Cough<br>◆ Bronchitis<br>◆ Asthma |
| **Comfrey**<br>*Symphytum officinale*<br>Knitbone | ◆ *Topically:* broken bones, wounds, burns, sores, bruises, skin rashes or irritations<br>◆ *Note: Avoid internal use.* |
| **Cranberry**<br>*Vaccinium macrocarpona* | ◆ Urinary tract infection or irritation<br>◆ Bladder infection<br>◆ Gout |
| **Crampbark**<br>*Viburnum prunifolium* | ◆ Menstrual cramps<br>◆ Uterine and afterbirth sedative |
| **Dandelion**<br>*Taraxacum officinalis* | ◆ Weak liver<br>◆ Urinary tract infection<br>◆ Fluid retention<br>◆ High blood pressure<br>◆ Premenstrual syndrome<br>◆ Loss of appetite<br>◆ Kidney or gallbladder stones |
| **Devil's claw**<br>*Harpagophytum procumbens* | ◆ Arthritis<br>◆ Inflammatory conditions<br>◆ Stiff joints<br>◆ Loss of appetite<br>◆ Liver or gallbladder complaint |

## Traditional Usage

| | |
|---|---|
| **Echinacea**<br>*Echinacea purpurea or*<br>*E. angustifolia*<br>Purple coneflower | ◆ Most types of infection<br>◆ Colds, flu, sore throat<br>◆ Blood impurities<br>◆ Weak immune system<br>◆ Skin wounds |
| **Ephedra**<br>*Ephedra sinica* | ◆ Respiratory infections<br>◆ Asthma, bronchitis, hayfever<br>◆ Headaches |
| **Evening primrose oil**<br>*Oenothera biennis* | ◆ Skin disorder, eczema, acne<br>◆ Premenstrual syndrome<br>◆ Inflammatory conditions<br>◆ High blood pressure or high cholesterol |
| **Eyebright**<br>*Euphrasia officinalis* | ◆ Conjunctivitis, pink eye<br>◆ Inflammation of blood vessels in eyes<br>◆ Poor eyesight<br>◆ Allergies |
| **Fennel seed**<br>*foeniculum vulgare* | ◆ Coughs, bronchitis, lung congestion<br>◆ Flatulence, feeling of fullness<br>◆ Poor appetite<br>◆ Poor digestion |
| **Feverfew**<br>*Tanacetum parthenium*<br>Featherfew | ◆ Headaches<br>◆ Painful menses<br>◆ Migraines (acute and prevention)<br>◆ Arthritis |
| **Flax seed**<br>*Linum usitatissimu* | ◆ Skin disorder<br>◆ Constipation<br>◆ Cardiovascular disorder<br>◆ Irritable colon, diverticulitis |
| **Garlic**<br>*Allium sativum* | ◆ Common cold, sore throat<br>◆ *Externally* for ear infection in child<br>◆ High triglycerides (blood fats)<br>◆ Yeast infections<br>◆ High blood pressure or high cholesterol<br>◆ Conditions requiring antibacterial, antifungal, antiviral, antibiotic treatment |
| **Gentian root**<br>*Gentiana lutea*<br>Bitter root | ◆ Poor digestion, low stomach acid<br>◆ Poor appetite<br>◆ Flatulence |

## Traditional Usage

| | |
|---|---|
| **Ginger root**<br>*Zingiber officinale*<br>African ginger | ◆ Nausea, motion sickness<br>◆ Flatulence<br>◆ Poor digestion<br>◆ Poor appetite<br>◆ Arthritis, bursitis, general inflammation |
| **Ginkgo**<br>*Ginkgo biloba* | ◆ Poor memory or mental function<br>◆ Hearing loss or ringing in ears<br>◆ Poor circulation |
| **Goldenseal root**<br>*Hydrastis canadensis*<br>Yellow root | ◆ Bacterial and viral conditions<br>◆ Infections<br>◆ Skin inflammation |
| **Gotu Kola**<br>*Centella asiatica* | ◆ Poor memory<br>◆ Poor circulation |
| **Gymnemma**<br>*Gymnemma sylvestre* | ◆ Diabetes mellitus. |
| **Hawthorn leaf**<br>*Crataegus oxycantha*<br>English hawthorn | ◆ High blood pressure<br>◆ Poor circulation<br>◆ Angina or heart disease<br>◆ Hypothyroidism |
| **Horse chestnut**<br>*Aecsulus hippocastanum*<br>Spanish chestnut | ◆ Venous condition, including varicose veins, hemorrhoids<br>◆ Leg ulcers<br>◆ Eczema |
| **Horseradish**<br>*Armoracia lapathifolia* | ◆ Sinusitis<br>◆ Respiratory problem<br>◆ Fluid retention<br>◆ Rheumatism |
| **Horsetail**<br>*Equisetum arvense* | ◆ Bladder or kidney stones<br>◆ Urinary tract infection<br>◆ Problem nails or hair<br>◆ Bed-wetting |
| **Kava kava**<br>*Piper methysticum* | ◆ Anxiety, stress<br>◆ Depression<br>◆ Insomnia<br>◆ Muscle tension |

## Traditional Usage

| | |
|---|---|
| **Kelp**<br>*Fucus vesiculosus*<br>Bladderwrack | ◆ Hypothyroidism<br>◆ Arteriosclerosis<br>◆ Digestive disorders |
| **Licorice root**<br>*Glycyrrhiza glabra or uralenses* | ◆ Herpes, eczema, psoriasis<br>◆ Inflammatory and viral conditions<br>◆ Menstrual or menopausal disorder<br>◆ Blood sugar imbalance<br>◆ Chronic indigestion, heartburn, stomach ulcers |
| **Marshmallow root**<br>*Althea officinalis* | ◆ Inflammation or irritation of mucosal tissue, such as sore throat<br>◆ Ulcers, colitis<br>◆ General inflammation |
| **Milk thistle**<br>*Silbum marianum*<br>Holy thistle | ◆ Liver conditions<br>◆ Hepatitis<br>◆ Poor fat digestion |
| **Mullein**<br>*Verbascum thapsus* | ◆ Chest congestion; dry, bronchial cough<br>◆ Ear infection<br>◆ Asthma |
| **Myrrh**<br>*Commiphora molmol* | ◆ Cough and cold<br>◆ Sores in mouth<br>◆ Stomach flu |
| **Oat seed**<br>*Avena sativa* | ◆ Weak nerves<br>◆ Anxiety, stress<br>◆ Insomnia<br>◆ Connective tissue disorder<br>◆ Opium or tobacco withdrawal |
| **Onion**<br>*Allium cepa* | ◆ Coughs<br>◆ Poor digestion<br>◆ High blood pressure<br>◆ Antiparasitic, antifungal, antiseptic<br>◆ Cardiovascular problems |
| **Oregon grape root**<br>*Mahonia aquifolium* | ◆ Skin disorder, acne, cold sores, eczema<br>◆ Liver or gallbladder problems<br>◆ High blood pressure<br>◆ Blood impurities |

## Traditional Usage

| | |
|---|---|
| **Passion flower**<br>*Passiflora incarnata* | ♦ Anxiety, nervousness, stress<br>♦ Insomnia<br>♦ High blood pressure |
| **Peppermint**<br>*Mentha piperita* | ♦ Cramps<br>♦ Poor digestion, such as heartburn or indigestion<br>♦ Intestinal problems, such as irritable bowel syndrome or diverticulitis<br>♦ Nausea<br>♦ Flatulence |
| **Phytolacca**<br>*Phytolocca americana*<br>Pokeroot | ♦ Swollen glands, tonsillitis, mumps<br>♦ Throat infection<br>♦ *Note: Fresh plant is poisonous.* |
| **Plantain leaf**<br>*Plantago lanceolata* | ♦ Insect bites and stings<br>♦ Poison ivy, poison oak<br>♦ Cuts |
| **Red clover**<br>*Trifolium pratense* | ♦ Cancer<br>♦ Cough, bronchitis, whooping cough<br>♦ Skin eruptions, including eczema and psoriasis |
| **Red raspberry leaf**<br>*Rubus idaeus*<br>Wild red raspberry | ♦ Diarrhea<br>♦ Menstrual cramps<br>♦ Sore throat<br>♦ Morning sickness<br>♦ Motion sickness |
| **Sarsaparilla**<br>*Smilax officinalis* | ♦ Blood impurities<br>♦ Enlarged prostate<br>♦ Rheumatism<br>♦ Skin conditions, such as psoriasis |
| **Saw palmetto berries**<br>*Serenoa repens* | ♦ Enlarged prostate<br>♦ Ovarian cysts<br>♦ Male pattern baldness |
| **Scullcap**<br>*Scutellaria lateriflora*<br>Scutellaria | ♦ Anxiety<br>♦ Insomnia<br>♦ Nervousness<br>♦ Depression |

## Traditional Usage

| | |
|---|---|
| **Shiitake mushroom**<br>*Lentinus edodes* | ◆ Weak immune system<br>◆ HIV positive (Human Immuno Virus) (antiviral)<br>◆ Cancer<br>◆ High blood cholesterol |
| **Siberian ginseng**<br>*Eleutherococcus*<br>*senticosus* | ◆ Physical or mental stress<br>◆ Athletic performance enhancement<br>◆ Low stamina, lethargy, fatigue<br>◆ Radiation |
| **Slippery elm bark**<br>*Ulmus fulva* | ◆ Sore throat<br>◆ Cough (suppressant)<br>◆ Diarrhea<br>◆ Intestinal irritation, including irritable bowel syndrome and colitis |
| **St. John's Wort**<br>*Hypericum perforatum*<br>Hypericum | ◆ Inflammation<br>◆ Depression, seasonal affective disorder (SAD)<br>◆ Virus infection<br>◆ Insomnia |
| **Stinging nettle**<br>*Urtica dioica*<br>Nettle | ◆ Anemia<br>◆ Hayfever<br>◆ Allergics<br>◆ Arthritis, gout<br>◆ Eczema |
| **Thuja**<br>*Thuja occidentalis*<br>White cedar | ◆ Skin problems, such as warts<br>◆ Bronchitis (expectorant) |
| **Tumeric**<br>*Curcuma longa* | ◆ Inflammatory, microbial, carcinogenic problems<br>◆ Arthritis, gout, tendonitis<br>◆ Insufficient bile secretion |
| **Valerian root**<br>*Valeriana officinalis* | ◆ Nervousness<br>◆ Stress<br>◆ Insomnia<br>◆ Headaches<br>◆ Depression<br>◆ Seizure disorder |
| **White willow bark**<br>*Salix alba* | ◆ Fever, headaches<br>◆ Pain, inflammation<br>*Note: Works similar to aspirin.* |

## Traditional Usage

| | |
|---|---|
| **Wild cherry bark**<br>*Prunus serotina* | ◆ Coughs.<br>◆ Bronchitis.<br>◆ Diarrhea. |
| **Witch hazel**<br>*Hamamelis virginiana* | ◆ Minor cuts and abrasions (disinfectant)<br>◆ Hemorrhoids, anal irritation<br>◆ Vaginitis<br>◆ Insect stings, sun and wind burn<br>◆ Poison ivy blisters<br>◆ Skin care, cleansing, toning and refreshing |
| **Wild yam root**<br>*Dioscorea villosa* | ◆ Hormone imbalance<br>◆ Premenstrual syndrome |
| **Yarrow**<br>*Achillea millefolium* | ◆ Cold and fever (promotes sweating)<br>◆ External bleeding<br>◆ Heavy menses<br>◆ Inflammation |
| **Yellow dock root**<br>*Rumex crispus* | ◆ Skin eruptions<br>◆ Anemia<br>◆ Blood impurities |

# Appendix C: Food Allergies & Sensitivities

*Food allergies and sensitivities*

Food allergies and sensitivities have become much more common in today's fast-paced world. Because of the complexity of diagnosing food allergies, their possibility is often completely overlooked when a health problem arises. The most common way to test for food allergies is with an "elimination and reintroduction diet", in which certain foods are totally eliminated from the diet, then slowly reintroduced.

To perform this test, choose a suspected food or group of foods, and avoid completely for three weeks. In order to perform this test properly, read the labels on food containers, and question the contents of prepared foods both purchased and eaten out. Even small amounts of a suspected food can alter the test results if eaten before the three-week period ends.

Avoiding suspected foods gives the body a chance to completely clear them from the system. After three weeks, reintroduce the foods, one at a time. For example, if you eliminated wheat, citrus and corn, start by reintroducing only one of those foods. Eat that food throughout the day, along with other non-allergic foods, paying attention for a noticeable reaction. If you have a reaction, you know that is a food you are sensitive to, and should avoid for the next 60 to 90 days. Wait three more days before reintroducing the second food, and so on.

Common allergy-causing foods include wheat, corn, milk, and other dairy products, as well as soy, sugar, citrus, eggwhites, shellfish, coffee, food dyes, and additives. The best place to start with food elimination is with the foods you eat most often and crave. To make the test easier, look for replacement foods for the ones you will be avoiding. For example: soy, rice, or nut products, instead of dairy. Grains: rice, spelt, quinoa, or kamut instead of wheat. Sweeteners: honey, maple syrup, stevia, or fruit instead of sugar. For many people, this test forces them to learn about a whole new world of foods.

Another way to test for food allergies is to perform the "pulse test", which is measuring the pulse rate prior to eating, then again afterwards. First, sit in a relaxed position, and rest for 1 or 2 minutes to bring the pulse to a stable rate. Find the pulse (the heart beat) on the underside of a wrist. Using the first two fingers of the opposite hand, press lightly on the wrist in alignment with the base of the thumb. (If you have difficulty finding the pulse, bend your hand back away from where you are trying to feel the pulse; this will bring the heart beats closer to the surface.)

Using a watch with a second hand, count the number of beats felt in one minute. A normal pulse rate is 60 to 100 beats per minute. Now eat the food you wish to test. Wait fifteen minutes before once again relaxing, then count your pulse rate again for one minute. During the duration of this test, be sure to eat only the one food you are testing.

If your pulse rate increased more than ten beats per minute, remove this food from your diet for 90 days. After the suspected food has been removed for an extended period of time, you should be able to reintroduce it to your diet without any problem. Be careful, however, not to get back into the habit of eating that food daily.

*Note: Do not self-test any food that causes known severe allergic reactions.*

After testing for suspected food allergies, it may be advisable to do a "rotation diet," which is eating a suspected food on one day, and not eating it again for the next four days. The body is often capable of handling small amounts of food which are slightly allergic; however, the accumulation of foods eaten regularly causes an overload, which then is seen as a reaction. By rotating suspected foods, the body is allowed to clear the food out of your system, thus enabling you to tolerate small amounts a few days later. This should only be done with foods that do not cause severe reactions. An example is to eat apples on Monday, and not eat them again until Saturday. You may eat wheat one day and, as with the apples, not again for four more days. This rotation may include chicken, different types of fruit and vegetables, grains and any other type of food eaten.

It is recommended to keep a chart of which foods to eat on which days. Your local library may have books written specifically on this subject, and include charts and recipes. Food rotation is an excellent way to help your body recover from food allergies.

If either of these methods of food allergy testing have failed, or your results are uncertain, consult a physician specialized in this area. One of the most effective methods of allergy testing is provocation-neutralization. This procedure involves the injection of whole food extracts under the skin, which may produce a skin reaction and/or a reaction in the body such as headaches, fatigue, or mild nausea. The dose is diluted to a level that no longer produces a reaction, and then used as treatment for the offending food. Many food compounds can be tested in addition to environmental chemicals, dusts, and molds. Contact the American College for the Advancement in Medicine (ACAM) or the American Academy for Environmental Medicine (AAEM), to locate a physician specialized in this procedure. An alternate method of testing is the ELISA food test. This lab study involves a blood screen to detect major antibodies to food compounds. This test has the advantage of requiring only one blood draw, but is disadvantaged as it only screens for the main allergenic components of a food and may not detect smaller, but important components causing allergy.

# Appendix D: Hydrotherapy

*Hydrotherapy*

Note: Avoid hot baths if suffering from heart problems or diabetes

## Heating Compress

Traditionally used for: colds, congestion, sore throats, and upper respiratory infections.

This is a cold application placed on a specific body part and left there until the body warms it. This procedure requires an active response from the body, which stimulates the immune system to react, causing an increased blood flow to that particular area.

### Sore Throat

Make sure you are warm before starting.

1. Wet and wring out a small towel in cold tap water.

2. Apply to throat and wrap snugly with a dry wool or cotton cloth or towel.

3. Keep the compress in place several hours, overnight, or until dry.

### Colds, Congestion, Upper Respiratory Infections

When treating congestion, cold or upper respiratory infection, the "cold sock treatment" is very effective. It works especially well for children with colds. By placing a cold, wet cloth on the feet, blood flow increases into the lower part of the body and therefore decreases congestion to the upper area of the body.

1. Soak feet in warm water for several minutes.

2. Take out of water, dry off.

3. Wring out a pair of cotton socks soaked in ice water and immediately place on the feet.

4.  Cover those with a pair of wool socks, and go to bed.

5.  In the morning, the socks should all be dry.

## Sitz Bath

Traditionally used for complaints of the pelvic area.

Sitz baths can be hot, cold, or an alternation of both, as a condition requires. Which temperature variation is most suitable in a given case will vary among individuals. The idea is to fill the tub to the appropriate level and remain in water for length of time described below. After the bath, dry and rest for a minimum of thirty minutes.

**The hot sitz bath** is generally performed for 3 to 8 minutes, with the water temperature between 106°F and 110°F, and the water level ½ inch above the naval. Feet are generally placed out of the tub, or can be placed on top of an over turned bucket in order to keep them out of the water. A cold compress can be applied to the forehead and back of neck to keep cool. After the required time has elapsed, cold water is poured over the areas that have been soaked. An alternative is to use a cold, wet washcloth over the same area.

**The cold sitz bath** is generally performed for 3 to 8 minutes, and has a water temperature between 55°F and 75°F with the water level ½ inch below the naval. In order to enhance reaction to the cold stimulation, the cold sitz bath should be preceded by a 2 to 4 minute warm sitz bath. To help prevent chilling, the water level of the cold sitz bath should be 1 inch less than that of the hot, and the feet should be placed in a basin of hot water. During the cold sitz bath, the hips and lower abdominal region should be briskly rubbed with a dry wash cloth to support circulatory reaction to the cold. **Note***: Seriously ill or debilitated individuals should avoid cold sitz baths, unless employed under the guidance of a physician.* Sitz baths can be used 1 to 2 times daily or several times weekly as required.

**The neutral sitz bath** is generally performed for thirty minutes to two hours. The water temperature is between 92°F and 97°F with the water level at the navel. Additional water may need to be added in order to maintain the desired temperature. Be careful that adding additional water does not raise level above desired height.

## Alternating Hot and Cold Extremity/Foot Bath

Traditionally used for healing specific body parts. Causes an increase in blood flow to the particular area being treated.

1.  Fill one basin with hot (not scalding) water, approximately 103°F.

2.  Place the body part to be treated in the hot bath for 3 to 5 minutes.

3.  Fill a second basin with cold water (40-70° F); ice in the water may intensify the treatment.

4.  Place the treated body part in the cold water for 30 to 60 seconds.

5.  Repeat these steps four to eight times. Each time, increase the hot bath one to two degrees Fahrenheit, not to exceed 110°F. Maintain this temperature once it is reached.

6.  Finish with a cold bath—except when treating rheumatoid arthritis.

7.  Thoroughly dry the treated part.

**Do not use with:**
♦ Cancer
♦ Vascular disease
♦ Decreased sensation/neuropathy
♦ Hemorrhage
♦ Diabetes


## Head Vapor (Stream Inhalation)

Traditionally used for coughs, congestion, sinus infection.

Bring a quart of pure water to a boil in a glass or stainless steel pot; remove from the heat. When the water has cooled below boiling point, add the recommended amount of essential oils (if required) to the water, and quickly replace the lid. Place the pot on a table. Sit in a tall chair so you are positioned above the steam. Make a "tent" with a large bath or beach towel draped over your head and to below the waist, and covering the pot and the area around it; the "tent" should be closed on all sides.

Once under the "tent," remove the pot lid. Inhale deeply through the nose and exhale through the mouth. Continue for several minutes until the respiratory passages are thoroughly steamed and the face and chest have begun to perspire. DO NOT OVERDO. Dry well and dress. *Note:* It may be advisable to undress down to the waist or wear old clothing to avoid perspiration, and any possible damage to good cloths.

## Steam Pack (Hot Pack)

Traditionally used for muscle spasms, cough, congestion, and to encourage blood flow.

Steam packs are hot applications used to bring heat and warmth to specific parts of the body. They can be made from commercially purchased packs or by heating wet towels. To prepare, heat the steam pack to approximately 120° F. Place the heated pack within several layers of towels, then position on the area to be treated. Leave the pack in place 5 to 20 minutes, depending on the desired results. If the pack is too hot or too cool, adjust the number of layers of towel around the pack. The pack may need to be re-heated to obtain the desired level of warmth.

Alternative: Wet a towel using hot tap water. Apply directly to the skin without protective layers. As with any steam pack, be cautious to be sure that the heat is not excessive and would burn the skin. Take special care with children and with adults who have decreased sensation.

*Note: Never take a steam pack directly from a microwave or other heating device and apply directly to the skin.*

## Alternating hot and cold therapies

**Alternating Hot and Cold Leg Spray** –Sit on edge of tub, keeping feet inside tub. Use a hand-held shower attachment to spray legs (beginning at toes and moving upward to knee), first with very warm water for 2 minutes, then with cold water for 10 seconds. Alternate in this manner for 4 to 5 repetitions. Pat the legs dry, then massage in the Essential Oil as described under appropriate remedy.

**Alternating Hot and Cold Contrast Baths** to affected joints. Begin by immersing the affected part (e.g., hand) in a basin of hot (110°-115°F) water for up to 6 minutes. Then, immerse it in a basin of cold (55° to 60°) for 1 to 3 minutes. Alternate back and forth for 20-40 minutes. Add hot and cold water to the respective basins or as required for maintaining the appropriate temperature. Add 5 drops of an undiluted aromatherapy blend (i.e., not the massage blend diluted with jojoba or emu oil) as described under the appropriate remedy to both the hot and cold water. *(When treating arthritis always begin and end with hot.)* After completing the hydrotherapy, dry and gently rub one of the aromatherapy massage blends around the affected area. Traditionally used for: muscle spasms, encourage blood flow, stimulate immune system, and stimulate nervous system.

**Alternating Hot and Cold Shower**. While in shower, aim a strong stream of water at affected area. Begin with 2 minutes of tolerably hot water, then switch to 20 seconds of cold water. Repeat one more time, finishing with cold. Degree of hot and cold is determined by individual tolerance. To increase the benefit of this therapy, do not dry after the shower. Instead, perform an Aromatherapy Rub (as described under the appropriate remedy section) while the skin is still wet.

**Epsom Salts Bath:** Avoid hot baths if suffering from heart problems or diabetes. If suffering from a serious illness, check with your physician regarding the advisability of hot baths in your case. Add 2 pounds of Epsom salts to a full tub of warm water. Essential oils may also be added, if desired. Before entering tub, drink a cup of a diaphoretic (sweat-inducing) herb tea such as peppermint (Mentha piperita), yarrow (Achillea millefolium) or thyme (Thymus vulgaris) prepared by infusion (see Appendix). Use 1 Tbsp. of herb to 2 cups pure water. Continue drinking while in the tub. Soak in tub for up to 20 minutes, until perspiring freely. Then rinse briefly with cold water, wrap body in a sheet, go to bed and cover up well. Remain in bed for 1 hour, until perspiring has stopped. Then take a tepid shower. Do not dry. While still wet, massage body with essential oil as described under appropriate remedy section. This procedure may help the body rid itself of impurities and superfluous fluids.

# Appendix E: Homeopathy

## *Homeopathy*

Homeopathy is a medical system based on the principal that "like cures like." This means that the same substances that can produce a symptom also can be used to treat the symptom when given in much smaller doses. Homeopathic medicines are recognized by the FDA as official drugs; therefore, the manufacturing, use, labeling, and dispensing are regulated, as with pharmaceutical drugs. Homeopathic medicines are prepared from plant, animal, and mineral sources in extremely dilute amounts.

These remedies are specific to each individual's set of symptoms, which may include emotional, physical, and/or mental. To select the right homeopathic remedy for your condition, find the description given that most closely matches your own symptoms. Not every aspect of a definition will match; however, the closer the fit, the better chance of success. Often, there are key parts of a description that may help direct you to the appropriate remedy; for example, thirsty versus thirstless, or chilly versus hot.

Homeopathic medicines are most commonly found in two different scales of potency. "X" potencies are lower than "C" potencies. The "X" potency means the first dilution is equal to 1 part of the original substance to 9 parts of the solvent. So, a 3X potency equals 1 part of the original substance to 1,000 parts of the solvent; and a 6X potency equals 1 part of the original substance to 1,000,000 parts of the solvent. The "C" potency refers to a first dilution that is equal to 1 part of the original substance to 99 parts of the solvent. Although seemingly contradictory, the more dilute a homeopathic medicine, the more potent may be its action; thus, a 6X or 6C potency may act more deeply than a 3X or 3C potency. In general, while not a hard and fast rule, the lower potencies (e.g., 6X and 6C) are used for acute treatments; and the higher potencies (e.g., 30C and 200C) are used for treating longer-standing, chronic disorders.

Examples:

| | | |
|---|---|---|
| Weakest | = | Nux Vomica 3X |
| Stronger | = | Nux Vomica 6X |
| Even Stronger | = | Nux Vomica 6C |
| Strongest | = | Nux Vomica 30C |

The label on the bottle may carry a medicine's full name or abbreviated name. In either case, it should be the same medicine.

Examples:

| | | |
|---|---|---|
| Rhus Toxicidredon | = | Rhus Tox |
| Kali Bichromium | = | Kali Bich |
| Magnesium Phosphorica | = | Mag Phos |
| Natrium Muriatricum | = | Nat Mur |

## *Basic rules of homeopathic administration:*

1. Look for a remedy that most closely matches your symptoms.

2. Choose only one remedy at a time, unless otherwise instructed.

3. In acute cases (e.g., cold, flu, bruises, stings), if after a few days no results are apparent, select another remedy. With chronic cases (e.g., arthritis, asthma, eczema), give a remedy at least several weeks to a month before changing the remedy.

4. Pour pellets into the cap or a plastic spoon. Never touch the pellets with your fingers.

5. Sometimes, during homeopathic treatments, symptoms initially may become worse. This is called *homeopathic aggravation*, which may be considered a sign that the remedy is working. This reaction usually passes quickly and is often followed by marked improvement of symptoms. However, an aggravation that persists may indicate that the wrong remedy was selected, or the potency chosen was too high or too low, or the doses are being administered too frequently, or you are hypersensitive and may not be a good candidate for homeopathic self-treatment. *Always discontinue use of a homeopathic medicine if a severe or persistent aggravation of symptoms occurs.*

6. Avoid strong smells, such as eucalyptus, mint, and camphor. Also avoid eating or drinking substances that contain caffeine, camphor, or mint (including mint toothpaste). These substances will render the homeopathic remedy useless.

7. When administering homeopathic medicines to a young baby, who is not yet able to hold pellets in the mouths and let them dissolve, proceed as follows: Crush 3 pellets (use a mortar and pestle if available). Then, using

a plastic teaspoon, dissolve the powder in 2 tbsp. pure water. Administer 1/2 to 1 tsp. of this solution, as indicated under the remedy description. Stir the solution well before each successive dose. Make a fresh solution daily. *When treating a baby, discontinue use of any homeopathic medicine if there is any abnormal reaction, and always work with the pediatrician before, and during treatments.*

Homeopathy is a very sophisticated science. Consider consulting a professional homeopath when addressing serious or complex health disorders.

# Appendix F: Chelation and Prolotherapy

*Chelation and Prolotherapy*

### Chelation Therapy

While chelation remains controversial in conventional medical circles, over 800,000 people have benefited from this therapy. The treatment involves the intravenous infusion of vitamins, magnesium, and ethelene diamine tetra-acetic acid (EDTA) given on a regular basis to improve blood flow. According to a study by Chappel and Stahl, approximately 80% of patients will benefit from the treatment. Patients receiving chelation therapy may experience a reduction in angina, blood pressure, cholesterol, and circulatory problems. Chelation removes toxic heavy metals such as lead, cadmium, arsenic, aluminum, and mercury and helps rid the body of free radicals. Free radicals can directly harm the lining of the arteries, contributing to plaque buildup. Patients who undergo chelation therapy have been able to cancel heart surgery, angioplasty, and limb amputations.

For more information on chelation therapy, contact the American College for Advancement in Medicine (ACAM) – (see Appendix G )

### Prolotherapy

Prolotherapy (proliferative therapy), also known as ligament reconstructive therapy or sclerotherapy, is a recognized orthopedic procedure that stimulates the body's natural healing processes to strengthen joints weakened by trauma or arthritis.

Joints weakened when ligaments and tendons are stretched, torn, or fragmented, become hypermobile and painful. Traditional approaches with anti-inflammatory drugs and surgery often fail to stabilize the joint and relieve pain permanently. Prolotherapy has the unique ability to directly address the cause of instability and repair the weakened sites, resulting in permanent stabilization of the joint. When precisely injected into the site of pain or injury, prolotherapy creates a mild, controlled inflammation, which stimulates the body to lay down new tendon or ligament fibers, resulting in a strengthening of the weakened structure. When the joint becomes strong, pain will be relieved. Prolotherapy can be used to relieve a broad spectrum of conditions, including arthritis, back pain, neck pain, herniated discs, TMJ disorder, tennis elbow, shoulder pain, sciatica, wrist and hand pain, and ankle disorders.

# Appendix G:  Resource Guide

*Resource Guide*

www.urhealthy.com
The official website of Self-Care Anywhere. Telehealth Cards can be ordered at this site.

The Magaziner Center for Wellness and Anti-Aging Medicine
1907 Greentree Road
Cherry Hill, NJ 08003
(856) 424-8222
www.drmagaziner.com
The official website of Scott R. Greenberg M.D. Information on alternative medical procedures such as allergy testing, chelation therapy, and prolotherapy; also featuring the free Nutrition and Allergy hotline on Tuesday and Wednesday evenings, from 5PM-6PM EST., at (856) 424-0707.

## *Aromatherapy Essential Oils*

A Woman of Uncommon Scents
P.O. Box 103
Roxbury, PA 17251
(800) 377-3685
Excellent quality, pure, unadulterated essential oils, many of which are either derived from organically-grown, ethically wildcrafted plants.

## *Herbal Products*

Frontier Natural Products Co-op
3021 78th St.
P.O. Box 299
Norway, IA 52318
(800) 669-3275
Large selection of quality herbal products, many of which are organically grown or wildcrafted.

Starwest Botanicals
11253 Trade Center Drive
Rancho Cordova, CA 95742
(800) 800-4372
Large selection of quality herbal products, many of which are organically grown or wildcrafted

### Homeopathic Medicines

Dolisos
3014 Rigel Ave.
Las Vegas, NV, 89102
(800) 365-4767
Quality homeopathic medicines and cell salts in a wide range of potencies.

Hahnemann Laboratories
1940 Fourth St.
San Rafael, CA 94901
(888) 427-6422
Excellent C-potency homeopathic medicines produced by traditional methods.

### Natural Foods Suppliers

Gold Mine Natural Food Company
7805 Arjons Drive
San Diego, CA 92126
(800) 475-3663
Excellent organic grains, flours, legumes, seeds, oils, miso, umbeboshi paste, tamari, seaweeds, pasta, fresh sauerkraut, as well as cooking utensils.

SunOrganic Farm
P.O. Box 2429
Valley Center, CA 92082
(888) 269-9888
Top quality organically grown food products including: Grains, flours, beans, seeds, nuts, seed and nut butter, oils, dried fruits and sprouting seeds.

### Nutritional Supplements

Allergy Research Group/Nutricology
30806 Santana St.
Hayward, CA 94544
(800) 545-9960
www.nutricology.com

Biotics Research NW
PO Box 7027
Olympia, WA 98507
(800) 636-6913
Superior products including: emulsified Vitamins A, D and E. Also, emulsified Co-Q 10, hydrochloric acid capsules, proteolytic enzyme formula, bile extract, glandular extracts and fatty acid products.

Douglas Laboratories
600 Boyce Road
Pittsburgh, PA 15205
(800) DOUGLAB
www.douglaslabs.com

Ecological Formulas
1061 B Shary Circle
Concord, CA 94518
(800) 888-4584
Specialty nutritional products including sialic acid; calcium and magnesium butyrate; amino acids, glandular extracts; proteolytic enzyme formula; progesterone cream.

Lanc Labs
110 Commerce Dr.
Allendale, NJ 07401
(800) 526-3005

Metagenics
971 Calle Negocio
San Clemente, CA 92673
(800) 692-9400
www.metagenics.com

Nature's Design
PO Box 3001
Lynwood, WA 98046
(800) 832-8488
Excellent quality vitamin and mineral supplements including: beta-carotene; mixed mineral ascorbate Vitamin C; B-Complex with co-enzyme B-vitamins; emulsified vitamin E; amino acid chelated minerals as well as unique herbal formulas.

NutriSupplies
2695 North Military Trail Suite 7
West Palm beach, FL 33409
(800) 388-8808
Complete line of vitamins and minerals, including: vitamin A, vitamin D, and individual B-vitamins such as folic acid, niacin, and sublingual vitamin B12. Amino acids, glandular extracts, digestive aids and herbal capsules.

Pure Encapsulations
490 Boston Post Rd.
Sudbury, MA  01776
(800) 753-CAPS
www.pureencapsulations.com

The Taurence Company
(800)327-0722
High quality Acidophilus

Thorne Research
PO Box 25
Dover, ID  83825
(800) 228-1966
www.thorne.com

Tyler Encapsulations
2204-8 NW Birdsdale
Gresham, OR  97030
(800) 869-9705
www.tyler-inc.com

## *Reference Laboratories*

AccuChem Labs
900 N. Bowser Rd.
Suite 880
Richardson, TX  75081
(800) 451-0116
www.accuchemlabs.com

Antibody Assay
1715 E. Wilshire #715
Santa Ana, CA  92705
(800) 522-2611
www.antibodyassay.com

Diagnos-Techs
6620 S. 192$^{nd}$ place, Building J
Kent, WA  98032
(800) 878-3787

Doctors Data
3755 Illinois Ave.
Charles IL 60174-2420
(800) 323-2784
www.doctorsdata.com

Great Smokies Diagnostic Laboratory
63 Zillicoa St.
Asheville, NC  28801-1074
(800) 522-4762
www.greatsmokies-lab.com

ImmunoLaboratories
1620 W. Oakland Park Boulevard
Fort Lauderdale, FL  33311
(800) 231-9197
www.immunolabs.com

Immunosciences Lab
8730 Wilshire Blvd.
Suite 305
Beverly Hills, CA  90211
(800) 950-4686
www.immuno-sci-lab.com

## *Personal Air Purifier*

BreatheFree.com
Sales (888)434-8313

Environmental Purification Systems
Sales (415) 682-7231

National Ecological and Environmental Delivery System (NEEDS)
Sales (800) 634-1380

## *Support*

AIDS Action Committee
131 Clarendon Street
Boston, MA   02116
(617)437-6200

Alzheimer's Association
919 North Michigan Avenue
Chicago, IL  60611
(800)272-3900
(312)335-8700

American Academy of Allergy and Immunology
611 Wells Street
Milwaukee, WI  53202

American Cancer Society
1599 Clifton Road
Atlanta, GA  30329

American Dental Association
211 East Chicago Avenue
Chicago, IL 60611
(312) 440-2500

American Diabetes Association
1660 Duke Street
Alexandria, VA 22314
800-232-3472
(703)549-1500

American Heart Association
7272 Greenville Avenue
Dallas, TX 75231
(214) 373-6300

Cancer Information Service
National Cancer Institute
Building 31, Room 10A24
9000 Rockville Pike
Bethesda, MD 20892

AIDS Hot Line
English: (800) 342-AIDS (all times)
Spanish: (800) 344-7432 (8:00am – 2:00 pmEastern time)
Sponsored by the Centers for Disease Control and Prevention. HIV and AIDS related information and educational services as well as medical and support group referrals.

Alcohol and Drug Helpline
(800) 252-6465

American Anorexia/Bulimia Association
(212) 501-8351
Information. referrals and outreach programs for those affected by on eating disorders.

Cancer Information Service
(800) 4-CANCER
Sponsored by the National Cancer Institute. Provides information on cancer treatment and prevention.

Cocaine Hot Line
(800) COCAINE
Provides referrals to hospitals, counseling centers, and docotors specializing in cocaine treatment.

Dial a Hearing Test
(800) 222-EARS
(800) 345-EARS (Pennsylvania)

Lung Line Information Service
(800) 222-5864
(303) 355-5864
Information on respiratory diseases and immune disorders. Specialist available to answer specific questions.

National Institute on Drug Abuse
(301) 443-6245
Information on health hazards of and safety precautions against pesticides.

Prostate Information Hot Line
(800) 543-9632

Sexually Transmitted Diseases Hot Line
(800) 227-8922

### Schools, Physicians & Practitioners

American Academy of Environmental Medicine
American Financial Center
7701 East Kellogg, Suite 625
Wichita, KS 67207-1705
(316) 684-5500
Referrals for physicians specializing in Food Allergy, Environmental Medicine and Detoxification.

American College for Advancement in Medicine (ACAM)
23121 Verdugo Drive, Suite 204
Laguna Hills, CA 92653
(800) 532-3688
www.acam.org
Referrals for physicians practicing holistic medicine, chelation therapy and orthomoleculer medicine.

American Holistic Medical Association
4101 Lake Boone Trail, Ste 201
Raleigh, NC 27607
(919) 787-5181
Provides referrals for licensed professionals practicing holistic health care.

American Society of Clinical Hypnosis
2200 E Devon Ave, Ste 291
Des Plaines, IL 60018-4534
(847) 297-3317

American Association of Naturopathic Physicians (AANP)
601 Valley Street
Suite #105
Seattle, WA 98109
(206) 298-0125
AANP
www.infinite.org/Naturopathic.Physician

Association for Applied Psychophysiology and Biofeedback
10200 W. 44$^{th}$ Ave., #304
Wheat Ridge, CO 80033-2840
(800) 477-8892
Provides referrals for local biofeedback practitioners.

Homeopathic Academy of Naturopathic Physicians
P.O. Box 69565
Portland, OR 97201
(503) 795-0579

International Foundation for Homeopathy (IFH)
P.O. Box 7
Edmonds, WA 98020
(206) 776-1499
National Certification Board for Theraputic Massage & Bodywork
(800) 296-0664

# References

Abehsera, Michael. The Healing Clay. New York: Citadel Press, 1979.

Airola, Paavo. Every Woman's Book. Phoenix: Health Plus Publishers, 1980.

Airola, Paavo. How To Get Well. Phoenix: Health Plus Publishers, 1974.

Auerbach, Paul S., Medicine For The Outdoors. Boston: Little, Brown and Company, 1986.

Benjamin, Harry. Everybody's Guide To Nature Cure. London: Health For All Publishing Company; 1936.

Berkowsky, Bruce. Aromatherapy Synthesis Materia Medica. Mount Vernon, WA: Joseph Ben Hil-Meyer Research, 1999.

Berkowsky, Bruce. Dr. Berkowsky's At-Home Natural Health Science Spa Program. Nature's Therapies Journal (5) 3, 1996.

Binding, G.J. and Moyle, Alan. About Kelp. Wellingborough,England: Thorsons Publishers, 1974.

Birch, Beryl Bender. Power Yoga New York. Simon & Schuster 1995

Boericke, W. Homeopathic Materia Medica and Repertory. New Delhi: B. Jain Publishers, 1994.

Boericke, W. and Dewey, W.A. The Twelve Tissue Remedies. Philadelphia: Hahnemann Publishing House, 1888.

Boston Women's Health Book Collective. The New Our Bodies, Ourselves. New York: Simon and Schuster, 1984.

Boyle, Wade and Saine, Andre. Lectures in Naturopathic Hydrotherapy. East Palestine, Ohio: Buckeye Naturopathic Press, 1988.

Bragg, Paul and Bragg, Patricia. Bragg Apple Cider Vinegar System. Santa Barbara, CA: Health Science, 1980.

Brown, O. Phelps. The Complete Herbalist. Jersey City, N.J., O. Phelps Brown, 1878.

Buchman, Dian, D. The Complete Book of Water Healing. New York: Instant Improvement, 1994.

Buegel, Dale, Lewis, Blair and Chernin, Dennis. Homeopathic Remedies For Health Professionals and Laypeople. Honesdale, PA: The Himalayan International Institute of Yoga Science and Philosophy of the U.S.A., 1991.

Carper, Jean. Miracle Cures. New York: HarperCollins 1997

Chapman, Esther. How To Use The 12 Tissue Salts. New York: Jove Publications, 1979.

Chapman, J.B. and Perry, Edward, L. The Biochemic Handbook. St. Louis: Formur, 1976.

Charmine, Susan, E.  The Complete Raw Juice Therapy. New York: Baronet Publishing, 1977.

Christopher, John, R.    School of Natural Healing.    Springville, Utah: Christopher Publications, 1976.

Curtis, Susan and Fraser, Romy. Natural Healing For Women.   London: Pandora Press, 1991.

Clarke, John, H.   The Prescriber. Saffron Walden, England: C.W. Daniel Company, 1972.

Clarke, John, H.   A Dictionary of Practical Materia Medica Volumes 1-3. New Delhi: B. Jain Publishers, 1993.

Das, Rai B. B., Select Your Remedy. New Dlehi: Vishwamber Free Homeo Dispensary, 1993.

Davis, Martha and Elizabeth Robbins Eshelman and Mathew McKay  The Relaxation & Strcs Reduction Workbook. California: New Harbinger Publications 1988

Davis, Patricia.  Aromatherapy An A-Z.  Saffron Walden, England:  C.W. Daniel Company, 1988.

Dorland's Medical Dictionary. Philadelphia: The Saunders Press, 1980.

Ellingwood,    Finley.   American   Materia   Mcdica,   Therapeutics   and Pharmacognosy.  Portland: Eclectic Medical Publications, 1985.

Felter,  Harvey W. and Lloyd, John U. King's American Dispensatory Volumcs I and II. Portland: Eclectic Medical Publications, 1983.

Fischbach, France. A Manual of Laboratory Diagnostic Tests.  New York: J.B. Lippincott Company, 1984.

Garrison, R.H. and Somer, Elizabeth.  The Nutrition Desk Reference.  New Canaan, Ct.: Keats Publishing, 1990.

Haas, Elson, M. Staying Healthy with Nutrition.  Berkeley, CA: Celestial Arts, 1992.

Jarvis, D.C., Folk Medicine. New York: Fawcett Crest, 1958.

Johns Hopkins Medical Institutions Johns Hopkins Symptoms & Remedies. New York Random House 1995

Keville, Kathi. Herbs for Health and Healing.  U Pennsylavania: Rodale Press 1996

Kirchheimer, Sid. The Doctors Book Of Home Remedies II.  Pennsylvania: Rodale Press 1993

Kirschmann, John D., Nutrition Almanac.  New York: McGraw-Hill, 1979.

Kloss, Jethro. Back To Eden. Washington, D.C.: Jethro Kloss, 1939.

Kowalchik,   Claire   and   Hylton,   W.H.   (Editors).   Rodale's   Illustrated Encyclopedia of Herbs. Emmaus, PA: Rodale Press, 1987.

Lavabre, Marcel. Aromatherapy Workbook.   Rochester, Vermont: Healing Arts Press, 1990.

Lipski, Elizabeth. Digestive Wellness. New Canaan, Ct.: Keats Publishing, 1996.

Lust, John and Tierra, Michael. The Natural Remedy Bible. New York: Pocket Books, 1990.

Mabey, Richard. The New Age Herbalist. New York: Collier Books 1988

Magaziner, Allan. Total Health Handbook. New York: Kensington Books, 1999.

Magaziner, Allan. The Complete Idiots Guide to Living Longer and Healthier. New York: Alpha Books, 1999.

Market House Books The Bantam Medical Dictionary. New York: Bantam Books 1900

Mindell, Earl. Earl Mindell's Herb Bible. New York: Simon & Schuster 1992

Mojay, Gabriel. Aromatherapy For Healing The Spirit. New York: Henry Holt and Company, 1996.

Morrison, Roger. Desktop Guide To Keynotes and Confirmatory Symptoms. Albany, CA: Hahnemann Clinic Publishing, 1993.

Moyers, Bill. Healing And The Mind. New York: Doubleday 1993

Murray, Michael and Pizzorno, Joseph. Encyclopedia of Natural Medicine. Rocklin, CA: Prima Publishing, 1991.

Mowrey, Daniel B. Herbal Tonic Therapies. New York: Wings Books, 1993.

Mowrey, Daniel B. The Scientific Validation of Herbal Medicine. Cormorant Books, 1986.

Murphy, Robin. Homeopathic Medical Repertory. Pagosa Springs, CO: Hahnemann Academy of North America, 1993.

Olshevsky, M, Noy, S, Zwang, M and Burger, R. The Manual of Natural Therapy. New York: Citadel Press, 1990.

Passwater, Richard, A. and Cranton, Elmer, M. Trace Elements, Hair Analysis and Nutrition. New Canaan, Ct.: Keats Publishing, 1983.

Pedersen, Mark. Nutritional Herbology. Bountiful, Utah: Pedesen Publishing, 1987.

Potterton, David (Ed.). Culpeper's Color Herbal. New York: Sterling Publishing Company, 1983.

Powell, Eric. Biochemistry Up To Date. Devon, England: Health Science Press, 1963.

Rose, Jeanne. Jeanne Rose's Herbal Body Book. New York: Perigee Books, 1976.

Sarno, John. Healing Back Pain. New York: Warner Books 1991

Sellar, Wanda. The Directory of Essential Oils. Saffron Walden, England: C.W. Daniel Company, 1994.

Sheppard-Hanger, Sylla. The Aromatherapy Practitioner Reference Manual. Tampa: Atlantic Institute of Aromatherapy, 1995.

Smith, Trevor. Homeopathic Medicine For Women. Rochester, Vermont: Healing Arts Press, 1989.

The Burton Golderg Group. Alternative Medicine The Definitive Guide. Washington: Future Medicine Publishing 1995

Thrash, Agatha. and Thrash, Calvin. Natural Remedies. Sunfield, Michigan: Family Health Publication, 1983.

Thrash, Agatha. and Thrash, Calvin. Home Remedies. Seale, Alabama: Thrash Publications, 1981.

Thrash, Agatha. and Thrash, Calvin. Rx: Charcoal. New Lifestyle Books, 1988.

Ullman, Dana. Homeopathic Medicine for Children and Infants. New York: G.P. Putnam's Sons, 1992.

Valnet, Jean. The Practice of Aromatherapy. New York: Destiny Books, 1980.

Vermeulen, Frans. Synoptic Materia Medica. Haarlem, The Netherlands: Merlijn Publishers, 1992.

Vermeulen, Frans. Synoptic Materia Medica II. Haarlem, The Netherlands: Merlijn Publishers, 1996.

Vogel, A. Swiss Nature Doctor. Teufen, Switzerland: A. Vogel, 1980.

Walker, Norman W. Raw Vegetable Juices. New York: Jove Publications, 1970.

Weil, Andrew. Natural Health, Natural Medicine Boston: Houghton Mifflin Company 1990

Werbach, Melvyn R. Nutritional Influences on Illness. New Canaan, Ct.: Keats Publishing, 1987.

Yeung, Him-che. Handbook of Chinese Herbs and Formulas. Los Angeles: Institute of Chinese Medicine, 1985.

# Index

# About the Authors

To contact authors, visit the Independently Healthy website at: www.urhealthy.com

**Gary Skole**
Gary Skole is a nationally certified personal trainer and founder and president of 4EverFit Wellness Centers and Family Choice Home Services, a company dedicated to helping senior citizens and disabled individuals live independently in their own homes. He is a member of the Private Care Association, Tri-State Holistic Health Association and Home Health and Staffing Association. He has helped numerous individuals take control of their health-care needs and live healthy, independent lives.

**Scott R. Greenberg, M.D.**
Dr. Scott Greenberg is a practicing physician at the Magaziner Center for Wellness & Anti-Aging Medicine in Cherry Hill, NJ. He specializes in natural approaches to family practice problems, with a particular focus on nutrition, cancer therapies, preventive medicine, anti-aging strategies and the use of prolotherapy for pain management.

Dr. Greenberg holds a BA in biology from Rutgers College in New Brunswick, N.J., and an MD from Hahnemann University in Philadelphia, where he achieved many academic honors, as well as community service awards.

Dr. Greenberg is board certified in family practice and chelation therapy, a diplomate of the American Board of Family Practice, and a member of the American College for the Advancement in Medicine. He is also a diplomate of the National Board of Medical Examiners, and is a recipient of the Physicians Recognition Award from the American Medical Association. Dr. Greenberg has been a featured guest on the syndicated health program "On Call" and is a published author who has been featured in both medical journals and the lay press.

**Michael Gazsi, N.D.**
Dr. Michael Gazsi is a graduate of National College of Naturopathic Medicine in Portland Oregon. He is medical director of the Center for Integrative Medicine, with offices in Ridgefield and Stamford Connecticut. Dr. Gazsi specializes in the use of meridian and blood analysis and the use of herbal and homeopathic medicine. Dr. Gazsi is editor of the newsletter *Shangrila*, and lectures regularly on subjects of health and nutrition.

*Medical Editor*

**Vivienne Matalon, M.D.**
Dr. Matalon is the medical director of TLC Healthcare in Marlton,N.J. She specializes in Internal Medicine, Diabetes, Bariatrics(weight control), and Holistic Medicine. Dr. Matalon is the international medical consultant for McLeods,U.K.; Innovex Inc, and Novartis Pharmaceuticals, member of the board of Trustees for Beaver College , Clinical Instructor UMDNJ Medical School. She has numerous publications and national medical speaking engagements to her credit.

# Other Books From
# New Century Publishing 2000

*A Doctor in your Suitcase*                                      $7.95 US
Natural medicine for self-care when you are away from home.      $11.95 CA

*Velvet Antler, Nature's Superior Tonic*                         $9.95 US
Amazing health breakthroughs from this powerful                  $14.95 CA
rejuvenating tonic.

*The Fitness for Golfers Handbook*                               $14.95 US
Taking your golf game to the next level.                         $19.95 CA

*Plant Power Revised, by Laurel Dewey*                           $19.95 US
The Humorous Herbalist's guide to finding, growing,              $29.95 CA
gathering and using 30 great medicinal herbs.

*Nutritional Leverage for Great Golf*                            $9.95 US
How to improve your score on the back nine.                      $14.95 CA

---

TO ORDER CONTACT (877) 742-7078 TOLL FREE
(905) 471-5711

SHIPPING $4.00 PER BOOK

NEW CENTURY PUBLISHERS 2000

| CANADA | UNITED STATES |
|---|---|
| 60 BULLOCK DR., UNIT 7 | P.O. BOX 36 |
| MARKHAM ON LP3 3P2 | EAST CANAAN, CT 06024 |